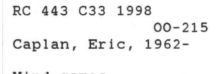
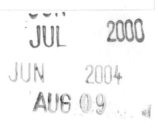
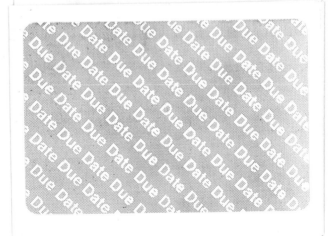

Mind Games

Mind Games

American Culture and the Birth of Psychotherapy

Eric Caplan

UNIVERSITY OF CALIFORNIA PRESS

Berkeley / Los Angeles / London

University of California Press
Berkeley and Los Angeles, California

University of California Press
London, England

© 1998 by the Regents of the University of California

Library of Congress Cataloging-in-Publication Data

Caplan, Eric, 1962–
    Mind Games :   American culture and the birth of
psychotherapy / Eric Caplan.
        p.   cm.
    Includes bibliographical references and index.
    ISBN 0–520–21169–3 (alk. paper)
    1. Psychotherapy—United States—History—19th century.
    2. Psychotherapy—Social aspects—United States.   3. Mental
healing—United States—History—19th century.   4. United
States—Social life and customs—19th century.   I. Title.
    RC443.C33   1998
    616.89′00973—dc21   98–16999
                                                                CIP

Printed in the United States of America

1 2 3 4 5 6 7 8 9

The paper used in this publication meets the minimum requirements
of American National Standard for Information Sciences—Perma-
nence of Paper for Printed Library Materials, ANSI Z39.48-1984 ⊗

For Elise

Psychotherapy is a most terrifying word, but we are forced to use it because there is no other which serves to distinguish us from Christian Scientists, the New Thought people, the faith healers, and the thousand and one other schools which have in common the disregard for medical science and the accumulated knowledge of the past.

—Richard C. Cabot, M.D. (1908)

Contents

Acknowledgments

I owe much to many. Over the past several years I have accrued more personal and intellectual debts than I could possibly hope to repay. Good friends in Ann Arbor, Boston, New York, Washington, D.C., Chicago, and elsewhere not only provided me with places to stay during my frequent visits but more important, offered me vital encouragement and much-needed advice.

As a graduate student at the University of Michigan I received generous support from the Horace Rackham School of Graduate Studies. Moreover, I was blessed not only with a brilliant but also an actively engaged dissertation committee. Athena Vrettos, who agreed to join my committee midway through the ordeal, provided an insightful reading of my chapters and offered a number of excellent comments about how I might improve the manuscript. Ruth Leys, of Johns Hopkins University, gave more of her time and energy than I thought possible. Sharing her wide-ranging knowledge of the history of psychiatry, she prevented me from making a host of embarrassing errors and helped me to hone my analysis at several critical points. Having guided this project from its inception to its completion, David Hollinger provided me with an unparalleled model of scholarly integrity and professional commitment. His unflagging support throughout the entire course of my graduate studies and beyond has provided me with a source of inspiration that I shall remember for the remainder of my career. Marty Pernick was unquestionably my most "hands-on" adviser. Having read every word I wrote not once, not twice, but several times, he continually pushed me to clarify my thoughts and to hone my analysis. A true fountain of knowledge, he pointed me to scores of books and articles that I might otherwise have overlooked. Never allowing me to content myself with easy answers to difficult questions, he singlehandedly, albeit gently, coerced me into improving virtually every aspect of this work.

Here at the University of Chicago I have benefited immensely from the intellectual camaraderie of Andy Wallace, Peter Miller, Nancy Yousef, David Vanmill, Paul Seeley, Robin Derby, David Brent, Ralph Austin, Ann Lorimar, Bill Sewell, Bert Cohler, Roger Gould, Tracy Teslow, Becky Roiphe, Moishe Postone, Bob Richards, Jan Goldstein, George Stocking, Daniela Barberis, and Shirley Martin. Moreover, the history of human sciences workshop has provided me with a splendid source of intellectual inspiration over the course of the past three years.

While living in Washington, D.C., and working at the National Library of Medicine and the Library of Congress I enjoyed the intellectual comradeship and friendship of Cathy Kerr, Carla Yanni, Ada Ferrer, Tami Hager, and Molly Pyle—each of whom was completing a dissertation of her own. I cannot express strongly enough my thanks to George Markoli, Nathan Kravis, Jacques Quen, Leonard Groopman, Lawrence Friedman, and other members of the History of Psychiatry Section at the New York Hospital–Cornell University Medical College. On two separate occasions they provided me with an opportunity to discuss earlier versions of chapters 2 and 6. More important, they offered a congenial, albeit critical, analysis of my work.

I am particularly grateful to Sander Gilman, Edward Shorter, Andy Scull, and Gerald Grob for their careful readings and critical advice regarding all aspects of this book. I owe a special debt of gratitude to the respective staffs of the Countway Medical Library of Harvard University Medical School, the Library of Congress, and the Historical Division of the National Library of Medicine—in particular, to James Cassedy for extending my first invitation to present my research in a formal setting. Over the course of the project I have benefited immensely from the support and advice of Mark Micale and Paul Lerner as well as Eugene Taylor, Ellen Herman, Hans Pol, Rachel Rosner, Michelle Fleischer, and other members of Cheiron. I also owe a great debt to Michael Goldsmith and to my stellar research assistant, Sarah Waxman.

As a historian, I have developed a newfound fondness for sociology, or to be more precise, for sociologists. Two stand out: Andy Abbott and Andy Scull. Were it not for their respective contributions this book would never have been completed. Andy Abbott singlehandedly revived my scholarly career when he offered me the chance to teach at the University of Chicago. Andy Scull, who solicited this manuscipt for his series, has been an extraordinarily gracious mentor, a careful and critical reader, and a good friend.

I would also like to thank my editor, Stan Holwitz, my anonymous reviewers, and my many splendid and engaging students here at the University of Chicago. My most enduring debts are to my family—to my parents, Mark and Gloria Caplan, and to my wife, Elise. Elise has been with me since the beginning of this work. She is my best friend and most ardent supporter. My final acknowledgment is to my daughter, Yael. She arrived in this world when this project was essentially completed. Watching her take her first steps has made the final steps of this project all the more satisfying.

CHAPTER I

Introduction

The truth is that medicine, professedly founded on observation, is as sensitive to outside influence, political, religious, philosophical, imaginative, as is the barometer to the changes of atmospheric density. Theoretically it ought to go on its own straightforward inductive path, without regard to changes of government or to fluctuations of public opinion. But . . . actually there is a closer relation between the medical sciences and the conditions of society and the general thought of the time, than would at first be suspected.

Oliver Wendell Holmes (1891)

My original intention was to write a history of the image of the psychotherapist in the United States. Such a work, I believed, would offer a number of significant insights concerning both American medicine and American culture. But in preparing a background chapter for that project, I soon discovered that a vital secondary source was not merely difficult to locate but impossible to find—that is to say, it did not exist. Much to my dismay I came to the conclusion that no one had yet written a history of the origins of psychotherapy in the United States. I do not mean to suggest that no work has been done on the subject. On the contrary, I was able to compile an extensive bibliography of valuable secondary sources examining both the history of institutional psychiatry and the history of psychoanalysis. Absent from virtually all of this literature, however, is any serious effort to explain the origins of psychotherapy.

1

In a nation that currently employs tens of thousands of licensed psychotherapists and perhaps an equal, if not greater, number of unlicensed practitioners, it struck me as odd that no historian had tackled this subject.[1] Indeed, throughout the past five years of research and writing I have remained continually fearful that someone might point me to a book or an article that explores this topic. In many respects the discovery of such a work would come as a welcome relief since, like many young historians, I suffer from the perverse fear that a subject that has not already been addressed may in fact be a subject not worth addressing at all, particularly when that subject is so large.

Over time I have come gradually to realize that the absence of a book on this topic is largely attributable to a widely held, though often unstated, conception of what is meant by psychotherapy—namely, virtually any method of healing that does not rely on somatic agents. There are several problems with this definition. The most obvious is one of semantics. Shamanism is *not* psychotherapy. But there are far more substantive issues as well. I shall mention just one: the issue of anachronism. Whereas no historian would dare suggest that a medieval nostrum employed to treat mania constitutes a crude form of psychopharmacology, a substantial number have made analogous claims regarding psychotherapy and such practices as mysticism, faith healing, even crystal therapy. Proponents of this position interpret psychotherapy in functional rather than historical terms. In so doing they neglect to consider the meaning that these healers and their patients might have attached to these esoteric and diverse practices. Worse still, such an ahistorical rendering of psychotherapy, to say nothing of mysticism, faith healing, and crystal therapy, fails to address what is in fact distinct about each of these systems of healing. Moreover, it leaves unanswered the most salient question about the late-nineteenth- and early-twentieth-century origins of the practice: Why, after decades of resistance, were mainstream physicians finally willing to embrace a system of mental therapeutics?

In the discussion that follows I argue that questions concerning the American origins of psychotherapy—by which I mean the *deliberate and systematic* effort to relieve nervous and mental symptoms without recourse to somatic agents—are best framed within the context of American medicine and American culture. My work rests on the proposition that an understanding of the invention of American psychotherapy requires not only a thorough grounding in the relevant medical and cultural matrices but also an awareness of the interaction between the two. This observation—as I hope is evident by the Holmes quotation that precedes my analysis—is neither novel nor surprising. It is, however, crucial to the story that I tell.

——————————

As late as 1907 Americans knew little of psychotherapy. The word itself was virtually nowhere to be found.[2] Talking cures were not talked about. Despite growing medical and cultural awareness of mental suffering, few physicians made any effort to treat such states by appealing to the mind.[3] Those who did frequently incurred the wrath of their colleagues. In a little-read book on the subject of psychology applied to medicine, David Wells captured the prevailing attitude of his medical colleagues regarding psychotherapy: "It takes courage and self-reliance to openly advocate and practice it."[4] Courage? Self-reliance? Why such trepidation? In our own therapeutically aware, talk show-driven age, Wells's fear seems bizarre indeed. But in 1907, when he offered these remarks, such circumspection was not only understandable, it was professionally imperative. For more than three decades American physicians—particularly those who specialized in the treatment of nervous and mental disorders—had scoffed at anything even remotely resembling mental therapeutics. Mind was to medicine what vinegar was to oil. The two did not mix well.

Prevailing neurological theory held that mental states were merely concomitants of physical states. Proponents of this doctrine, known as psychophysical parallelism, interpreted psychical symptoms as signs of some underlying but not yet discernible physical lesion.[5] Wounded minds were products of wounded bodies. Diseases fell into two categories: structural and functional. The former implied a known cause; the latter, an unknown cause. As a prominent neurologist explained, "Whatever the microscope can see, we call structural—what the microscope cannot see, we call functional."[6] The therapeutic implications of this position were clear. Because all symptoms, be they physical or mental, were attributable to physical irregularities, mental therapies could never hope to address the root of the problem. Successful therapies needed to be aimed at the body, not the mind. How such therapies might produce a positive mental outcome remained unclear. What mattered is that they did. As celebrated Philadelphia neurologist S. Weir Mitchell proclaimed, "You cure the body, and somehow find that the mind is also cured."[7]

In the context of this rigorously materialistic framework, psychotherapy seemed, at best, superfluous and, at worst, thoroughly misguided. The overwhelming majority of American physicians, regardless of their school or specialty, had ceased even to consider the possibility that psychological factors might play a role in exciting, maintaining, or treating mental and nervous disorders. Such views were not without a cogent foundation. As the respective discoveries of the microscopic organism responsible for syphilis and the nutritional deficiency responsible for pellagra soon revealed, materialistic agents did indeed have the capacity to generate a wide array of nervous and mental symptoms that no system of mental therapeutics, no matter how sophisticated it might be, could possibly hope to relieve.[8]

But it was not somatic ideology alone that prevented specialists in nervous diseases from considering psychotherapy. Practical concerns were equally significant. Of these, perhaps none was more important than the desire of American physicians to maintain a sense of professional and scientific credibility. In the final decades of the nineteenth century this meant, among other things, avoiding at all costs anything that even remotely resembled the practices of their nonmedical rivals. In large measure this reluctance lay at the core of mainstream medicine's antipathy to mental therapeutics.[9] That is to say, many late-nineteenth- and early-twentieth-century American physicians eschewed mental healing precisely because it already occupied a prominent position in the larger culture.

Fearing that any association in the public mind with such unsavory characters as Christian Scientists, faith healers, and proponents of the New Thought might compromise their hard-won professional standing, American physicians were understandably reluctant to adopt what many rightly considered the identical methods of their lay rivals. As Harvard psychologist Hugo Münsterberg explained, "Physicians do not like to touch a tool that has been misused so badly."[10] Indeed, the decision to invoke the word *psychotherapy* was in part an effort to address this latter issue. In a fascinating admission, Boston neurologist Richard C. Cabot wrote, "Psychotherapy is a most terrifying word, but we are forced to use it because there is no other which serves to distinguish us from Christian Scientists, the New Thought people, the faith healers, and the thousand and one other schools which have in common the disregard for medical science and the accumulated knowledge of the past."[11]

As Cabot's remarks make clear winning professional support for psychotherapy would require a long and arduous battle. American physicians who promoted the clinical use of mental therapeutics confronted substantial opposition—particularly from the ranks of their professional colleagues. To meet this resistance they had to address two separate but related issues. First, they had to establish a cogent scientific and theoretical rationale for addressing their therapies to the mind rather than to the body. Against the backdrop of prevailing somatic theories of disease, to say nothing of compelling clinical and laboratory evidence, this task was particularly arduous. Second, and perhaps even more daunting, they had to address an even more practical concern—that of distinguishing their "scientific psychotherapy" from the disreputable methods to which their more somatically inclined colleagues frequently and not implausibly compared it.[12]

In the face of such obstacles what one historian has recently referred to as the "sudden appearance" of psychotherapy in the United States soon after the turn of the century is surprising, to say the least.[13] Previous historians have traced this transformation in medical attitudes to the role of elites. In perhaps the most respected interpretation of this medical-cultural episode, Nathan G. Hale, Jr., relying on Thomas Kuhn's model of scientific revolutions, has argued that beginning in the mid-1880s a small cohort of prominent neurologists, psychiatrists, and psychologists began to argue "that the somatic style, as then defined, had exhausted its actual possibilities."[14] Building on Hale's analysis, George Drinka has declared, "[In] placing less emphasis on the brain and giving new credence to personal emotions, ideas, and symbols, a few doctors inched toward a more subtle comprehension of how to listen to human sufferers, how to feel compassion for their symptoms, how to confront their pain."[15]

But rather than adding clarity to their respective analyses, Kuhn's model of scientific revolution needlessly constricts Hale's and Drinka's otherwise trenchant observations by compelling them to assume that which they need first to prove—namely, the presence of a crisis in the somatic paradigm. But the facts do not necessarily point to such a conclusion.[16] Indeed, while a number of physicians did in fact isolate several cracks in its foundation, the somatic paradigm proved to be more durable and adaptable than either these authors or those who have built on their arguments suggest.

In the pages that follow I argue that the birth of psychotherapy in the first decade of the twentieth century had little to do with a crisis in the somatic paradigm. On the contrary, the medical embrace of psychotherapy was only partially attributable to internal medical affairs. Far more significant was a host of nonmedical factors that impinged directly on the practice of medicine. Of these, some of the more prominent were a growing legal and popular recognition of accident-induced traumatic neuroses, a begrudging recognition that somatic therapies could not by themselves explain the results they yielded, a rapidly expanding indigenous mind-cure movement and with it the creation of a new type of "patient," and, finally, a mainstream pastoral healing movement that physicians realized they could ignore only at their own peril. Psychotherapy emerged at considerable odds and in the face of considerable opposition—much, indeed most, of which was generated by the medical profession itself. Its arrival signified a begrudging acceptance on behalf of both medical elites and rank-and-file physicians that their allegiance to the somatic paradigm compromised their capacity both to treat effectively and to compete effectively in a rapidly expanding mental-medical marketplace.

A contemporary observer of the American medical and cultural landscape during the final decade of the nineteenth century would be hard-pressed to locate any signs of the emergence of modern "psychotherapy." Prior to the medical revolution of the late nineteenth century the capacity of physicians to distinguish with any certainty the respective roles of material and mental factors in sickness and in health was virtually nonexistent. Both medical theory and practice were, in the words of Charles E. Rosenberg, "necessarily and ubiquitously 'psychosomatic.'"[17] The extent to which either the mind or the body contributed to a particular disease was impossible to discern.[18] Each no doubt played a role, and the responsible physician endeavored to treat both accordingly.

The work of the great nineteenth-century neuroscientific and bacteriological pioneers destroyed this holistic medical paradigm. Out of its ashes emerged not one but two competing theories of disease—each of which had its origins in the older psychosomatic order. One was psychological, the other somatic.[19] Whereas the latter quickly achieved dominion across the entire medical spectrum, the former remained a potent cultural influence.[20] In contrast to previous generations of physicians, somatically inclined medical doctors of the late nineteenth century focused primarily on material factors. Earlier in the century a physician might explain the presence of an illness by appealing to nonmaterial agents, but by the 1870s doing so was out of the question.

Physicians no longer considered mental and behavioral symptoms on their own terms and for their own sake. On the contrary, they now interpreted such clues only insofar as they enabled them to infer "the [diseased] physical conditions [of the central nervous system] implied by the psychical states."[21] Support for this somatic perspective increased substantially soon after Robert Koch's 1876 discovery of the microbe responsible for anthrax and the subsequent acceptance of germ theory.[22] In keeping with the somatic zeitgeist, many physicians, including those who specialized in the treatment of nervous disorders, abandoned their preoccupation with what might be considered psychosocial factors.[23]

Jettisoning the mind from medicine in no way signified declining interest in nervous and mental symptoms, however. If anything, the opposite was true. That is to say, somatically inclined physicians devoted an unprecedented amount of attention to the psychical symptoms of those for whom there existed no clearly discernible anatomical or organic irregularities. What they did not do, however, and what distinguished them from physicians of an earlier generation, was to consider the possibility that psychosocial factors might play a role in the healing process. Instead, they relied almost exclusively on somatic therapies. Rest cures, diet cures, electrical cures, and water cures abounded. Indeed, during the final three decades of the nineteenth century only a tiny minority within the American medical community gave credence to the possibility that mental healing, either by itself or in conjunction with one of many available somatic therapies, offered much hope. Despite a growing medical recognition of mental suffering, few physicians displayed any concomitant commitment to mental therapeutics.

Paradoxically, acceptance of the somatic paradigm proved to be a critical precondition for the advent of an epistemologically meaningful conception of "psychotherapy."[24] Simply put, what came to be known as psychotherapy was inconceivable within the context of mid-nineteenth-century psychosomaticism. Its implausibility was attributable not to the practical or theoretical limitations of this holistic paradigm but rather to its expansive scope. After all, what need was there to explain that which was readily assumed—namely, a correspondence between mind and body, on the one hand, and environment and health, on the other? With the ascension of the somatic paradigm this logic no longer held, and psychical factors came to be regarded merely as the products of certain yet-to-be-determined neurophysiological processes. Without this profound theoretical reorientation the emergence of psychotherapy would have been inconceivable. In making this claim I do not mean to suggest that prior to the late nineteenth century physicians were oblivious to the role of mental factors in healing. On the contrary, the role of the mind (and of the body) was ubiquitous—but by default rather than design. In all but the most obvious ailments there was no possible way for a physician to disentangle the mental from the physical components of a particular disease.

The moral therapy practiced in nineteenth-century European and American asylums provides a splendid illustration of this phenomenon.[25] That both moral therapy and psychotherapy share certain assumptions regarding the impact of environmental, experiential, and behavioral phenomena cannot be denied.[26] But more significant than the apparent similarities between these two therapeutic systems is their fundamental difference.[27] Moral therapy was the therapeutic complement to the expansive environmental ethos that pervaded Jacksonian America and post-Enlightenment Europe. By way of contrast, psychotherapy was a highly contested response to the science-engendered materialism of the late nineteenth and early twentieth century that had no brief for mental considerations.

Having shared my findings with several scholars and many well-read friends, I have begrudgingly accepted the fact that those reading a book about the origins of psychotherapy in the United States expect, indeed demand, to find Sigmund Freud occupying a prominent place in this story. They will be disappointed—though I hope not for long. Odd as this may sound, Freud has little role to play in this early chapter in the history of American psychotherapy. Prior to 1910 there are virtually no references to his work in American medical periodicals and none whatsoever in popular cultural sources.[28] Simply put, the primary factors that compelled physicians in the United States to embrace psychotherapy had little to do with ideas emanating from Vienna or, for that matter, from any other European city. American doctors had little reason to look across the Atlantic. The germs of psychotherapy could be found much closer to home.

In the chapters that follow I seek to explain the causal paths linking culture, profession, and knowledge in the formation of psychotherapy in the United States. The invention of American "psychotherapy," as I make clear, was not simply an internal medical affair but rather the product of a host of interlocking social and cultural discourses endemic to late Victorian America.[29] Where my analysis departs from others that have acknowledged the cultural dimensions of American psychotherapy is in its capacity to locate discrete nodal points at which medicine and culture actually intersect. By focusing on specific "medical-cultural" discourses such as railway spine, industrial liability, functional nervous disorders, psychical research, mind cure, and pastoral counseling, I reveal the extent to which psychiatric theory itself and, more particularly, the practice of psychotherapy have been shaped by influences that on the surface appear to have little or no relationship to professional medicine. Moreover, I demonstrate that on the eve of Freud's historic visit to the United States in September 1909, mental therapeutics was already integrally woven into the fabric of American medicine and culture.

This work is composed of six chapters, each of which examines a distinct element in the formation of American "psychotherapy." The first examines the medical-legal controversy generated by the proliferation of railway accident-induced traumatic neuroses during the late nineteenth century. Here I argue that almost half a century before the shell shock experienced by veterans of the First World War legitimized the existence of psychoneuroses, several European and American physicians had explored the possibility that certain traumatic experiences might induce otherwise healthy, hereditarily untainted men and women to take on the symptoms of a wide variety of physical ailments that had no apparent somatic basis.

The second chapter assesses the cultural and medical significance of neurasthenia, a functional nervous disease commonly believed to affect upper-class men and women. I argue that prior to 1900 virtually all medical therapies designed to treat so-called functional nervous disorders were somatically based. Although common sense suggests that there might be some causal relationship between the discovery of functional nervous/psychical diseases and the advent of psychological therapies, little evidence exists in support of this position.[30] Of the more than two hundred books and articles concerning the treatment of neurasthenia that appeared in the 1906 issue of the *Index Catalogue of the Library of the Surgeon-General's Office,* a paltry sixteen were included under the heading, "Treatment by Hypnotism," and only four of the sixteen were published by American authors.[31] Moreover, in contrast to previous scholars who focus almost exclusively on the cultural components of neurasthenic discourse, I concentrate instead on its medical features and, in so doing, reveal the profound somatic bias that informed both the medical and the cultural response to this disease. In addition, I es-

tablish that certain elite physicians, deducing from the variegated experiences of a wide array of somatic treatments, began to speculate that a
single factor, the psychical element, might be common to them all.

In the third chapter I focus on what William James termed the
"mind cure movement" and explore its impact on American religion,
medicine, and culture. I argue that because of its unique ideas concerning the capacity of mental therapies to cure all diseases, the American
mind-cure movement differed substantially from other nineteenth-
century health reform and antimaterialist campaigns. Moreover, I suggest that the movement not only tapped into but also stimulated the
growth of a huge and potentially limitless market of "nervous" men
and women who, for a variety of reasons, possessed great faith in the potential efficacy of nonsomatic therapies—thereby enticing and antagonizing different factions within the American neurological and psychiatric communities.

In the fourth chapter I explore the impact of the somatic paradigm
on late-nineteenth- and early-twentieth-century psychiatry and neurology. I argue that the ascendance of the somatic paradigm did not completely abolish medical interest in psychological matters. During the
1890s, when the neurological critique of asylum psychiatry had finally
succeeded in convincing most American asylum superintendents of the
need to consider the role of physiological factors alone in diagnosing
and treating insanity, elites within the American neurological profession were just beginning to call attention to the role of mental factors
in certain functional nervous disorders.

Within less than two years this scenario had changed dramatically.
The reason for this change is the subject of my fifth chapter. Here I provide a case study of the first popular psychotherapy movement in the
United States, the Boston-based Emmanuel movement, which lasted
from 1906 to 1910. This church-sponsored psychotherapy venture was
the primary agent responsible for the efflorescence of psychotherapy in
the United States. Whereas decades of vigorous internal professional
debates had failed to generate a consensus among American physicians
regarding the scientific legitimacy and clinical efficacy of mental therapeutics, in two short years the Emmanuel movement forced the American medical community to confront squarely and publicly a subject that
it had long avoided. In the final chapter I consider briefly the impact of
psychoanalysis and other psychiatric modalities that have marked the
landscape of twentieth-century psychiatry and culture.

CHAPTER 2

Trains, Brains, and Sprains

Railway Spine and the Origins of Psychoneuroses

In what has come to be one of the most conspicuous cinematic metaphors of sexual intimacy, directors have readily seized on the image of a train passing into a tunnel. This image, of course, owes itself to the psychoanalytic theories of Freud. That a train, the great nineteenth-century symbol of technology and progress, is the vehicle commonly used to connote unconscious sexual desire is more appropriate than most people have ever dreamed. For it was an experience with trains themselves that unwittingly drove a host of prominent nineteenth-century physicians to discover the human unconscious.

The relationship among trains, brains, and the unconscious is by no means readily apparent. The discovery of the nexus that links these apparently disparate items was more the result of serendipity than design. Train accidents gave rise to what many surgeons regarded as a novel spinal ailment. Further investigation led some to theorize that the brain, not the spine, was the source of the disorder. Eventually, even this brain-based model was discarded for a mind-centered one. My contention that the discovery of traumatic neuroses figured prominently in inspiring psychotherapy will come as little surprise to anyone well versed in the history of psychoanalysis. But the notion that traumatic experience might give rise to psychoneuroses did not originate with Sigmund Freud and Joseph Breuer's *Studies on Hysteria*.[1] Indeed, what is rightly regarded as the beginnings of psychoanalysis can likewise be seen as a significant contribution to an already vibrant debate concerning the effects of traumatic experience.

11

One of the great ironies in the development of psychotherapy in the United States concerns the vital role played by economically and culturally conservative railway surgeons. It was these surgeons—not liberal psychiatrists or even progressive neurologists—who were the leading exemplars not only of a revised psychogenic paradigm but also of a crude form of psychotherapy itself. Spurred by a rising tide of costly litigation resulting from an increasing incidence of railway accidents, they began to question the limitations of the somatic paradigm.

The professional discourse regarding the origins of traumatic neuroses, while not a sufficient cause, was nonetheless a necessary prerequisite for the emergence of what came to be known as psychotherapy.[2] More than fifty years before the horrors of the First World War brought to light the traumatic origins of various psychoneuroses, a number of prominent physicians on both sides of the Atlantic had acknowledged the possibility that fright itself might give rise to myriad physical and psychological symptoms. Modern travel, not modern warfare, engendered a novel and hitherto unfathomable ailment, the railway spine. Born in 1866 as an exclusively somatic disease, railway spine entered its adolescence in the 1880s as a confusing psychical ailment, began its adulthood in the 1890s in a state of somatic-psychic flux, and suffered an early death in the first decade of the twentieth century. In its short life railway spine contributed both to a fundamental restructuring of the somatic paradigm and to the relegitimation of psychogenic notions of causality.

Railroad track in the United States had grown from 3,000 miles in 1840 to almost 52,000 in 1872.[3] This was by no means an unmitigated blessing. With the expansion came accidents, injuries, and death.[4] Walter Licht reports that for every 117 trainmen employed in the United States in 1889, one was killed; for every 12, one was injured.[5] Workers and their families were not the only parties to be adversely affected; passengers and bystanders were also at risk.[6] Although the majority of train-wreck victims experienced commonly expected ailments such as broken bones, concussions, and contusions, other victims appeared to escape physically unscathed. But some who literally had walked away from a high-speed wreck soon displayed a host of seemingly inexplicable symptoms. Cases of full or partial paralysis, headaches, and various aches and pains often emerged at a later date. While the immediate cause of these and other apparently somatic symptoms remained a mystery, physicians were often able to trace certain symptoms back to the traumatic experience of the railroad accident itself. But rather than provide a psychological explanation for what were indisputably post-traumatic symptoms, the overwhelming majority of physicians offered instead a compelling materialistic rationalization for the disorder. The very name of the condition, railway spine, was indicative of late-nineteenth-century medicine's materialistic orientation.[7]

Not all physicians accepted this somatic interpretation, however. Some argued that those suffering from this disease were in fact conniving malingerers who had feigned their symptoms for the purpose of suing the railroads. Others dissented vigorously from this line of argument. Railway spine, they proclaimed, while perhaps a misnomer, was a mentally induced affliction that could be treated best by psychological intervention. By the 1890s a consensus among physicians regarding railway spine was nowhere to be found. Morton Prince charged that there were "two different and almost radically opposed views."[8] Proponents of the first insisted that railway spine was an organic disease that would in time reveal itself by way of microscopic inquiry. Advocates of the second maintained that the symptoms associated with railway spine were psychologically induced and bore a stark resemblance to those commonly associated with such functional diseases as neurasthenia and hysteria. This conflict was more than merely an academic matter. It was a much smaller part of a fierce medicolegal debate that had its origins in a now-forgotten 1866 series of lectures delivered by distinguished English surgeon John Eric Erichsen.

The publication of Erichsen's brief 144-page volume set into motion a process that swiftly moved beyond the capacity of any single individual to control. As a later commentator proclaimed, "[To] John Eric Erichsen, of London, belongs the credit of being the first to describe a group of symptoms, mainly nervous, that frequently occurred after a concussion of the spine, even though no demonstrable lesion was inferable antemortem, or discoverable postmortem."[9] The eminent American neurologist Charles Dana did not exaggerate when he later asserted that Erichsen's lectures had been "epoch-making."[10] While Erichsen had no way of anticipating the full impact of his doctrines, as the first author to write extensively on the topic of railway spine he had unwittingly defined the parameters of an ensuing medicolegal discourse that would persist long after his death. His thesis became the sole referent against which his critics were forced to respond, and as a contemporary commentator noted, it propelled railway spine into "the public mind as one of the *expected events of railway travel*."[11]

That Erichsen's name is rarely found in the history of psychiatry, neurology, or psychotherapy is not surprising, however. From a scientific perspective his work contained little that could be considered novel. His book's notoriety was attributable not to its contents but to the response it generated.[12] In offering his lectures, Erichsen's aim appeared modest enough. "My object," he wrote, "has been to describe certain forms of Injury of the Nervous System that commonly result from Accidents of Railways, to which I believe the mind of the Profession has not been directed with that amount of attention which their frequency and the important questions involved in them, appear to demand."[13]

Erichsen offered a systematic demonstration of an increasingly common ailment that he claimed was primarily, though not uniquely, attributable to railroad accidents. He presented no anatomical or pathological evidence in support of his diagnosis but argued instead by way of analogy and according to clinical observations. Like the brain, the spine, Erichsen argued, was susceptible to a concussion that induced "molecular changes" in the spinal cord and gave rise to a wide variety of subjective symptoms.[14] In many respects his analysis bore a striking resemblance to George Miller Beard's soon-to-be-articulated conception of neurasthenia.[15] Like Beard, Erichsen sought to apply a single label to a wide variety of symptoms. But whereas Beard could only speculate as to what factors of modern civilization might cause neurasthenia, Erichsen was able to pinpoint a single, dominant variable that gave rise to what he termed "concussion of the spine." "It must . . . be obvious," Erichsen charged, "that in no ordinary accident can the shock be so great as in those that occur on Railways. The rapidity of the movement, the momentum of the persons injured, the suddenness of its arrest, the helplessness of the sufferers, and the natural perturbation of the mind that must disturb the bravest, are all circumstances that of necessity greatly increase the severity resulting to the nervous system, and that justly cause these cases to be considered as somewhat exceptional from ordinary accidents."[16]

Erichsen's causal analysis joined together an unequivocal physical element, spinal concussion, and certain nonexclusive physical agents, helplessness and mental unrest. Railway spine could be properly diagnosed only by paying careful attention to the patient's symptoms, which included the following: "defective memory; confused thoughts; diminished business aptitude; ill temper; disturbed sleep; hot head; impaired vision; impaired hearing; perverted taste and smell; impaired sense of touch; attitude changes; gait changes; loss of limb power; loss of motor power; modification or diminution of sensation in the limbs; numbness; coldness; weight loss; sexual impotence; variable pulse."[17] Erichsen's decision to attribute these symptoms to some underlying somatic irregularity can be traced to the prevailing scientific climate of Victorian England. But science alone did not inspire Erichsen's interpretation.

Issues of gender likewise figured prominently in his analysis.[18] Railway accidents affected women as well as men. But since men were more likely to travel by rail, they were far more likely to be victims of accidents. Of the six cases of railway accident-induced spinal concussion that Erichsen discussed in his work, only one involved a woman. Erichsen was not surprised to observe that following such accidents men and women displayed similar physical symptoms—excepting, of course, disruption of the menstrual cycle. What shocked him, however, was his discovery that both sexes exhibited extreme emotional volatility. Given the prevailing sex-specific views regarding hysteria, the presence of apparently hysterical symptoms in men, more than any other single factor, convinced Erichsen that railway accidents and other traumas that elicited similar symptoms must be indicative of some serious organic disturbance.[19] Like most other physicians of his day, Erichsen simply could not fathom the possibility of a big, strapping man falling victim to what he and others of his generation held to be an almost exclusively female malady.[20] To support this view Erichsen included the case of a forty-five-year-old male victim of a railroad accident.[21] After recounting this man's sordid tale Erichsen asked,

Is it reasonable to say that such a man has suddenly become "hysterical," like a lovesick girl? . . . To me, I confess, the sight of a man of forty-five, rendered "hysterical," not for a few hours or days even, but by some sudden and overwhelming calamity that may for the time break down his mental vigor, not permanently so but for months or years would be a novel melancholy phenomenon, and is one that I have neither seen described by any writer with whose works I am acquainted, nor witnessed in a hospital experience of twenty-five years.[22]

Erichsen's views on these matters were neither unorthodox nor a source of serious contention among his colleagues. In fact, they were simply a reiteration of widely accepted medical views on the subject. Hysterics, as Carroll Smith-Rosenberg observes, were typically denied "the sympathy granted to sufferers from unquestionably organic ailments."[23]

Whereas prevailing assumptions regarding gender seemed to confirm Erichsen's doctrines, those concerning class appeared to negate them. Unlike neurasthenia, which initially appeared to affect only upper-class men and women, accident-induced spinal injuries transcended class boundaries. Indeed, the overwhelming number of railroad passengers were from the upper and middle classes. Physicians did not, however, regard the apparent presence of railway spine in all social classes as further evidence of its legitimacy. On the contrary, the apparent frequency of the condition among lower-class victims caused many to question whether some other agency might better explain these cases. "Those who suffer most," a skeptical British physician sarcastically asserted, "are notoriously occupants of the third-class carriages."[24] That there were neither figures to support these claims nor any consideration of the possibility that third-class carriages might be more dangerous than first- or second-class ones made little difference to those who were intent on discrediting Erichsen's analysis.

Long after he first promulgated them, Erichsen's views remained a source of irritation for the railroad companies and for the lawyers and surgeons who represented them on both sides of the Atlantic. "It would hardly be stating the case too broadly," charged railroad advocate D.R. Wallace, "to say that it is doubtful if there has ever been a damage suit brought against a railroad company for any obscure nervous trouble, real or pretended, either in this country [the United States] or in Great Britain, for the last quarter of a century, in which the book has not figured."[25] "The extravagant estimate of the money value being 'shaken,' as it is called in England," explained a prominent American surgeon, "is largely due in this country at least to a single work, the only one in our language which enters into a detailed discussion of the so-called symptoms of concussion of the spinal cord."[26] Criticism was not confined to the British surgeon's writings; it also extended to his character and integrity. "The ingenuity and plausibility with which his book was written," commented railway surgeon John G. Johnson, "spoke more to his skill as a partisan" than it did to his desire to seek the truth.[27] "I think him worse, and he has done railway corporations infinitely more damage," charged another, "than the fellow who takes his life in his hands and holds up and robs a stage-coach or railroad train."[28]

Erichsen denied the charge that he had written his book to benefit the interests of the public at the expense of the railroads. In a letter to the *British Medical Journal,* he challenged the claims of a reviewer who asserted that the "title of Erichsen's little volume is calculated to mislead the casual reader":[29] "I must add that this particular title—the 'lettering' as it is called—was devised by the publisher and the bookbinder and was arranged with a view to space rather than to accuracy. With it I had nothing to do."[30] That his book might occasionally play into the hands of unscrupulous dissimulators and their attorneys, he continued, was hardly his fault. "If the public . . . 'believes that there is a specialty in the injuries produced by railway accidents,' that," said Erichsen, "is none of my doing."[31]

Psychosomatic Backlash

For fifteen years Erichsen's work remained the only book-length study of the topic. Translated into several languages, it sold thousands of copies throughout Europe and North America. Finally, in 1880, Boston surgeon Richard Manning Hodges offered the first serious English-language challenge to Erichsen's somatic doctrines. In contrast to Erichsen's claim regarding the unique capacity of railway accidents to elicit the many symptoms he listed, Hodges argued that railway accidents were just one of several possible mishaps that might give rise to virtually identical symptoms.[32] Hodges did not dispute the capacity of traumatic experiences to cause a wide array of physical and mental symptoms. What he questioned was why the symptoms attributable to railway accidents were considerably more durable than those caused by other traumatic events. The answer, he wrote, "is due, not to the specific peculiarities of train accidents, but to the annoying litigation and exorbitant claims for pecuniary damage that are constantly the grave result of their existence."[33] In other words, railway accidents were unique because they alone had the capacity to make their victims instantaneously wealthy.

Soon after the publication of Hodges's article Herbert W. Page, surgeon to the London and North-West Railway, received the prestigious Boylston Prize from Harvard University for an essay on the topic of spinal injuries.[34] Two years later Page expanded his findings and published the first book that explicitly challenged Erichsen's doctrines.[35] Building on Hodges's analysis, Page argued that while railway accidents might immediately give rise to a host of subjective symptoms, those that emerged at a later date could only be explained by psychical factors.

In formulating his conception of nervous shock Page relied on the work of his British surgical colleague Thomas Furneaux Jordan, who in 1866 had published his prize-winning essay, "Shock after Surgical Operations."[36] This article established Jordan's reputation as one of the world's foremost authorities on shock. But it was not Jordan's discussion of surgical shock that Page found intriguing. Rather it was his specific references to railway accidents: "The incidents of a railway accident contribute to a form of a combination of the most terrible circumstances which it is possible for the mind to conceive. The vastness of the destructive forces, the magnitude of the results, the imminent danger of the lives of numbers of human beings, and the hopelessness of escape from danger, give rise to emotions which in themselves are quite sufficient to produce shock or even death." [37] Although Jordan's analysis did not directly refute Erichsen's conception of spinal concussion, it provided a compelling alternative that Page readily adopted. "Purely psychical causes," Page argued, "[could explain] the very remarkable fact that after a railway collision the symptoms of general nervous shock are so common, and so often severe, in those who have received no bodily injury, or who have presented little sign of collapse at the time of the accident." [38]

Following Hodges's and Jordan's lead, Page identified fright as the primary agency responsible for the trauma-induced symptoms that Erichsen had earlier attributed to spinal concussion. Page then combined their analyses with the recent findings of distinguished British surgeon James B. Paget. In 1873 Paget had delivered a series of lectures on the topic of neuromimesis, which, he explained, was a phenomenon that arose under certain infrequent circumstances and induced patients to present symptoms that mimicked those of actual structural diseases. [39] Fright itself, Page thus extrapolated from his reading of Hodges and Paget, was capable of eliciting neuromimetic symptoms by way of some willful hypnotic state.

And, as of the hypnotic state, so of other neuromimeses also, the patients may voluntarily submit themselves to their exhibition, and the manifestations thereof become in themselves not less real. The existence of a certain amount of control is shown moreover by the disappearance of the mimicries, when all cause for their representation is removed. The matter of compensation as we have seen, exerts in many cases a very favorable influence on the symptoms of general nervous shock. It does so in these cases also, and examples are not few in which the typical neuromimesis came to an end shortly after settlement of claim had secured for the patients complete repose of mind, and had freed them from the necessity of any longer *allowing* themselves to be victims of the mimetic phenomena. [40]

In suggesting that something akin to a hypnotic state explained not only the persistence of neuromimetic symptoms but also their disappearance following settlements, Page had provided one of the first exclusively psychological explanations for both the cause and the cure of functional ailments.

Page's synthesis was both original and compelling. But despite its many virtues it contained a fundamental contradiction that contemporary commentators could not fail to recognize. His assertion that neuromimesis was a product of human will directly contradicted Paget's original presentation of the subject that emphasized the "unwilling" participation of the victim.[41] Moreover, Page's statements concerning voluntary submission to hypnotic states likewise failed to consider the most recent French investigations of the subject that had emphasized the possible role played by unconscious factors. For Page, conscious forces, not unconscious ones, were the dynamic variable.

The implications that could be drawn from this volitional model, Page asserted, could not be more clear: "The lesson to be learned from this is very obvious, that the sooner any cause for the representation of the phenomena is removed, the better, and that the patient should as far as possible be freed from the hurtful sympathy of friends."[42] As a surgeon Page simply could not fathom the possibility of unconscious, involuntary submission to psychical forces. But much to his chagrin Page's volitional model of accident-induced neuromimesis provided the foundation for a newly emerging and increasingly respectable psychogenic paradigm. Except for the element of human volition, the British railway surgeon's explanation for traumatic injuries remained fundamentally intact as it made its journey from the surgical to the neurological domain.

From the Spine to the Brain: A Functional Reassessment

Page had accomplished a remarkable feat. He had written a book that appealed to two distinct and significant constituencies. Both surgeons and neurologists were intrigued by his discussion of psychogenesis and his argument concerning the palliative effects of settlements. Neurologists were happy to see a railway surgeon who neither discounted the legitimacy of neuromimetic symptoms nor claimed that the overwhelming majority of plaintiffs in damage cases were frauds and malingerers. Surgeons, especially those who like Page were employed by the railways, also had cause to be pleased. A prominent member of their ranks had published a book that not only assailed Erichsen's doctrines but also appealed, so it seemed, to a wide range of medical specialties.[43]

Charles Dana noted that until the publication of Page's book the topic of railway spine had been exclusively "in the surgeon's hand and studied from a surgeon's standpoint." "It was not until after the appearance of Page's work," he added, "that neurologists took up the matter seriously."[44] When they did, it swiftly became apparent that there was little consensus to be found. Rather than usher in a new age of medical consensus, Page's work simply shifted the domain of the previously existing conflict from the realm of surgery to that of neurology.

By citing the role of mental factors in the production of accident-induced neuromimetic symptoms, Page unwittingly contributed to a renaissance of medical interest in psychogenesis. Page's work became a clarion call to both European and American neurologists. Initially, an overwhelming majority of neurologists looked favorably on the British railway surgeon's analysis. For instance, Harvard neurologist James Jackson Putnam considered it highly probable that psychical agency alone might produce the hysterical symptoms associated with railway accidents, and he praised Page's work for dwelling "particularly upon the important point that a rapid improvement after the settlement of legal claims is by no means proof that the patient's symptoms were imaginary or assumed, an inference which is often unjustly drawn."[45]

Still, more important from the medico-legal point of view, is the fact that even in chronic cases where the patient presents no symptoms that might not more or less readily be feigned, it is sometimes possible by careful searching to discover signs of so-called hysterical state, which, although not strictly objective, have almost the same value as if they were so as evidence against malingering. So far as I know, this fact has not previously been noticed, certainly it has not found its way into the literature of the "railway spine."[46]

But the definition of hysteria to which Putnam and other neurologists subscribed was in many respects dissimilar to the one held by Page. As Putnam's fellow Bostonian, George Walton, explained, when American neurologists spoke of hysteria they meant "not the vague hysteria of former times, but the functional disturbance of the cerebral centers which modern research, as set forth by Professor Charcot, has shown to follow given laws, and to offer pathognomonic characteristics."[47] It was precisely this physiological interpretation of hysteria that the British medical profession, in general, and railway surgeons, in particular, found so distasteful.[48]

Page's imprecise conception of railway accident-induced male hysteria and the subsequent American reception of his doctrines figured prominently in Jean-Martin Charcot's analysis of the subject.[49] According to Mark Micale, "In the period 1885–88, Charcot's work on masculine hysteria was practically synonymous with the investigation of traumatic hysteria."[50] Moreover, like most physicians of his day Charcot saw little reason to challenge the sanctity of the somatic paradigm and the prevailing medical wisdom concerning the physiological foundation of all diseases. His investigation of hysteria was resolutely somatic in its orientation.[51] Given his neurological expertise, this perspective was not the least bit surprising. In many respects his doctrines bore a striking resemblance to Erichsen's spinal concussion and Beard's neurasthenia. All three presupposed what Edward Shorter refers to as "a hidden organicity."[52] Hysteria was exceptional in one critical respect, however. Of the three, it alone was believed to be almost exclusively a matter of heredity.[53]

Throughout the 1870s Charcot remained committed to his somatic doctrines but acknowledged that "clinical and pathological research is necessary (in the case of the human subject) to a final judgment and the furnishing of proof."[54] In 1878 he took an audacious step and began a formal investigation of hypnotism.[55] But rather than consider the possible psychical effects of hypnotism, Charcot concentrated on what he perceived to be its predominant physiological implications.[56] Just as he had maintained that the presence of hysterical symptoms was itself indicative of some underlying neurological irregularity, he likewise proposed that "hypnosis itself involved physiological changes in the nervous system."[57] Indeed, the ability to be hypnotized was itself, Charcot insisted, evidence of some underlying hysterical, that is, cerebral, disturbance. Hypnotizing nonhysterical individuals was, by definition, impossible.[58]

Charcot's reputation added a hitherto absent credibility to the study of both hysteria and hypnotism. Of particular significance in this respect was his conception of male hysteria. Charcot was not the first physician to acknowledge the presence of male hysteria.[59] Indeed, when he first turned his attention to hysteria in the early 1860s, the notion of masculine hysteria already possessed a long history. But, as Micale notes, "[it] consisted mostly of passing, programmatic statements with little theoretical elaboration, clinical illustration, or academic recognition."[60]

Charcot's first diagnosis of male hysteria took place in February 1879—only two years before Page submitted his prize-winning essay. Over the next fourteen years Charcot recorded an additional sixty cases of male hysteria, many of which involved working-class men.[61] More significantly, however, Charcot did not present his first paper on male hysteria until the spring of 1882.[62] Although Charcot had earlier insisted that female hysteria was almost invariably a product of heredity, the majority of cases of male hysteria that he recounted during the 1880s were triggered by the destructive influence of a physical trauma.[63] Charcot himself commented,

Quite recently, male hysteria has been studied in America by Putnam and Walton, principally in connection with and as a sequel of traumatisms, and more especially of railroad accidents. They have recognized along with Page, who has also interested himself in this question in England, that many of those nervous accidents designated under the name of *railway spine*, which, in his opinion, might better be called *railway brain*, are in reality, whether appearing in man or in woman, simply hysterical manifestations.[64]

Charcot did not fail to acknowledge the practical questions that such circumstances posed: "The victims of railroad accidents quite naturally claim damages against companies. The case goes to court [and] thousands of dollars are at stake."[65] Not surprisingly, therefore, the significance of male hysteria, he noted, had itself become a source of legal controversy and a subject of great interest to the medicolegalist "for he is often called upon to give his opinion, in matters concerning which pecuniary interests are at stake, before a tribunal which would likely be influenced (and this circumstance renders his task the more difficult) by the disfavor which is still attached to the word hysteria on account of prejudices profoundly rooted."[66]

But to Charcot the medicolegal ramifications of traumatic hysteria were not nearly so significant as the neurological ones. Neither Page's status as a railway surgeon nor his desire to refute Erichsen's somatic doctrines was especially relevant to him. What intrigued the French neurologist about the Anglo-American discourse on the subject was the compelling evidence it offered in support of his view concerning the psychical origins of male hysteria and nothing more. By 1885 Charcot had come to accept Page's psychical conception of the agency responsible for traumatic hysteria. But his willingness to acknowledge the possible mental etiology of the disease did not induce him to abandon a physiological interpretation of its nature. On the contrary, mental traumas, he speculated, in some yet-to-be-comprehended fashion, induced an indiscernible physiological disturbance in the nervous system.[67] "It is always necessary, alongside of the traumatism," he charged, "to take account of a factor which very probably has played a more important part in the genesis of these accidents than the wound itself." In language that virtually mimicked Erichsen's original discussion of railway accidents, Charcot maintained, "I refer to the terror experienced by the patient at the moment of the accident, and which found expression shortly afterwards in loss of consciousness."[68]

Charcot explained this process by expanding on Page's earlier example concerning the apparently hypnotic effect of railway accidents on certain weak-minded individuals. He likened traumatic hysteria to states of drunkenness, drug intoxication, and what he had earlier defined as the somnambulistic state of the hypnotic trance. But unlike Page, who was chary about the possibility of psychical traumas evoking physiological disorders, Charcot insisted that the evidence of somatic disturbances was indisputable. Like Erichsen's spinal concussion and Beard's neurasthenia, Charcot's hysteria was known exclusively by its symptoms. " 'What, then, is hysteria?' Charcot asked in his last essay on the subject in 1893. 'We know nothing of its nature, nor about any lesions producing it. We know it only through its manifestations and are therefore only able to characterize it by its symptoms, for the more hysteria is subjective, the more it is necessary to make it objective in order to recognize it.' "[69] Hysteria, Charcot insisted, revealed itself by way of four factors: emotional volatility, sensory stigmata, motor disturbances, and an "hysterogenic zone."[70] Charcot's ability to isolate particular physiological symptoms unique to hysteria attracted neurologists in precisely the same manner as Beard's earlier description of neurasthenia. Both men had provided their newly emerging specialty with compelling nosological schemes that promoted their professional development and enabled them to compete more effectively with other segments of the increasingly specialized medical profession.[71]

Charcot's willingness to ascribe etiological significance to the psychical effects of traumatic experiences in no way diminished the importance he attached to the hereditary and physiological aspects of the disease. Traumatic experiences, he insisted, merely triggered preexisting hysterical tendencies and gave rise to what he maintained was "unquestionably one of those lesions which escape our present means of anatomical investigation, and which, for want of a better term, we designate dynamic or *functional* lesions."[72] As Ola Anderson explains, "Charcot conceived of the dynamic lesion as localized in the nervous system in the same manner as the structural lesions that had been observed in connection with a number of organic diseases."[73] The most striking feature of these so-called dynamic lesions was not their elusive nature, however. Rather it was that unlike structural lesions they were neither permanent nor incurable.

Despite its initial allure Charcot's analysis of traumatic male hysteria failed to arouse the same degree of interest in other lands as in his native France. Its inability to catch on elsewhere was attributable in part to a pervasive resistance to the concept of male hysteria.[74] Much of the opposition to Charcot's doctrines was rooted in age-old prejudices regarding the exclusively feminine nature of the disease.[75] Other factors were also at play—especially those related to national pride and cultural prejudice.[76] As an eminent American neurologist explained, "The Latin races, the French especially, are much more prone to these impressionable disorders, than is the composite race of this country that has come together from all nations of the world to form a new stock. I don't think we ought to apply the deductions of the Salpêtrière too absolutely."[77]

Leading German neurologists were equally critical of Charcot's findings. As early as 1878, Carl F. Westphal attributed the symptoms of railway spine to small foci of myelitis or encephalitis caused by the trauma.[78] Westphal's students, R. Thomsen and Hermann Oppenheim, initially disputed their teacher's somatic interpretation, but further investigation compelled Oppenheim to reconsider his mentor's theory.[79] "The traumatic neuroses," Oppenheim insisted, "are the result of *psychic and physical shock*. Both act mostly upon the cerebrum and evoke molecular alterations in the same areas which govern the higher psychic and the motor and sensory functions and those of the special senses."[80]

The most outspoken Anglo-American proponent of Oppenheim's theory was Philip Coombs Knapp, a Boston neurologist and clinical instructor of diseases of the nervous system at Harvard University.[81] Knapp detested Page's book. He claimed it "read like the work of a special pleader for the railway companies."[82] "Most of the cases that I have reported," Knapp proclaimed, "had no pecuniary interest whatever."[83] Similar views were expressed by several of Knapp's American neurological colleagues. Describing the case of a former hotel waiter who had saved a drowning man but then lost his mental composure, Landon Carter Gray declared, "Now, if he was suing a railroad, the question would come up at once, 'Is he shamming?' But you cannot sue the Atlantic Ocean, and there is no basis for suspicion in this case."[84] Philadelphia neurologist Francis X. Dercum carried Knapp's and Gray's analyses one step further. "In regard to the disappearance of so-called 'litigation symptoms,' made so much by Page and others," Dercum explained, "my observation has been that when a claim for damages has been settled, the mental condition improves very much. . . . After a while, however, I have seen the old mental condition partly reestablish itself while the physical condition has undergone no change save that which could be accounted for by the slow repair of time."[85]

The competing theories of Page, Charcot, Knapp, Dercum, and others not only inspired a novel neurological discourse but also heightened the stakes in a fifteen-year medicolegal controversy. The role of expert testimony had become a serious bone of contention among physicians who now had two contradictory sources on which they could base their claims. American neurologist Edward Spitzka explained,

The great difficulty under which both the legal and medical gentlemen, connected with trials growing out of real and alleged injuries to the spinal cord, labor seems to be a belief on the part of the plaintiffs that it is necessary to prove the existence of coarse organic disease of the spinal cord and its membranes in order to convince a court or jury that damage has really been done. On the part of the defense a similar impression prevails, and is aided by an excessive zeal to prove simulation on the part of the plaintiff.[86]

Writing in the *Medical Record* soon after the publication of Page's work, Dana began his article on railway spine with the following observation.

The physician who is called into court to testify in a case of spinal injury witnesses a curious spectacle. The lawyer for the prosecution waves before the jury a volume of "Erichsen Upon Spinal Concussion." He reads to them, in impressive accents, the statement that every injury to the spine, however slight, is full of danger to the sufferer. He asks, with sonorous emphasis, if Mr. Erichsen is not a surgeon of world-wide fame; and if he does not say that slight injuries to the back may cause chronic spinal disease of the most serious character. He sneers at the work of a certain Mr. Page, who is known to be professedly only a railway surgeon. He shows that his client has paralysis, anemia, meningitis, in fine, "spinal concussion." On the other hand, the lawyer for the defense brandishes triumphantly a larger work, by Mr. Herbert Page, on "Injuries to the Spine"; he reads to the jury cases of malingering therein related, shows that Mr. Erichsen has for years made a business of being an expert for people with injured spines, but that he has never yet found a case that proved fatal. He quotes Mr. Page's two hundred and thirty four cases of spinal concussion, in most of which recovery resulted, and shows, through his medical expert, that the spinal cord is so admirably protected that it could never possibly be injured by anything so utterly trivial as a railway collision.[87]

Given these two mutually exclusive and highly antagonistic perspectives, it is no wonder that over the course of the 1880s there emerged not one but several competing explanations and classification schemes for the symptoms that frequently followed railway accidents.

Railway Surgeons Respond

The evolving medical awareness of the possible psychical nature of railway and other traumatic injuries went largely unnoticed in the greater community.[88] In many respects the internal medical discourse on the topic was rendered superfluous by the social and cultural circumstances endemic to the rapidly industrializing United States, to say nothing of the overwhelming impact of Erichsen's doctrines in courts of law. In the first decade following the publication of his book, the English railway companies paid over $11 million in damages.[89] Similar figures were cited for the United States. Of these claims, hundreds came from those seeking compensation for spinal concussion or what an eminent physician soon termed Erichsen's disease.[90]

Finding for an alleged victim of spinal concussion was one of the few ways that ordinary men could vent their frustration against what many believed to be a rapacious and pernicious industry.[91] In the eyes of the overwhelming majority of American men and women of the 1890s and beyond Erichsen's original doctrines were alive and well. Harold N. Moyer, writing shortly after the turn of the century, asserted that "the term spinal concussion, as used by Erichsen nearly forty years ago, has served as a foundation for an extraordinary superstructure and one that has maintained itself decade after decade in spite of the advances in our knowledge of neural pathology."[92]

The role played by juries was a source of special irritation to railway surgeons and the corporations they represented. "Juries," asserted the Philadelphia surgeon Thomas G. Morton, "usually sympathize with the plaintiff and can hardly be said to carefully weigh evidence when their sympathies are aroused by the plea of mental and physical suffering or by the sight of bodily injury or deformity which is always made as prominent as possible."[93] Moreover, they were, according to John Punton, almost universally unreceptive to the efforts of railway surgeons to attribute an accident victim's symptoms to psychological rather than to physiological factors: "We try to explain what the psychologico-pathogenic idea is, and as a result we lose our case."[94] The rising populist impulses that were spreading across the mid- and southwestern portions of the United States and the growing labor unrest in the Northeast merely exacerbated the railroad corporations' image as rapacious demons. "Unfortunately, in our section," wrote Georgia surgeon Hugh Burford, "the average juror views railway corporations as a great octopus subject to public prey."[95] Railway spine, charged D.R. Wallace, was merely a symptom of the present "epidemic of madness and insane furor against the railroads and other corporate enterprises."[96]

Statistics appear to confirm these observations. At trial plaintiffs won almost 70 percent of their cases against the railroads.[97] Such findings were rarely overturned on appeal.[98] Keeping cases of this nature out of the hands of juries thus became a central preoccupation for railroad owners, executives, shareholders, and attorneys. Fortunately for the railroad industry most mid- and late-nineteenth-century American judges shared many of its concerns.[99] By midcentury, in fact, a majority of American judges had become convinced that a jury could not be depended on to handle most negligence cases "fairly"—particularly when those cases concerned injured workers.[100] The same, however, could not be said of cases involving injured passengers.[101] As Philadelphia attorney Christopher Stuart Patterson explained in his 1886 treatise, *Railway Accident Law*, different standards applied to each category.[102] Indeed, most American judges readily acknowledged that common carriers owed a higher duty to their passengers than to their employees: "When carriers undertake to convey persons by the powerful but dangerous agency of steam, public policy and safety require that they be held to the greatest possible care and diligence. And whether the consideration for such transportation be pecuniary or otherwise, the personal safety of the passengers should not be left to the sport of chance or the negligence of careless agents."[103]

Given the pervasiveness of this view and the almost ubiquitous hostility expressed by most jurors, railroad companies concluded early on that they had little to gain by contesting the claims of passengers with broken bones, missing limbs, and other similarly conspicuous injuries in courts of law. As the physician Henry Hollingsworth Smith explained,

So generally is this liability for injury caused by negligence admitted, that most corporations or employers do not hesitate at prompt settlement of a just and reasonable claim, being influenced thereto not only by a proper regard for the suffering induced, but also as an acknowledgment of "the Majesty of the Law"; it being a well settled principle "that they are liable for past and future physical and mental suffering, together with the loss of earning power where the consequences are such as in the ordinary course of nature may be reasonably expected to ensue."[104]

Not every passenger-injury case was black and white, however. With potentially large sums of money at stake, the possibility of fraudulent claims needed to be taken seriously. Cases of alleged railway spine proved to be especially suspect.[105]

Prior to the publication of Erichsen's lectures an accident victim who failed to display any clearly discernible anatomical or physiological symptoms was not likely to fare well in a court of law. Erichsen's book forever altered this situation. It lent a hitherto absent credibility to the plaintiff's claims and greatly enhanced the prospects of financial compensation. As Erichsen's surgical colleague Dr. James Syme declared,

A victim of a train accident [need only] to go to bed, call in a couple of sympathizing doctors, diligently peruse Mr. Erichsen's lately-published work on Railway Injuries, go into court on crutches, and give a doleful account of the distress experienced by his wife and children through his personal sufferings, which have resulted from the culpable negligence that allowed him to leave his seat prematurely. Who can doubt that in such circumstances the jury would give large demands?[106]

Many railway executives rightly feared that the answer to this question was almost no one. "That cities and corporations are robbed of vast sums of money yearly by malingerers, aided by unscrupulous legal talent, and by ignorant or dishonest surgeons," charged an angry American physician, "we all know to be true."[107]

Had Erichsen written a treatise that advanced the interests of the railways and denounced past, current, and future plaintiffs as conniving malingerers, he might very well have put an end to the controversy. But in choosing the opposite track, he greatly heightened the stakes of an already contentious issue. While railroad accidents were not the only source of spinal injuries, they were, said Erichsen, the most frequent cause. And what made spinal injuries so baffling, Erichsen wrote, was "the disproportion that exists between the apparently trifling accident that the patient has sustained, and the real and serious mischief that has occurred."[108] It was precisely this claim that infuriated the railroad companies, who refused to accept the possibility that a "trifling accident" could give rise to so severe an injury as Erichsen described. The only merit in Erichsen's argument, they claimed, concerned the alleged "serious mischief" that such accidents might cause, but this mischief concerned not the spine but the deliberate efforts of alleged railway-accident victims to defraud the corporations.

The growing incidence of alleged cases of spinal concussion and the frequent willingness of juries to find for the plaintiffs in such cases contributed to the formation of several regional associations of railway surgeons throughout the 1880s. Local associations of railway surgeons were established as early as January 1882—before the publication of Page's book.[109] Over the course of the decade more than fifty additional local organizations were established. Finally, on June 28, 1888, more than two hundred members representing several of these organizations met in Chicago and founded the National Association of Railway Surgeons (NARS). Later that year the association issued the first volume of the *National Association of Railway Surgeons Journal*.[110]

A number of factors motivated the formation of the NARS. But among the primary causes were medicolegal issues arising from Erichsen's analysis.[111] Years of costly settlements and damage awards forced the North American railroad industry to take action. As Milton Jay asserted, "There is nothing that is probably of so much importance as the medico-legal aspects of spinal injuries. Out of twenty cases of law suits brought to recover damages from railway injuries, fifteen of them will claim to have sustained injury to the spine, even if the spinal cord has not been touched."[112]

One of the primary goals of the NARS was to provide its members with information and material that they could employ when testifying on behalf of their lines to assure that surgeons were "better equipped to go on the witness stand and protect the company's rights in courts of justice, and thus increase their annual dividends."[113] Given proper information, railway surgeons hoped to neutralize the expert testimony offered by neurologists and other medical experts who frequently sided with plaintiffs. R. Harvey Reed elaborated:

The Association does not propose to stop at the mere treatment of the patient, which, to relieve promptly and permanently, is a decided benefit to the company, but they propose to study how to protect the company from impositions at court by studying medico-legal aspects of their cases, and thereby seek to discourage malingery in all its multiplicity of forms, whereby tens of thousands of dollars are fraudulently wrung from our railroad companies usually by so-called courts of justice.[114]

The association had done nothing radical in denying the reality of spinal concussion. If anything its position in this regard was well in keeping with the one of the predominant strands of the American neurological discourse. In fact, some of America's most distinguished neurologists contributed to the cause of railway surgery.[115] But examples of harmony between neurologists and railway surgeons were the exception rather than the norm. And in this war of words neurologists had a decided advantage. Their insistence on the somatic nature of traumatically induced injuries found a receptive home among juries throughout the nation.

Leaders of the National Association of Railway Surgeons were not naive. They realized that the public was little inclined to support their point of view. Public hostility to powerful corporations—particularly to the railroad industry—was a fact that few failed to acknowledge. Efforts to influence public perception regarding the psychical nature of railway spine were therefore largely worthless. Acquiring professional support from the larger medical profession was a different matter, however. If an overwhelming majority of American physicians could be convinced not only of the folly of Erichsen's doctrines but also of the legitimacy of psychogenesis, public opinion would cease to be so significant.

The leader of the NARS's crusade to convert the medical profession to this position was not a physician but an attorney. Clark Bell proved to be one of the most formidable advocates for the railroad industry.[116] A far more accomplished polemicist than most physicians, Bell delivered one of the most widely quoted speeches in the organization's short history.[117] Railway spine, he asserted,

is the Nemesis of the modern railway. It is the veritable Old Man of the Sea, that it is on the shoulders and is an ever-present, ever-to-be-dreaded terror to railway commerce and railway managers. Invented by one of the most clever English surgeons as a means of procuring enormous verdicts from the railway corporations in accident cases, it has baffled both railway surgeons and counsel, and, vampire-like, sucked more blood of the corporate bodies and railway companies than all other cases combined. It is the ready refuge of the malingerer, the weapon always burnished bright and sharpened, of the unscrupulous attorney and his partner in profit, the medical expert, and affords advantages for the scheming, avaricious claimant who has suffered an actual injury unparalleled by any other cause of injury known in railway damage cases.[118]

Bell called on the nation's railway surgeons to take matters into their own hands and put an end to this mockery of justice. "Has not the time come," Bell asked rhetorically, "when the profession of surgery should define this injury so that courts, counsel, and juries may know and locate and apply to it those tests which are insisted upon in regard to all other physical injuries?"[119] Bell then posed this challenge: "Why should the railway surgeons of the nation hesitate in forming such a consensus of surgical thought as would present an insurmountable barrier to the further spread and advancement of an everywhere recognized evil?"[120]

What Bell neglected to consider, however, was that such an "evil" was by no means recognized everywhere.

While several physicians were sympathetic if not actually supportive of the NARS's endeavor, they expressed little enthusiasm for Bell's analysis, which, in their eyes, reflected old thinking. The majority of American physicians, including neurologists and railway surgeons, were not nearly so interested in exposing frauds or serving as expert witnesses as they were in treating their patients and discovering the true nature of their ailments. In the eyes of the medical profession—particularly neurologists—attacking Erichsen was simply beating a dead horse.

The only significant issue remaining to be resolved concerned not the etiology of railway spine but its pathology. Several questions still needed to be answered: Did psychic traumas merely trigger some pre-existing *nervous diathesis?* Did they give rise to some unique functional disturbance irrespective of a patient's prior personal and hereditary roots? Or did they simply elicit a psychopathological response with no underlying somatic disturbance? The answers to these questions had substantially greater legal than therapeutic significance. In fact, from a purely therapeutic perspective they were, prior to the first decade of the twentieth century, inconsequential. Nervous disorders, regardless of their perceived etiology and pathology, were treated in virtually identical manners. Legally, however, these distinctions were fundamental. John E. Parson, Esq., commenting on the role of mental distress as an element of damage in cases to recover for personal injuries asserted,

The general principle is well established that in actions of tort, where for the wrong, there is a right to recover damages, mental distress may be taken into consideration in fixing the amount. But the weight of authority seems to establish that when the injury consists in distress of mind alone, or where the mental distress is separate from and independent of the wrong, it does not constitute an element of damage and may not be considered in determining the amount of recovery.[121]

Given Parson's analysis, it was only fitting then that the National Association of Railway Surgeons would begin promoting a purely psychical conception of railway spine. Rather than expend their energy on the thankless and publicly derided task of exposing fraudulent spinal cases in an effort to increase dividends, railway surgeons, like their fellow physicians, were now free to take such complaints seriously and offer such treatment as they saw fit without having to compromise their medical integrity or their employers' pocket.

Suggestion and American Railway Surgery

J. H. Greene, an Iowa railway surgeon, was one of the earliest American physicians to recognize the role of suggestion in fomenting traumatic neuroses. Citing the work of both Charcot and Hippolyte Bernheim, Greene proclaimed, "I believe with the modern views on this subject, a greater importance will be attached to this doctrine of hypnotic suggestion in the cure [of traumatic neuroses] and that it will eventually come up in the courts."[122] "This doctrine," Greene added, "reconciles in great part the opposing views of surgeons in these cases and that with the acceptance of the theory of hypnotic suggestion they can meet on common ground, without being regarded one as the tool of the corporation, the other as preparing a case for a prospective fee. It also explains the peculiar efficacy of the 'golden cure,' without throwing the comparatively few people in with the perjurers."[123] In Bernheim's suggestive therapeutics Greene found exactly what he and other railway surgeons had been seeking.[124]

While Greene provided a plausible theoretical rationale that supported the power of suggestion, Warren Bell Outten offered a more practical example. Among the most powerful figures in the NARS, Outten had devoted more than thirty years of his professional life to his duties as chief surgeon for the Missouri Pacific Railway. Over the course of his career Outten observed that railway employees and passengers were not equally susceptible to traumatic neuroses.[125] Outten attributed this difference to two separate, albeit related, factors. Both the employees' "familiarity and experience with dangerous elements" and "the social surroundings of the respective classes" figured prominently in his analysis.[126] In support of this contention he offered the following example.

A man has been in a collision. He was perfectly conscious that he met with no blow; knows, in fact, exactly what occurred to him when the accident happened; and yet he finds that within a few hours, occasionally much sooner, he is seized with a pain in his back, gets worse, and summons a physician. Cause, railway collision! The physician expresses doubt, and suggests grave consequences. Railway injury; nervous patient; *suggestion on suggestion* continued; and then there is the development of a serious case— psychic influences possibly leading to traumatic hysteria or neurasthenia.[127]

A sympathetic surrounding composed of friends and loved ones, Outten continued, merely aggravates the patient's condition by fixing his mind on his ailments and his suffering. Outten offered the following qualification, however: "All, of course, depends upon the mental strength and integrity of the individual himself, and the integrity of his surroundings."[128]

The role of the attending physicians figured prominently in Outten's analysis of traumatic neuroses. "It seems rather startling," Outten explained, "that a physician, by virtue of mental superiority, prejudice, and suggestion could create an essentially serious condition, but we candidly believe that it is possible in a weakened and receptive mind to suggest and develop consequences of a very serious nature."[129] Neurologists, Outten added, were among the greatest culprits in this respect: "When a wreck upon a railway train occurs near a large city, you invariably have railway spine simply for the reason that the neurologists or nerve doctors are always present in the cities, while we can show twenty times the number of accidents occurring upon a road away from a popular center never to have them."[130] During a neurological examination "the mind of the patient," he charged, "is fed with suggestions to the intensification of the neurotic state, while the principle or rest is ignored."[131]

Outten and other American railway surgeons had inadvertently generated a novel synthesis regarding hypnosis and suggestion. Not surprisingly, this interpretation favored the interests of the railway corporations. Borrowing from Charcot they argued that traumatic neuroses, while legitimate medical ailments, were typically the afflictions of the hereditarily tainted and morally suspect. The so-called neuropath, charged David Booth, "possesses a susceptibility to suggestion and liability to exaggeration."[132] Of course, claims that railway accidents merely triggered preexisting tendencies were nothing new. But the further assertion of American railway surgeons that doctors themselves frequently aggravated and, on certain occasions, unwittingly inspired these cases by their suggestive influences reflected not Charcot's physiological doctrines, but a perverse and self-serving reading of Bernheim's psychical ones. "The psychic, suggestive, and auto-suggestive element," asserted R. S. Harnden, "enters so largely into these cases, and in fact into all except graver traumatisms accompanied by objective symptoms, that the nicest degree of skill and tact becomes necessary upon the part of the surgeon."[133]

Virginia Railway surgeon George Ross captured the extent to which railway surgeons had, in fact, fused the conflicting theories of Charcot and Bernheim in a manner that served their own interests. "Suggestion," Ross maintained, "is a tremendous factor, and I believe the doctor into whose hands the patient first goes can materially influence the patient in any manner he pleases."[134] Ross's choice of words revealed far more than he realized and captured the prevailing sentiments of his fellow railway surgeons. For Ross, suggestion operated on both a psychical and a physiological plane. The physician's authoritative stature, not the patient's ancestral or acquired vices, served as the dynamic variable in Ross's confused analysis. What the physician did and, more importantly, what he said "materially" rather than psychically influenced the patient for better or ill.

From Charcot, American railway surgeons learned that a state akin to hypnotic suggestion had the capacity to trigger certain traumatic neuroses among a particular class of hereditarily or environmentally tainted men and women. Their often dismal plight, railway surgeons insisted, bore little or no relationship to any train wreck. To the contrary, men and women of this nature were like dry powder in search of a match. The virtue of Charcot's explanation was that it exculpated the railroads in those instances in which it could be unequivocally applied. Such cases were the minority, however. The overwhelming number of victims suffering from traumatic neuroses were free of any demonstrable ancestral or acquired vices.

In these cases Bernheim's psychical doctrines, despite their failure to stigmatize the victim, were far more enticing. They could be used to shift the blame from the accident itself to the attending physician, sympathetic friends, loved ones, and lawyers. Together, these respective, albeit unwitting, suggestive influences could not help but evoke a full-fledged case of traumatic neurosis. Few railway surgeons denied that the shock of the initial accident might itself have contributed to the patient's heightened suggestibility. But the significance of shock, they insisted, could be greatly mitigated provided that certain safeguards were taken—the most important of which involved removing the victim from the harmful influences inevitable in an overly sympathetic environment.

American railway surgeons argued that the most effective treatment of traumatic neuroses involved a combination of the rest cure, especially its emphasis on isolation, and suggestive therapeutics.[135] But unlike S. Weir Mitchell and other neurologists who conceived of this therapy in somatic terms, the surgeons argued that it operated on a purely psychical level.[136] Simply removing the patient from ill-advised sympathizers yielded beneficial therapeutic results. Isolation itself, rather than rest per se, had the primary therapeutic value. A successful cure required neither the production of Weir Mitchell's much-heralded "fat and blood" nor the reduction of what he termed "wear and tear." All it entailed was directing the patient's mind away from hurtful suggestions.

"The law of isolation should be so binding in the treatment of these functional nervous affections due to trauma," Punton asserted, "that failure of its enforcement, in the incipient states, at least, should be sufficient ground to excuse any railroad company from further responsibility of any claims made against them for any subsequent nervous disease."[137] Punton likewise acknowledged the efficacy of suggestive therapeutics but begrudged the fact that "not all physicians can reap positive results with suggestion and thus choose not to avail themselves of this powerful therapeutic tool."[138] The final word on the subject came from the most eminent of all railway surgeons, Outten, who in a single sentence captured the prevailing psychogenic and psychotherapeutic synthesis achieved by the NARS: "I maintain that many of these cases are made by suggestion and can be treated by suggestion."[139]

In advocating the clinical use of suggestive therapeutics and emphasizing the psychological features of the Weir Mitchell Rest Cure, American railway surgeons had unwittingly become the first American medical specialty to achieve a consensus regarding the therapeutic value of what would soon be known throughout the world as psychotherapy. Whereas neurologists and psychiatrists were only just beginning to debate seriously among themselves the possible costs and benefits of directing their therapies toward the mind rather than the body, American railway surgeons, by the turn of the century, had become committed to the theory, if not actually the practice, of pursuing such a course. That their motivation was in large measure dictated by the material interests of their employers did not diminish their considerable accomplishment. More than three decades of conflict had generated a novel and compelling psychical synthesis that would provide the future foundation for the birth of American psychotherapy.

Epilogue

Shortly before his death in 1896 an elderly and long since retired John Eric Erichsen took time to pen a letter to R. M. Swearingen. Earlier that year the Texas physician had defended Erichsen against a series of ad hominem attacks appearing in a variety of NARS publications. An old man now, Erichsen expressed little desire to become engaged in what he termed "surgical polemics," let alone to defend himself from any personal attacks. Instead, he preferred to reflect on the "most hospitable and friendly reception" he received from his surgical brethren in the United States during a visit some twenty years ago. But despite his statements to the contrary, Erichsen could not resist the temptation to express himself one final time on the subject he had almost single-handedly created.

Nearly thirty years have passed since I first brought the subject of railway and other injuries of the nervous system to the notice of the profession. At that time (1866), the pathology of the nervous system and injuries was very imperfectly understood, and even the nomenclature had not been invented. "Neurosis" and "neurasthenia" even, were unknown terms, and what I then, for want of a better name, called "concussion of the spine," is now universally recognized and described under the more modern appellation of "traumatic neurasthenia." The morbid states are the same, and the symptoms identical; but the name has been changed, and the modern designation is probably more in accordance with modern views than was the older one. In all my writings on this subject, I have pointed out that symptoms arising from railway shocks are identical with those that occur from other and more ordinary accidents of civil life, and that these symptoms so occurring had been described by surgeons many years before railways were dreamt of, and fully a century before I had written a line on the subject.[140]

What Erichsen failed to consider was that a constellation of ideas and interests vastly beyond his or anyone else's capacity to control had combined to render his original intent nothing more than an interesting historical footnote.

CHAPTER 3

Avoiding Psychotherapy

*Neurasthenia and the Limits
of Somatic Therapy*

What Erichsen referred to as neurasthenia was as much a
product of nineteenth-century medicine's somatic orientation as it was
a contribution to it.[1] Popularized by George Miller Beard, a New York
neurologist, neurasthenia was held to be a culturally and hereditarily
derived disease primarily, though not exclusively, confined to "brain
workers."[2] Beard was neither the first physician to discuss neurasthenia
nor the only one of his day to pay close attention to the many symptoms by which it could be identified. In fact, in 1869, the very year that
Beard had first announced his discovery, E. H. Van Deusen, a Michigan
asylum superintendent, had already published an original article on the
subject.[3] Neurasthenia, Van Deusen proclaimed, "may with propriety
be regarded as a distinct form of disease."[4] Its primary cause was "excessive mental labor, especially when combined with anxiety and deficient
nourishment."[5]

Beard's conception of neurasthenia differed from Van Deusen's in
one significant respect. Unlike the Michigan asylum superintendent,
who did little more than offer a clinical description of neurasthenia,
Beard made a considerable effort to establish a legitimate pathological
foundation for it. "In regard to the pathology of neurasthenia," he
wrote, "we are compelled, in the absence of definite knowledge, to reason from logical probability." Proof of his diagnosis, he felt sure, would
"in time be substantially confirmed by microscopical and chemical examination of those patients who die in a neurasthenic condition."[6] Until then the pathology of neurasthenia would remain a black box. As

one physician explained, "When we can know and understand the origin of a thought, and the molecular change of gray matter in the brain consequent upon that thought, then, and not till then may the pathology of neurasthenia be written."[7]

Prior to the 1880s what little attention Beard's doctrines received was mostly negative.[8] The early opposition that greeted Beard's "discovery" was not long-lasting, however. By the early 1880s neurasthenia's status as a distinct disease entity, while not universally embraced, received little challenge. W.A. McClain merely stated the obvious when he asserted that "the fact is now generally admitted that thought exhausts the nervous substance as surely as walking exhausts the muscles."[9] Acceptance of neurasthenia was attributable not only to its consistency with prevailing medical and scientific wisdom but also to its broader cultural resonance.[10] Regarding the former, the evidence, speculative as it was, seemed to be overwhelming. Especially promising was the recent discovery of specific microbes responsible for various infectious diseases. As Edward Cowles, superintendent of the prestigious McLean Asylum, explained, recent bacteriological discoveries "promise[d] to throw great light upon these mysteries of our problem."[11] But a physician need not posit a bacteriological basis of neurasthenia if he wished to exploit the novel germ theory; all he need do was seize its logic. "The influences which lead to nervous exhaustion," J.S. Greene maintained, "are all-pervasive. They permeate the atmosphere of our modern civilization as bacteria do the air we breathe. We are all to a greater or less degree impressible by them; but, like the living microscopic germs, they make their easiest victims of those whose powers of resistance are weakest."[12]

Cultural factors were equally significant. Beard argued that nervousness was confined almost exclusively to what he termed the "comfortable classes."[13] Moreover, he insisted that neurasthenia was itself a uniquely American disease. Brain workers, he insisted, were the most likely victims. Being neurasthenic afforded one the opportunity to "move in neurasthenic circles."[14] "Among the rich and well-to-do and especially among professional men and those who belong to the higher walks of life," one physician explained, "this disease is more often found in its most typical form."[15] The explicitly class-conscious rhetoric employed by Beard and others did far more than merely destigmatize nervousness and anxiety. It made them seem virtuous.[16] Neurasthenic men and women could, if they so chose, wear their diagnosis as a badge of honor. "Fifth Avenue," said Beard, "is in some features a very much better field for pathological study than Five Points."[17] Writing shortly after the turn of the century, a prominent Swiss physician proclaimed, "The name neurasthenia is on everybody's lips: it is the fashionable new disease."[18]

The disease was a tribute not only to the individual who contracted it but also to the very culture that produced it. In addition to its class components, neurasthenia possessed a peculiarly American flavor, which not only posed a great challenge to American medicine but also created special opportunities for private practitioners. Beard proclaimed, "Neurasthenia was modern and originally American; and no age, no country, and no form of civilization, not Greece, nor Rome, nor Spain, nor the Netherlands, in the days of glory, possessed such maladies."[19] "Extreme nervous tension seems to be so peculiarly American," added Annie Payson Call, "that a German physician coming to this country to practice became puzzled by the variety of nervous disorders he was called upon to help, and finally announced his discovery of a new disease which he chose to call 'Amercanitis.'"[20]

Few diseases could lay claim to such highbrow, to say nothing of patriotic, credentials. "We cannot, as in many other diseases," Beard charged, "look to Germany for light and information—for in Germany this condition is comparatively unknown, and in France and England is far more rare than with us. It is a disease almost exclusively of well-to-do classes and can, therefore, be satisfactorily studied only in private practice."[21] By framing neurasthenia in this manner, Beard was able to win the support of some otherwise skeptical colleagues who had grown frustrated with the failure of American medicine to keep pace with European research. Moreover, his assertions concerning the need to study the disease in private practice could not fail to please his fellow neurologists, whose livelihoods depended on their ability to attract private patients.[22]

Along with class and national concerns, issues of sex and gender occupied a prominent position in the discussion of neurasthenia.[23] Whereas the source of nervous fatigue in men was held to lie in the male-occupied public sphere, the source of such fatigue in women was attributed to the female-occupied private sphere.[24] Each contained a set of intrinsic perils. But whereas the factors that gave rise to neurasthenia in men were typically regarded as serious matters, those that engendered the disease in women were commonly looked on as mere trifles. Male victims of neurasthenia were held to be "active professional business men who do much brain work"; female victims were seen as suffering "under a monotonous strain of domestic life."[25] "The chief

causes of the neurasthenic condition in women," H.C. Sharpe explained, "are due to the domestic surroundings and social life of the
patient."[26]

The actual number of late-nineteenth-century American men and
women who suffered from nervous exhaustion is difficult, if not impossible, to ascertain. American physicians differed greatly in their estima-
tions of the disease's impact. The significance of their dispute was not
to be found in its resolution but in the popular notions it engendered—in what T. Jackson Lears asserts was the "the *belief* of contemporary observers that nervousness was on the rise."[27] Of all the assumptions that informed neurasthenic discourse none was more important
than Beard's claims concerning the proliferation of nervousness: "The
development of nervousness and the increase of functional nervous diseases, under whatever names they may be known, have been so great in
modern times, especially in the Northern portions of the United States,
that there is no need of statistics—the facts can be demonstrated by the
general observations of those who have opportunities to observe, and
improve those opportunities as to be able to draw correct conclusions."[28] Few challenged the veracity of Beard's claims. "No physician
can practice medicine and not meet with it," said J.S. Jewell.[29]

The Significance of Patient-Centered Therapeutics

Prior to Beard's efforts to popularize neurasthenia, the
symptoms by which he identified the disease were rarely accepted by
the medical community as signs of a legitimate illness. In most cases
a man or woman displaying the wide array of symptoms that Beard
grouped under the heading of neurasthenia was either dismissed altogether or labeled a hypochondriac or hysteric. Beard put an end to this
situation; he added medical dignity to what Donald Meyer asserts had
previously been "a whole set of experiences, forms of behavior and
states of mind that medicine had not accepted."[30] Beard's list of symptoms was vast. Among other things, it included,

insomnia, flushing, drowsiness, bad dreams, cerebral irritation, . . . neurasthenic asthenopia, . . . atonic voice, . . . nervous dyspepsia, . . . sweating
hands and feet, . . . fear of lightning, or fear of responsibility, of open places
or of closed places, fear of society, . . . fear of fears, . . . fear of everything, . . .

lack of decision in trifling matters, . . . pains in the back, . . . cold hands and feet, . . . a feeling of profound exhaustion unaccompanied by positive pain, . . . vague pains and flying neuralgias, . . . involuntary emissions, . . . dryness of the hair.[31]

Such symptoms, Beard insisted, "are not in any way imaginary, but real; not trifling, but serious; although not usually dangerous." "In strictness," he continued, "nothing in disease can be imaginary. If I bring pain upon by worrying, by dwelling upon myself, that pain is as real as though it were brought upon by an objective influence."[32] Thomas Stretch Dowse, a respected British physician who originally eschewed Beard's work and challenged his conception of neurasthenia as a distinct disease entity, eventually embraced Beard's doctrines. "I found the term [neurasthenia] vague and unscientific, and I expected the scalpel and the microscope to reveal to me the cause of any arrest of nerve function. I am happy to say, that as I have grown older so have I grown wiser in this respect: and I am therefore now very glad to have recourse to a term, which is in every way most applicable to a number of nervous arrangements."[33]

Beard excoriated his medical colleagues for failing to take such symptoms seriously. Others joined his attack. John P. Savage lamented the fact that "great sufferers, therefore, are frequently dismissed as they were in former years 'possessed by the devil,' without sympathy, advice, or any attempt at treatment, other than the simple injunction, 'Go thy way, thou art mad at thyself.'"[34] Beard's colleague Alphonse David Rockwell pointed out that "[one] reason why neurasthenia has been so long neglected and so little understood is that in many cases the symptoms are so subtle, illusory, and difficult of analysis and classification. One who has not seen and carefully examined a large number of cases of this disease will hardly believe it possible that it can manifest itself in so many different ways."[35]

But not all physicians accepted the large list of symptoms offered by Beard, Savage, Rockwell, and others. C. P. Hughes argued that Beard "has recently given new emphasis to the study of this interesting subject, though his enthusiasm has led him into too indiscriminate a symptomatology, and into too voluminous and needless a symptomatic nosology."[36] Louis Faugeres Bishop maintained that "to the neurologist, neurasthenia as a diagnosis is too often a nosological dumping-ground for everything that is not something else."[37] One of Beard's harshest critics was the renowned British neurologist W. R. Gowers who, in his 1888 magisterial volume on nervous diseases, confined his discussion of neurasthenia to the final two pages. *"There is no more justification for regarding neurasthenia as a definite malady, to be distinguished from others and separately described,"* Gowers declared, *"than there is for adopting a similar course with regard to 'debility' among general diseases."* [38]

One of the more intriguing criticisms of Beard's elaborate symptomatology came from Philip Coombs Knapp, who had played a prominent role in the debates regarding railway spine. Knapp did not deny that neurasthenia constituted a distinct disease entity. What he questioned was the inclusion of mental factors among its symptoms. "The line between these normal conditions and conditions indicating actual disease" Knapp observed, "is no more definite than the line between ordinary mental depression and melancholia." [39] Knapp argued that Beard's inclusion of mental symptoms needlessly undermined the somatic integrity of Beard's doctrines. Although Knapp did not deny the legitimacy of either psychological symptoms or psychopathology itself, he questioned their relationship to neurasthenia, which he held to be a resolutely somatic disease with clearly discernible organic symptoms. The mental symptoms that Beard and others described, he maintained, did not rightfully belong on the list of neurasthenic symptoms.

The Role of Rapport

His critics notwithstanding, Beard had performed a remarkable feat. His inclusion of "subjective" mental symptoms had a powerful, if unintended effect, on the future course of American neurological and psychiatric medicine. Beard and his followers unwittingly added a new dignity to the doctor-patient interaction. [40] Unlike several other diseases that could be diagnosed on the basis of "objective" symptoms—for instance, smallpox or typhus—a diagnosis of neurasthenia required the establishment of a special type of relationship between doctor and patient. [41]

A hallmark of postbellum American medicine was the decline of patient-centered therapeutics. In an age in which elite physicians were devoting unprecedented attention to the bacteriological and pathological bases of disease, neurasthenia served as a continual reminder that physicians could ill afford to lose focus on their patients. The patient/ disease dichotomy that had always occupied a prominent role in American medicine tilted in favor of the latter, and disease entities supplanted suffering men and women as the primary source of medical attention.[42] This is not to suggest that the patient had been forgotten. On the contrary, few physicians lost sight of the human side of the medical equation. The desire to heal the sick remained a paramount concern, but the focus of healing, especially among elite, laboratory-trained physicians, shifted away from the patient and toward his diseased body— thereby reducing "the significance of the doctor-patient relationship as a source of professional legitimacy and an element of therapy."[43]

The focus on disease entities was fueled by two hotly contested theories: the "specific disease" concept and the "New Rationalism."[44] The former held that there was a large but finite number of specific diseases; the latter suggested that while people and diseases might vary widely, "the variations were always measurable and categorizable at some level of generality greater than the individual."[45] The clinical impact of these respective doctrines was not nearly so profound as it might have been largely because conservative physicians refused to embrace them wholeheartedly.[46] Many opposed the adoption of general therapeutic guidelines on philosophical and scientific grounds; others based their arguments on what appears to be little more than self-interest.[47]

Not surprisingly, medical efforts to grapple with the questions posed by functional nervous diseases captured both the enthusiasm for and the reaction against this trend toward generalizable diagnostic categories and therapeutic strategies.[48] In one of the earliest discussions of the disease T. W. Fisher proclaimed in 1872 that "the indications for treatment in cases of neurasthenia are fundamentally the same, whatever the variety of manifestation, with the addition of such special methods as the peculiarities of each case seem to require."[49] Within ten years Fisher's faith in generalizable methods of treatment had been shattered. "Just as no two artists can portray the same person in the same way," Howell T. Pershing asserted, "so no two physicians can treat the same case of neurasthenia in the same way."[50]

Emphasis on individualized treatment readily translated into a renewed awareness of the patient as a person. "Remember," declared William Broaddus Pritchard, "there are two parties to the transaction."[51] Few put the matter more succinctly than McClain: "The treatment [of neurasthenia] resolves itself into an effort to treat the individual and not the disease."[52] In part, advocacy for individualized therapeutics represented a retrograde step in the quest to establish generalizable medical laws.[53] Physicians who argued that the successful treatment of neurasthenia demanded individualized, patient-centered therapeutics thus unwittingly resurrected a therapeutic philosophy that, following the Civil War, had been increasingly called into question.[54] There was one critical difference, however. The revival of individualized therapeutics during the final decades of the nineteenth century took place in an utterly different medical-cultural context. Environmentalism no longer played so prominent a role in shaping either medical theory or practice. Materialism held the day. Although by no means incompatible with materialism, individualized therapeutics nonetheless helped to highlight some of materialism's deficiencies.

Physicians had long acknowledged that an important element in any individualized therapeutics scheme was the relationship that existed between them and their patients. An effective doctor-patient rapport, many believed, was a significant aid in the treatment not only of neurasthenia but also of virtually every aberrant physical and mental condition.[55] As Pritchard asserted, "[The] first step—the essential foundation of any plan of successful treatment in neurasthenia—is the establishment of a proper relation between physician and patient."[56] Central to this "proper relation" was the capacity of the physician to exert authority and the willingness of the patient to comply. "All authorities agree," explained Punton, "that the full control of the life and conduct of the patient while undergoing treatment is absolutely essential for success."[57] But attaining and maintaining such control was no simple task. The physician, explained homeopath William Harvey King, needed simultaneously to "create within the patient a sense of his sympathy, and at the same time rule her, as it were, with a rod of iron."[58]

Physicians who advocated this position realized that their arguments concerning the need to control the patient's mental as well as physical life were not widely shared. "It is this notion of the possibility of an outsider's assuming to exert an influence over regions and processes of the patient's mind which he himself is wholly unable to reach and explore," Putnam acknowledged, "that seems to many persons, so foreign, so obscure, and so unreasonable, and yet it is a notion of fundamental importance for securing to the physician the necessary confidence for dealing with neurasthenic patients."[59] "For the time being," Jeanne Cady Solis explained, "the patient's mind must be taken possession of, and dominated. The inability to make decisions must be met by the physician, the thoughts and feelings, as well as actions of the patient, must be controlled and directed."[60]

Physicians wishing to treat those whom they diagnosed as neurasthenic needed to acquire a good deal of personal information and constantly consider that their patient's nervous exhaustion was, as one physician observed, "compatible with the appearance of perfect health." [61] Beard himself was especially adamant on this particular point. A proper diagnosis, he declared, required "more than a few minutes conversation." [62] It demanded a meaningful discussion between doctor and patient. "We must make a diagnosis of the intellectual character as well as the disease," he insisted, "before we can make a prognosis or adopt a plan of treatment." [63] Other physicians echoed Beard's views. "The physician mainly depends upon the patient himself to tell how he feels," Cowles observed. [64] Both "must, in the highest degree, work together," asserted Anna Hayward Johnson. [65]

What Beard and his followers had no way of anticipating, however, was that the very same doctor-patient rapport needed to diagnose neurasthenia might ultimately hold the key to its treatment. While virtually all physicians agreed that the establishment of an effective rapport was a vital prerequisite for assuring patient compliance with what were often burdensome somatic therapies, a small but growing minority began to speculate that the significance of rapport lay not solely in its capacity to inspire submission but also in its potential to affect the patient's mental state. [66] Experience treating neurasthenic men and women pointed to the possibility that certain nonsomatic factors might also warrant therapeutic consideration. [67] How was it, certain physicians asked, that so many different modalities of somatic therapies ranging from electricity and hydrotherapy to diet, rest, nutrition, and medication could achieve virtually identical results? Might they not share a common ground? Deducing from the variegated experiences of a wide array of somatic treatments, the Boston neurologist Morton Prince declared, "I think if these treatments are carefully analyzed it will be found that there is one factor that is common in them all, namely, the psychical element." [68]

Neurasthenic Therapy: *Soma* not *Psyche*

Although common sense suggests that there might be some causal relationship between the discovery of functional nervous/ psychical diseases and the advent of psychological therapies, little evidence exists in support of this position. Prior to the first decade of the twentieth century the overwhelming number of therapies designed to combat neurasthenia were products of American medicine's growing fidelity to the somatic paradigm. Only a tiny minority of physicians who specialized in the treatment of neurasthenia considered the possible psychological dimensions of their various therapeutic schemes. Late-nineteenth-century physicians were driven by two distinct goals. The first was to treat diseases and restore their patients' health. The second was to understand the nature of the diseases they treated. While these goals were by no means mutually exclusive, they were not necessarily reinforcing—a point frequently missed by historians.[69] A physician's capacity to treat a disease did not require that he comprehend its pathology and etiology. More significantly, such knowledge did not guarantee an effective treatment. For instance, Koch's 1882 discovery of the microscopic organism responsible for tuberculosis neither slowed the progress of the disease nor altered its treatment. Indeed, the power of such knowledge might remain dormant for several decades.

In keeping with a long-standing, albeit rarely acknowledged, tradition, physicians did not allow their admitted ignorance to impede their therapeutic ambitions. Possessing only a remote comprehension of how a recommended therapy achieved its effects, physicians typically prescribed a wide array of somatic therapies. Despite assertions to the contrary neurologists and other physicians who treated victims of neurasthenia were guided by the same "crude" empirics that they had been so quick to condemn in others. Such sentiments were epitomized by William F. Hutchinson. While he had no desire to decry "the brilliant results of late pathological study," Hutchinson nonetheless proclaimed that in the case of functional nervous diseases, clinical observations and empirical therapeutics were of greater value: "It matters little if we fail to discover the exact morbific lesion in any case under treatment, if such treatment be followed by cure."[70] Many agreed. "The therapeutics of this disease, contrary to most diseased conditions," insisted another, "is far in advance of the etiology and pathology."[71] Even a physician who mistakenly diagnosed an "organic" disease as neurasthenia had little reason to worry. The therapeutic consequences of a mistaken diagnosis were deemed relatively trivial. "To mistake an organic for a functional condition is not, as a rule, so serious a matter," maintained Rockwell. "[It] is, indeed," he continued, "sometimes desirable to keep for a time the worst from a patient but to tell one afflicted only functionally that his disease is organic and incurable is a most serious matter. It takes away hope, shatters the *morale,* and materially lessens the chance of ultimate recovery."[72]

Physicians did not want for methods in their efforts to treat neurasthenia. They had many from which to choose. Some modes of treatment were the mirror opposites of others. Certain patients might be sent to bed; others would be encouraged to exercise. Along with rest cures and exercise cures physicians devised various therapies composed of certain combinations of diet, massage, electricity, hydropathy, medication, and even surgery. The central aim of all these therapies was to restore the patient's "vital nerve force."[73]

Restoration of nerve force typically required a multifaceted therapeutic regimen. Beard led the way in therapeutic innovation.[74] His zeal inspired a generation of American physicians seeking to treat neurasthenic patients and provided a foundation for subsequent innovations. But as Hale makes clear, what it did not do was generate any significant interest in mental therapeutics.[75] In fact, prior to the first decade of the twentieth century few American physicians gave much thought to the possible psychological dimensions of functional nervous disorder. Committed to the somatic paradigm, the overwhelming majority persisted in their faith that various material remedies such as hydrotherapy, diet, electrotherapy, medication, and rest remained the most efficacious methods for treating these vexing neurological diseases. By documenting the prevalence of these somatic therapies, I seek to demonstrate convincingly that prior to 1900 virtually all medical therapies designed to treat so-called functional nervous disorders were somatically based.

HYDROTHERAPY

Introduced to the United States during the 1840s, hydrotherapy quickly gained popularity among a wide cross-section of the populace—particularly among men and women who doubted the efficacy of prevailing drugs.[76] Although regular physicians condemned the hydropathists' environmentalism, they readily acknowledged the clinical efficacy of the water cure, or what they themselves soon termed hydrotherapy. Conspicuously absent in either the late-nineteenth-century hydropathic or medical literature concerning the hydropathic treatment of neurasthenia, however, was any mention of psychosocial factors. Among both hydropathists and physicians somatic explanations held sway. As L. Reuben explained, hysteria and other imaginary ailments typically involved a "*bodily something* grating upon the nerves, and thus producing those unhappy sensations, no matter whether we can or cannot see it—can or cannot name it!"[77] In defense of the hydropaths it should be added that the theoretical discourse concerning hydrotherapy among regular physicians was equally lacking in sophistication. Indeed, the primary issue under discussion in the mainstream medical literature concerned not the agency behind the method but the details that one needed to consider when applying it.

A host of questions regarding the proper application of hydrotherapy had yet to be answered: In what manner should water be applied to the patient? Was cold water preferable to hot water? What was the optimal water temperature? What was the best time of day to apply hydrotherapy? Bernard Sachs maintained that "trickling out of a sponge is the proper way to apply the cold water in the morning." "No matter what the origin of the neurasthenia may be," he continued, "it is best to begin it with this cold water treatment."[78] Regarding the proper method of application Harold N. Moyer asserted, "The most important [is] the application of a sheet wrung out of cold water each morning as the patient gets out of bed. If this is done promptly, and the patient vigorously rubbed after the application, producing a quick reaction, the benefit is very marked."[79] Jeanne Cady Solis recommended using salt water: "Hydrotherapy, in the form of cool salt sponges, the salt glow followed by alternating hot and cold pours in the morning, and a warm bath at bedtime at least three times a week, is most efficient."[80] G. Manley Ransom insisted on hot baths: "After a proper bath, the neurasthenic patient will always experience a feeling of relief or of a moderate well-being."[81]

"Cold water," James Jackson Putnam wrote, "is far more important than hot water for this purpose, but extremely cold water is not well borne by neurasthenic patients *until they have been gradually taught to bear it.*"[82] But Putnam did not say exactly how cold the water should be. Daniel Brower recommended beginning a program of hydrotherapy with sponge baths at 70° F, gradually lowering the water temperature to 50° F.[83] Most physicians agreed that hydrotherapy was ideally suited to the early morning hours. "The best time for the bath," Putnam added, "is in the morning, or at noon, but it is essential that the skin should be warm, even perspiring, and that the patient should not be exhausted."[84] H. C. Patterson was even more specific. Bathing, he insisted, should take place exactly at 9:00 A.M.[85]

Wharton Sinkler provided among the most highly detailed descriptions of what was involved.

The patient is placed in the hot-air cabinet until perspiration begins. He is then given the circular or so-called "needle bath" for one minute, beginning with a temperature of 95° and gradually reduced to 85°, with a pressure of twenty pounds. The Scotch douche is then applied to the spine.

This consists in the application of an alternate douche of hot and cold water of temperature of 105° and 80°, with a pressure of about twenty pounds. The treatment at first should last for only twenty-five or thirty seconds. After a few days the pressure is increased to twenty-five or thirty pounds and the extremes of temperature used are much greater, alternating for example, between 110° and 70°. After about two weeks' treatment, in addition to the circular and Scotch douche the fan douche may be used to the body, abdomen, and extremities.[86]

While such an elaborate procedure left little room for discretion, a physician who followed Sinkler's recommendations had little reason to fear his patients' skepticism. In treating a disease about which much still remained unknown scrupulous regard to detail proved to be an effective agent not only in inspiring patients' confidence but also in maintaining a physician's belief that he was master of the situation.

DIET AND NUTRITION

Like hydrotherapy diet figured prominently in the treatment of neurasthenia. Since faulty nutrition was believed to play a prominent role both in causing and in maintaining the disease, even those neurasthenic patients who appeared outwardly healthy were nonetheless deemed to be suffering from the effects of a poor diet. "Nervous exhaustion," Beard maintained, "is compatible with the appearance of perfect health."[87] "The neurasthenic patient looks so well," added Rockwell, "is frequently so plump and healthful in appearance, that we are accustomed to say that he is well nourished, that his nutrition is good. This, however, cannot be. The morbid fears, the strange and persistent sensory symptoms, the vacillation, the feeble powers of endurance—all point to a deficient nutritive activity."[88] Such tautological reasoning did little to undermine its credibility among the overwhelming majority of physicians.[89] What mattered most to most physicians was neither the circularity of the argument nor its plausibility but the opportunity it provided them to act. By attributing neurasthenia to something so remediable as faulty nutrition, physicians could with little difficulty recommend a wide range of dietary solutions.

The belief that faulty nutrition contributed to the maintenance of neurasthenia was not drawn out of thin air. Rather, it was derived by way of analogy. Both prior medical knowledge and recently conducted scientific investigations contributed to the widely held belief that poor nutrition contributed to the neurasthenic state. Beard himself had compared neurasthenia to anemia. Other physicians based their assumption regarding the connection of poor nutrition and nervous exhaustion on the much-touted animal experiments performed by Clark University neurologist C.F. Hodge.[90] A strenuous advocate of laboratory research, Hodge credited an 1889 paper by Podia Korybut-Daszkiewicz with posing what he considered the most critical question: "Is the activity of the central nervous system accompanied by changes recognizable with the microscope?"[91] From experiments that he conducted with frogs, cats, dogs, birds, and honeybees, Hodge was able to answer this question with a resounding yes. By microscopically examining the effects of electrical stimulation on the nerve cells of these various animals and insects, Hodge established the following conclusions:

Metabolic changes in nerve cells are certainly as easy to demonstrate, microscopically, as similar processes in gland cells. They may be demonstrated equally well, and are the same in character, either by artificial or natural methods. The principal changes thus observed are: *for spinal ganglion cells of frog, cat, dog, under electrical stimulation; for spinal ganglion and brain cells of English sparrow, pigeon, swallow*; and *for brain cell of honey-bee, under normal fatigue:*—

   A. For nucleus: 1. Marked decrease in size. 2. Change from smooth and rounded to a jagged, irregular outline. 3. Loss of open reticulate appearance with darker stain.
   B. For cell-protoplasm: 1. Slight shrinkage in size, with vacuolation for spinal ganglia; considerable shrinkage, with enlargement of pericellular lymph space for cells of cerebrum and cerebellum. 2. Lessened power to stain or reduce osmic acid.
   C. For cell capsule, when present: Decrease in size of nuclei.
   D. Individual nerve cells, after electrical stimulation, recover, if allowed to rest for a sufficient time. The process of recovery is slow, from five hours' stimulation, being scarcely complete after twenty-four hours' rest.
   E. Provisional curves have been constructed from direct observation of the nerve cell to represent the processes of fatigue and recovery. These curves indicate that the nerve cell tires or rests rapidly at first, then slowly, then more rapidly again.[92]

Reaction to Hodge's "discovery" was both swift and enduring.[93] His experiments appeared to confirm almost fifty years of speculation concerning the possible effects of fatigue on nerve cells and to add new legitimacy to Beard's doctrines. "We have now accurate anatomical descriptions by Hodge and his successors," wrote Robert T. Edes, "in the work of the appearance of exhausted nerve cells under the microscope, showing that they undergo decided changes after rest and action identical with those to be seen on other cells."[94] Edes's views were echoed by John T. Quackenbos: "We also know from experiments made on the lower animals that at the end of a day of active toil the nuclei appear small and shrunken, but after a night of rest the cells are turgid with large, well-rounded nuclei."[95]

Having apparently proved that neurasthenia resulted from some underlying nutritional deficiency, Hodge's experiments provided physicians with a novel incentive to devise new dietary schemes to restore vital nerve energy. Moses Allan Starr encouraged his patients to eat "healthful" foods. "Meat of all kinds," he wrote, "seems to me to agree very well with this type of patient."[96] "I look upon large, well-cooked steaks as a very important part of the diet," commented J. G. Biller.[97] One of the advantages of sending a man off on sea voyages, explained Archibald Church, was that he would be assured of receiving four or five meals a day as well as extra food.[98] Just before his death, Beard, after offering the observation that "cannibals are the strongest and healthiest savages," recommended that human beings consider eating the creatures closest to them on the evolutionary scale.[99]

Beard was not the only physician to acknowledge the importance of diet.[100] Others quickly added their voice to the call for greater nutritional knowledge. Dowse included a lengthy discussion of diet in his book on neurasthenia. His list included the following recommendations.

> *Soups.*—White, barley, à la julienne, macaroni, milk, rice, sago, semolina, vermicelli, calf's head, oyster.
> *Fish.*—Eels, flounders, mullet, oysters, soles, brill, whiting, smelts, fresh cod.
> *Meat.*—Mutton in any form, beef, lamb, calf's head, sheep's head, ox-tails, sweetbread, bacon.
> *Poultry and Game.*—Fowl, pigeons, turkey, pheasant, partridge, etc.
> *Vegetables.*—Asparagus, spinach, sea kale, French beans, broccoli, beet root, stewed celery, Spanish onions, tomatoes, watercress, lettuce.
> *Wines.*—Amontillado, Manzanilla, Latour Claret, Château Lafitte.
> *Eggs.*—Boiled, poached, raw, yolk, white of.
> *Sweets.*—Farinaceous milk puddings, milk, fruit, and most kinds of jellies.[101]

While Dowse's dietary recommendations left room for a certain amount of discretion, they nonetheless reinforced the notion that the physician was in control. What patient could doubt the authority of those who expressed not only conviction but details as well? Like Sinkler's elaborate description of hydrotherapy, Dowse's discussion of diet revealed a physician's effort to cloak his ignorance in a mask of copious details.

ELECTRICITY

By the time of Beard's discovery, electricity and medicine had a history that dated back to the seventeenth century.[102] The therapeutic application of electricity began with the discovery of the Leyden vial in 1746, and its use "became fashionable and was enhanced by the discovery of the Voltaic pile in 1800 and by Faraday's discovery of induced electricity in 1831."[103] Guillaume Duchenne "was most probably the first to use faradic current in medical research and treatment."[104] During the 1860s and 1870s the medical profession in America and Great Britain began to display a great interest in the possibilities of electrotherapy.[105]

The leading American proponents of electrotherapy were Beard and Rockwell.[106] In a work that the two men coauthored they acknowledged that a remarkable number of cures had been achieved by nonprofessional electrical practitioners. But, they said, the success of lay electrical healers was more a matter of luck than skill because their insufficient medical knowledge rendered them ill-equipped to apply proper diagnostic and therapeutic discrimination.[107] As medical professionals Beard and Rockwell proclaimed that they could do better.[108] They proposed two methods of electrotherapy, general faradization and central galvanization. The former involved the application of electricity across the entire body; the latter aimed to treat more localized conditions. Beard described the general procedure in great detail.

In this method of treatment the feet of the patient are placed on a sheet of copper to which the negation pole is attached, while the positive, either a large sponge or the hand of the operator, is applied over the head (the hair being previously moistened), on the back of the neck, down the entire length of the spine, down the arms, over the stomach, liver, bowels, down the lower extremities—in short, over the entire surface of the body, from the head to the feet, but with special reference to the head and spine.[109]

Other physicians recommended slightly altered versions of the practice. "My method of applying general galvanization," Francis Bishop wrote, "is to place a pad, at least twelve inches square, on the bed, table, or operating chair, and allow my patient to lie on this pad, which is placed so as to cover the lumbar and lower dorsal spine, then, with an interrupting hand electrode, I go over every muscle of the body and produce gentle contractions."[110] Brower was even more specific.

The electrodes I use are about three by seven inches. One is placed on the forehead, and the other at the nucha. The general characteristics of the mental phenomena determine the polarity; if one of depression, the negative is placed on the forehead; if excitement, then the positive. The currents used are of low amperage never exceeding 2 milliamperes, and rarely using more than one. The application should be continued for five minutes. This longitudinal galvanization is followed by transverse galvanization, using the same electrode, with a current-strength from 1/2 to 1 milliampere, and a five-minute *seance*. The transverse galvanization is to be followed by bulbar galvanization. The positive electrode of the size above mentioned is placed at the nucha, and a round electrode about one and a half inches in diameter (the negative) is moved up and down over the ganglia of the cervical sympathetic on both discs without breaking the current. This *seance* should be continued for five minutes. The treatment by galvanism is followed by static insulation and sparks from the spine. The static machine used should be one that will furnish a spark of at least ten inches. The electrical treatment should be given daily for the first ten days, then every other day will be sufficient.[111]

As was the case with both hydrotherapy and diet, medical advocates of electrotherapy were incapable of explaining exactly how this particular method yielded its desired results. "Because we do not understand the pathology of functional neurasthenia disease and are unable to appreciate the errors of nutrition that undoubtedly underlie all these cases," Rockwell maintained, "is no reason why we should not persist in the use of a remedy that has been of such splendid service in their relief."[112]

What mattered most to proponents of electrotherapy was that the method appeared to yield discernible and beneficial clinical results. "The rationale of general Franklinization," proclaimed Margaret Cleaves, "lies in its ability to set up processes resulting in the production of physiologic effects. Whether we regard the neurasthenic condition as due to exhaustion, starvation, or poisoning of nerve centers, its treatment by means of Franklinization is absolutely rational."[113] "Every current that passes through any portion of the human body," wrote W. F. Robinson, "has two actions: first, the local action upon the nerves or muscles lying immediately beneath the point where it enters; and secondly, a general or systemic action upon the system at large."[114] He recommended five-minute-long, daily doses of static electricity lasting for a period of a month, followed by a two-week break and then a subsequent month of treatment. He also encouraged physicians not to reveal too much about the nature of electrotherapy for the duration of the treatment. In response to questions concerning the length of treatment he asserted, "Instead of fixing a definite date, it is much better to say a few words as to the great uncertainty of this affection, and tell them, what is no more than the truth, that the length of time required for a cure will depend upon the rate of progress made."[115]

Like proponents of hydrotherapy and diet, advocates of electrotherapy emphasized details. More significant, they acknowledged the psychological dimension of their therapy. Putnam maintained that "most of the effects of electricity in neurasthenia are doubtless secondary to its power of exciting the peripheral nerves in various ways."[116] What Putnam had in mind was the treatment's psychological impact. W. B. Miller, after providing a lengthy description and positive appraisal of his own experience employing electrotherapy to treat neurasthenia, concluded: "Lastly, great psychic impressions are made by the wise look and curious machine upon the hysterical and hypochondriacs."[117] Physicians who employed electrotherapy not only adhered to the same highly detailed regimen of their fellow hydrotherapists and nutritionally inclined physicians but also possessed state-of-the-art scientific contraptions that could not fail to impress their patients and win their confidence.

MEDICATION

For several physicians, medication played an important role in the treatment of neurasthenia. As was the case with other functional diseases and, for that matter, with structural diseases as well, no specific drug existed for the treatment of neurasthenia. Physicians relied on a vast number of pharmaceutical options, many of which they also employed when treating a variety of other diseases. Medical reliance on drugs was attributable to a number of factors. Of these, tradition and cultural expectations played no small part. For years regular physicians had relied on drugs to treat their patients: administering drugs had become a central aspect of medical practice.[118]

By the final decades of the nineteenth century more than merely the pride of medical science was at stake. Regular physicians faced mounting competition not only from among their own increasingly specialized ranks but also from other medical sects such as homeopathy, osteopathy, and chiropractics. In addition, physicians were confronted with competition from myriad irregular practitioners: faith healers, Christian Scientists, and metaphysical healers. Abandoning the one feature of their practice that set them apart from their competition was therefore the last thing on the minds of regular practitioners. In his original article on neurasthenia Van Deusen had spoken of the therapeutic effects of using quinine, arsenic, strychnine, iron, and phosphorus in conjunction with open air, gentle exercise, and other relaxing activities.[119] Beard himself argued on several occasions for the necessity of employing certain drugs along with electricity and other somatic therapies.[120] Other physicians emphasized the beneficial effects of zinc, bromide, opium, cannabis, and valerian.[121] New drugs were continually being added to the list of prospective treatments.

The efficacy of the medical profession's multifaceted approach did not go unchallenged. American homeopathy—with its emphasis on minuscule doses and its law of similars—owed its success in large measure to a growing awareness that indiscriminate drugging often caused more harm than good. "May the day come and come quickly," wrote J. P. C. Foster, "when the medical man will not regard his profession as the giving of drugs, but will dare, when drugs fail, to use any and every agency to secure the relief for which his patient has sought his advice."[122] Some physicians relied on drugs far more heavily than did others. "Little need be said of the use of medicines," wrote J. S. Greene. "Their role is a subordinate one; their usefulness is incidental, but not therefore trivial. A typical case of neurasthenia in a healthy subject may sometimes be managed without scarcely any aid from drugs but such cases are, perhaps, exceptional."[123] "The use of drugs," commented another physician, "is not to be advised unless they are especially indicated."[124]

While many physicians agreed that drugs had at best a limited role in the treatment of neurasthenia, few were willing to dismiss their use altogether. Throughout much of the nineteenth century drugs had played a prominent role in American medicine. Both a physician's self-image and his public image were largely tied to his capacity to administer drugs. Abandoning their use not only threatened to compromise physicians' professional esteem, it also had the capacity to diminish their public appeal.

REST

Although hydrotherapy, diet, electricity, and medication were all considered crucial ingredients in the recipe designed to treat neurasthenia, few physicians emphasized exclusive reliance on any single therapy. Instead, they typically recommended applying a combination of therapies. Virtually all physicians, regardless of their particular area of expertise, emphasized one factor far more than others: rest. "Rest is the sheet anchor in the treatment of neurasthenia," Moyer proclaimed.[125] "The gospel of work must make way for the gospel of rest," Beard added.[126] Rest was prescribed for men as well as women.[127] But most neurasthenics, be they male or female, were not put to bed for any extended duration. Few physicians found such extreme rest necessary. Others readily acknowledged that the cost of this procedure vastly exceeded the financial means of most patients.

In a brief article appearing in an 1875 series of lectures published by neurologist Edward C. Seguin, Mitchell offered his first discussion of the therapeutic value of rest in treating nervous disorders.[128] He attributed his discovery of the "rest cure" to a host of factors. His experience working with wounded soldiers during the Civil War and his later efforts to treat men and women suffering from functional nervous diseases inspired him to combine a variety of hitherto disparate therapies with prolonged bed rest.[129] Speaking in 1904, he reflected on the origins of his almost three-decade-old method of treatment. "It may strike you as interesting," he explained, "that for a while I was not fully aware of the enormous value of a therapeutic discovery which employed no new agents, but owed its usefulness to a combination of means more or less well known."[130] Equally significant, perhaps, was the cure's economic value. At a time when few American physicians earned more than $1,000 a year, Mitchell's annual income exceeded $70,000.[131]

Mitchell recognized that the efficacy of this particular therapy demanded a "childlike obedience," and "yet we do get it, even from men," he maintained.[132] Knowing when to prescribe rest was no simple task: "Rest and unrest have had their days and fashions in medicine; but be you sure that he who can tell when the one is wanted, and when the other, is a man who is a master in the ways of healing."[133] Mitchell concluded his original 1875 paper with the following admonition: "Rest can be made to help. Rest also can hurt, and he who deals with it as a means of cure must not fail to bear in mind the modes by which we can secure the light without the shadow, the good without the harm."[134]

As was the case with hydrotherapy, electrotherapy, and nutritional therapy, details figured prominently in the administration of the rest cure. "The details in the use of rest cure are important," contended H. C. Patterson, "for on them rest largely its success or failure."[135] The rest cure in its unadulterated form was composed of five elements: seclusion, rest, diet, electricity, and massage. While Mitchell promoted this "radical" therapy for both men and women, he concluded early on that women typically achieved greater benefits. He recommended separating a patient from familiar influences and confining her to her bed for a period of four to six weeks.[136] A private nurse, one not previously known to the patient, attended to all of her basic needs. So long as a patient was under his treatment Mitchell would "not permit her to sit up, or to sew, or to write or read, or to use the hands in an active way except to clean the teeth."[137] He even arranged to have the patient's "bowels and water passed while lying down."[138] Mitchell did leave some room for discretion, however. "The intelligent physician," he insisted, "must, of course, know how far to enforce and when to relax these rules."[139]

Mitchell was acutely aware that prolonged bed rest posed certain dangers. A patient's muscles quickly atrophied, and what little physical vigor she might previously have possessed swiftly waned. Some form of physical stimulation was therefore vital. But physical exercise was out of the question. "You must get the effect of exercise," Mitchell maintained, "without its ills."[140] To achieve this end, he recommended both daily massage and electrotherapy. Of one of his earliest cases Mitchell wrote, "Every day she was [massaged], thoroughly; and skin, muscles, and belly kneaded until they flushed, and tingled with blood, and for the time rose in temperature two to four degrees. Every day each muscle was made to contract by faradic currents, and so she failed to feel the effect of disuse of the muscles. She was forbidden to exercise and yet had exercise, and she was fed largely but with a watchful eye."[141] Mitchell was pleased to recount that as a result of this therapy, "this sickly, feeble, wasted creature had become a handsome, wholesome, helpful woman, and remains so to this day, with only a constant gain in vigor."[142] But a rest cure designed for one patient might not do for another. Mitchell recommended tailoring the amount of feeding, massage, and electricity that a patient received according to her pulse, temperature, and appetite.

Mitchell took little notice of his patient's psychological state. Instead, he relied almost exclusively on somatic factors. Although he made no effort to disguise his belief that a doctor's personality, in particular his capacity to secure his patient's submission, played a prominent role in the rest cure, he nonetheless insisted that the efficacy of the cure was rooted in its underlying somatic foundation. As Mitchell made clear in the title of the book in which he popularized his famous rest cure, *Fat and Blood: An Essay on the Treatment of Certain Forms of Neurasthenia and Hysteria,* what mattered was not the state of his patient's mind but rather that of her body. In large measure the medical community's willingness to embrace Mitchell's doctrines was attributable to their somatic orientation. As Quackenbos explained, the somatic rather than the psychological benefits of rest were what mattered most: "I believe that if the rest be made long enough, the food stimulating enough, the sleep regular, the change of employment judicious, and all worry removed, most cases of neurasthenia may be greatly improved if not entirely cured."[143]

Several historians have failed to appreciate the somatic foundation of Mitchell's treatment regime. As a result of this misconception they have, depending on their perspective, either lauded or assailed Mitchell's efforts to employ what they deem to be a crude psychotherapy, particularly when treating powerless female patients.[144] That Mitchell and other physicians who treated female victims of functional nervous diseases were unable to escape the sex roles that existed in nineteenth-century society cannot be denied.[145] But the extent to which their culturally derived, sex-based prejudices affected their therapeutic endeavors—in particular the rest cure—is frequently exaggerated. In a perceptive rejoinder to recent critics of Mitchell's methods, Regina Morantz-Sanchez explains, "[It] is clear, above all, that medical men were unable to cure most diseases—not just those of women but of everyone. Indeed, they 'tortured' men and women indiscriminately."[146]

Moreover, it is worth noting that only a small number of physicians embraced Mitchell's doctrines regarding the rest cure, and fewer still applied them in their unadulterated form. As Walter Bromberg explains, "The ideas that Dr. Mitchell promulgated were combated by many physicians."[147] Mitchell himself acknowledged the early condemnation of his program: "Let me say that for a long time the new treatment was received with utmost incredulity. When I spoke in my papers of the people who had gained half a pound a day or more, my results were questioned and ridiculed in this city as approaching charlatanism."[148] In his earliest published work on the subject Mitchell warned that the rest cure was not without its perils. Many agreed. "I am of the opinion," Morton Prince wrote, "that the rest cure is a method that, when properly undertook in its real underlying principles, is capable of doing the greatest harm, and I do not hesitate to say that it is a most dangerous method in inexperienced hands."[149] Safe and effective administration of the cure, Prince continued, demanded a level of skill and expertise that only well-educated neurologists possessed. Coming from a neurologist, such words were neither surprising nor disinterested. Prince was by no means the only physician to express such concerns. "Unless we desire this useful measure to come into disrepute," Frederick A. McGrew wrote, "there must be a more definite knowledge of its proper use and limitations. And this means, first of all, the substitution of a working scientific basis in place of the prevailing haphazard fashion of disposing of troublesome neurasthenia patients."[150]

Administering the rest cure, as many physicians pointed out, was no simple matter—especially to uncooperative male patients. "I have tried it [i.e., rest for men] repeatedly," Church declared, "and have nearly always failed."[151] H.C. Patterson echoed Church's views: "Men do not take as kindly to the rest cure as women, but if they are sufferers from profound neurasthenia the plan for them must be as rigid."[152] Arthur E. Mink proclaimed that regardless of the patient's sex, "it is impossible to carry out the Weir Mitchell rest-treatment, as a rule, so I merely urge the patient to take as much rest as possible."[153] In one of the most revealing statements concerning the potential efficacy of the rest cure, Pritchard argued, "For women and feminine males it will do no harm; for men and masculine women it is an insult to intelligence."[154]

A prolonged bed stay, many physicians warned, often did more harm than good. "The idleness and indolence encouraged by the rest cure, to say nothing of the abnormal feeding," H.V. Halbert warned, "may lead to an unhealthy mental life. A patient should be taught that work is the best thing in life, and he should learn to employ his faculties without enervation or exhaustion. No neurasthenic should be encouraged in the idea that he is an invalid."[155] Pritchard added, "I can conceive of no more fitting nor important statement in conclusion than one of condemnatory criticism of the misapplication of the Weir-Mitchell plan of rest and isolation in these cases. It is to be condemned first, as involving the conception of a *routine system or plan* of treatment; second, as encouraging introspection; and third, as violating in principle all intelligent interpretation of the whole subject."[156]

Certain physicians feared that the rest cure would merely substitute one vice for another. Herbert J. Hall argued that "the great need seems to be to lift the neurasthenic out of his tangle of nervous symptoms, not by substituting another abnormality in the shape of unduly prolonged rest, but by bringing about by a gradual process the conditions of a normal life, a life of pleasant and progressive occupation, as different as possible from the previous life and resulting in self-forgetfulness."[157]

Perhaps the greatest problem with the Mitchell program was its deceptive simplicity. Few of Mitchell's followers, it seemed, had the skill, patience, or insight to apply his program as he intended. "There is nothing easier than for a nervous system to tear itself to pieces in bed while taking the so-called rest cure," proclaimed William Harvey King.[158] Landon Carter Gray, a prominent and well-respected neurologist, readily acknowledged that "the recognition by Dr. Weir Mitchell of rest as the key-note of treatment in these cases was a stroke of genius." But, he insisted, "the rough and ready application of it, since the popularization of his idea with profession and laity, has often been appalling. It is seldom necessary to put patients to bed for three to six weeks, as was first proposed. As a rule, it will suffice to keep them there ten or twelve hours out of the twenty-four, and to have them avoid fatigue when they are up."[159]

The significance of the rest cure was primarily, though by no means exclusively, attributable to its compatibility with the somatic paradigm. Like hydrotherapy, diet, electricity, and medication, rest was believed to exert a profound effect on the body. Any changes in a patient's mental condition that resulted from prolonged bed rest were interpreted by most physicians as deriving from some overriding physical transformation. While few denied that mental factors might play a role in the treatment, fewer still considered this fact to be worthy of further scrutiny.

———

That efforts to treat neurasthenia had little direct impact on the emergence of what came to be known as psychotherapy is a point frequently missed by historians.[160] The same cannot be said of the unwitting impact of those efforts, however. More than three decades of clinical experience with neurasthenia and other functional nervous diseases had provided American physicians with a good deal of information about these and other similar disorders. While the presence of neurasthenic patients in neurologists' offices was a boon to the profession during the 1880s and 1890s, in the longer term the largely futile efforts to treat neurasthenia by somatic means caused a number of prominent physicians to reconsider some of their most cherished assumptions regarding the relationship between mind and body.

CHAPTER 4

Inventing Psychotherapy

The American Mind Cure Movement,
1830–1900

Every new [medical] discovery or procedure is hated on sight and denounced; then it is endured from familiarity, afterward pitied and sympathized with, and finally embraced and accepted. Many are the remedies and methods which were scouted and denounced, and the advocates fined and imprisoned; after which some member of the dominant party perceiving merit in the innovation, and perhaps some hope of profit and reputation, ventured to "introduce" it to the "regular" profession. It then becomes "scientific," which, in conventional usage, means orthodox.

Alexander Wilder, M.D. (1900)

The remarkable vogue of certain pseudo-philosophic and pseudo-religious healing methods in America is not an unmixed evil; one of the benefits which may accrue to us as a people may be the awakening of so-called "regular" medicine and so-called "orthodox" religion to their sins of omission.

Lewellys Barker, M.D. (1910)

The American medical profession's recognition of the theoretical and practical limitations of the somatic paradigm can be attributed only in part to the issues raised by the discovery of and efforts to treat railway spine, neurasthenia, and other so-called functional nervous diseases. That the experience treating these disorders contributed to a growing awareness of psychogenic notions of causality and the possibility of treating certain "bodily" diseases by mental means cannot be denied. What they did not do, however, was generate any *widespread* consideration of employing mental therapeutics to the exclusion of somatic therapies. Acting more as catalysts than as causal agents, they were only indirectly responsible for the birth of psychotherapy in the United States. A more significant inspiration came from what William James termed "the mind cure movement." [1]

At its core mind cure was an effort to contest the growing hegemony of what James himself had disparagingly labeled "medical materialism" and to offer an alternative or, at the very least, a supplementary approach to questions regarding sickness and health.[2] Composed of a loosely organized collection of men and women who held that mental therapies were by themselves sufficient to cure all diseases, the American mind cure movement distinguished itself not only from Spiritualism, antivivisectionism, and other movements aligned against what Steward W. Holmes has termed "science-engendered materialism" but also from a host of other nineteenth-century healing sects including Thomsonism, homeopathy, and hydropathy.[3] All these trends "formed a link in a chain of organizations opposed to the scientific revolution in late nineteenth-century medicine, and to the growing power of doctors."[4] This opposition to materialism was not a rejection of science per se. On the contrary, it was an effort to preserve an older, more holistic, vitalistic, and Baconian science against the new reductionist materialist experimentation.[5]

Proponents of the mind cure movement came from a variety of walks of American life. Although they often held antagonistic views, to those not directly involved in the movement they appeared to agree more than they disagreed. James chose to treat the many different schools as a single entity because, he maintained, "their agreements are so profound that differences may be neglected."[6] In certain respects this interpretation was understandable. Throughout the ages outsiders have often been blind to the fierce, sometimes lethal, debates that have raged within the larger context of various religious and political movements. That the considerable efforts and energies expended by various proponents of mental healing to differentiate their practices from those of their competitors went largely unnoticed by those not intimately connected with the movement is yet another illustration of this phenomenon. Try as they might practitioners of mental healing—regardless of their cultural status, scientific credentials, and even their ability to free people from mental and physical distress—proved unable to make the case that they were not all of a single breed.[7]

The rapid expansion of the mind cure movement in the United States just before and shortly after the turn of the century compelled certain

segments within a hitherto hostile American medical profession to consider seriously the role that mental factors played in the etiology, pathology, and treatment of certain functional nervous diseases.[8] Indeed,
many who would soon champion so-called scientific psychotherapy
readily acknowledged their intellectual debt to the indigenous mental
healers. As early as 1894 James publicly assailed a proposal to proscribe
the practice of mental healing. "What the real interest of medicine requires," James proclaimed, "is that mental therapeutics should *not* be
stamped out, but studied, and its laws ascertained."[9]

Over the course of the next decade an increasing number of American physicians grudgingly embraced James's position. Chicago psychiatrist Richard Dewey declared,

[The] phenomena of mental healing are worthy of more attention than
they have received. Those of Eddyism (which is the proper name for so-
called Christian Science), of osteopathy, or "divine healing," whether by
saints' relics or waters of Lourdes, or the holy coat of Trier, have in them
lessons for our profession. . . . In mental therapeutics it is my belief that
psychiatry has a new and rich domain to conquer and annex by separating
the false from the true in the fads and frauds of the day, and by placing
upon a scientific basis the facts of mental influence upon physical states.[10]

Dewey was far from alone in his assessment. As Robert Edes later explained, "Considering the very prominent position which psychic treatment in one form or another occupies in the public mind and the extravagant claims made for it, . . . it is worthwhile to consider what
morbid processes can be beneficially affected by mental action."[11] "The
extraordinary popular and pseudo-scientific interest in matters relating
to the possible alleviation of disease by mental means," added another
prominent physician, had forced the medical profession to focus its
attention on the subject.[12]

Such views were by no means confined to elite northeastern psychiatrists and neurologists. While their motives doubtless differed, a growing number of physicians throughout the nation began questioning the
limits, if not the allure, of their somatic remedies. An Illinois Medical
College dean captured the frustration felt by many of his medical
brethren when he spoke of the threat posed by the mind curists.

It is preposterous to deny the profound influence of mental suggestion
over bodily functions; and the doctor is a fool who does not avail himself of
this means of treating his patients. . . . To avoid sending from our college a
lot of poor fellows to be driven into the poor house by these Christian Scientists, faith-curists, and the like, we have created a lectureship on psycho-

therapy, and promise to make them more proficient in all these *isms* than their professional exponents themselves.[13]

Arguments of this nature were becoming increasingly common. In an article appearing in an 1898 issue of the *Medical Record,* New York physician W.F. Hartford declared, "I see no good reason why we should allow the army of irregulars to carry away the best patients from our business."[14] Despite these and a host of similar admissions few historians of American psychiatry have examined this vital link between the American mind cure movement and what later became known as psychotherapy. Although there are a number of notable exceptions to this historiographical lacuna, most standard histories of American psychiatry and psychoanalysis make little or no mention of the indigenous mental healing movement and its subsequent impact on the American medical profession. Moreover, many of the most illuminating studies of mind cure in the United States fail to consider the movement's relationship to American medicine. Instead, most are limited to an analysis of the movement's religious and cultural significance.

This interpretive strategy is derived in large measure from James's initial characterization of mind cure as "a religious or quasi-religious movement."[15] For instance, in his illuminating study of the history of religion in America, Sydney Ahlstrom maintains that mind cure is yet another example of "harmonial religion," which "encompassed those forms of piety and belief in which spiritual composure, physical health, and even economic well-being are undertook to flow from a person's rapport with the cosmos. Human beatitude and immortality are believed to depend to a great degree on one's being 'in tune with the infinite.'"[16] More recent scholars have interpreted the movement as an example of "transcendental medicine," "Christian physiology," and "physical religion."[17] The last, declares Catherine Albanese, was "above all, *healing* religion—religion in which acts of caring and curing constituted the central ritual for believers."[18] The problem with these and other similar modes of interpretation is that they fail to take seriously the pressure that American mind cure discourse exerted on the American medical community.[19]

A similar shortcoming can be found in the literature that treats the mind cure movement as a form of protest against such sweeping social and cultural phenomena as industrialism, urbanism, and modernism. Examples of this line of analysis can be found in the writings of Donald Meyer and Gail Thain Parker. In a fascinating study of "religion as pop psychology" Meyer argues that mind cure was "a protest against an inadequate science of medicine. It was a protest against a theology no longer nourishing. It was a feminine protest against a society careless in meeting the needs of many of its members for worthy roles."[20] More recently, Parker has suggested that "it is more logical to see in the appeal of mind-cure ideas a reflection of those terrors which the developing economy held for middle-class Americans."[21] While these and other similar interpretations are not without their merits, in neglecting to distinguish mind cure from other middle-class responses to social and cultural upheavals they fail to capture what was in fact unique about this particular movement—namely, its ideas about mental therapeutics. The mind cure movement generated widespread enthusiasm in large part because of its enticing claims concerning its capacity to relieve both nervous and physical ailments that neither mainstream medicine nor traditional Protestantism proved capable of addressing.

Just as there were practical reasons to consult a physician if one fractured an elbow, there were practical reasons to seek out a metaphysical or Christian Science healer if one were experiencing anxiety, insomnia, or nervous distress, or—worse still—diagnosed as suffering from some incurable ailment. Sufferers, from time immemorial, have sought comfort where they could find it. "It is a suggestive fact," Horatio Dresser observed, "that a large proportion of the cases which come under the care of the mental practitioner are those which have been given up by the best physicians of the regular school."[22] That American victims of nervous distress and "incurable" diseases flocked in increasing numbers to the various mind cure movements thus comes as little surprise. Many had nowhere else to turn.[23]

Mental Healing in America: Controversies and Consensus

The origins of the American mind cure movement can be traced to the particular healing theories and practices of an eccentric and obscure clock maker, Phineus Parkhurst Quimby.[24] Writing in 1908, Richard C. Cabot, perhaps the leading American medical advocate of psychotherapy, conceded that "a great deal which physicians have now taken into their practice they really owe to Quimby and to Christian Science."[25] Born in Lebanon, New Hampshire, Quimby spent his formative years in a small coastal town in southern Maine. Like thousands of other Americans, Quimby had the opportunity to witness one of the scores of demonstrations of mesmerism performed by Charles Poyen, a Frenchman, during his visit to the United States in the late 1830s. Quimby witnessed a similar demonstration in 1839—this time by Robert Collyer.

Introduced in the United States during the 1830s, mesmerism had an immediate and profound impact on both professional and lay audiences. Initially believed to operate according to some underlying physiological mechanism involving the manipulation of certain invisible vital fluids, mesmerism was soon dismissed by respectable scientists and physicians as little more than mere psychic suggestion.[26] The rejection of mesmerism by the mainstream medical community was not solely attributable to the alleged psychological basis of the practice, however. Echoing their previous reaction to phrenological doctrines, many American physicians refused to sanction a practice that had been so readily exploited by myriad unsavory characters.[27]

Popular enthusiasm for the practice was especially evident in those caught up in one of the midcentury's most popular fads, Spiritualism.[28] The link between mesmerism and Spiritualism was the writings of the Swedish mystic Emanuel Swedenborg.[29] Although a small number of Americans had known of Swedenborg's work for some time, Whitney Cross suggests that his ideas did not achieve widespread popularity until the appearance of a new English edition of his work in 1845.[30] Swedenborg's writings, embraced by a wide range of Americans, appeared to confirm what many wished to believe—the existence of an "interaction between the physical and metaphysical orders of reality as a lawful occurrence."[31] No less a figure than the dean of American transcendentalism, Ralph Waldo Emerson, took it on himself to discuss Swedenborg's ideas in an 1850 collection of essays entitled *Representative Men.*[32]

One of the first Americans to connect mesmerism to Swedenborgianism was an apprentice cobbler from Poughkeepsie, New York, Andrew Jackson Davis. In 1843 Davis had the opportunity to participate in a lecture-demonstration conducted by the famed phrenologist and mesmerist J. Stanley Grimes.[33] This event proved to be a turning point in Davis's life, for it was from this experience that he discovered his capacity to enter an entranced state during which he was able to perform a number of "standard Mesmeric feats [such] as reading while blindfolded and reporting clairvoyant travels to distant locales."[34] The apparent connection between mesmerism and Swedenborgianism that

Davis had first articulated was soon taken up by Davis's contemporary, George Bush.[35]

A former Presbyterian clergyman and recent convert to Swedenborg's Church of the New Jerusalem, Bush sought to explore the nexus between mesmerism and Swedenborgianism that Davis had recently uncovered.[36] "The main phenomena of Mesmerism," Bush wrote, "are *mental*. They involve the laws of *mental communication* between one spirit and another. They bring us, therefore, into precisely the sphere of phenomena which Swedenborg professes to unfold."[37] Efforts to link mesmerism to Swedenborgianism peaked during the Spiritualist fad of the 1850s and 1860s. Through séances and other efforts to communicate with the spirits of the dead, proponents of Spiritualism sought to establish the existence of universal laws that might apply to both the physical and the metaphysical spheres.[38]

The seeds that the mesmerists planted in both American cultural soil and Quimby's head swiftly began to mutate. At first sprouting into an ever-increasing fascination with mesmerism itself, they soon blossomed into a vibrant mental healing movement—largely as a result of Quimby and his disciples. Following Collyer's performance, Quimby embarked on an intensive investigation of animal magnetism. Beginning in 1843 the former clock maker set out on a four-year tour of New England with Lucius Burkmar. With Burkmar's aid Quimby performed hundreds of public demonstrations in which he revealed the wonders of animal magnetism.[39] By 1847 Quimby's interest in the practice of mesmerism began to wane, and he embarked on what Dresser maintains was a twelve-year investigation of "Science and Health."[40] Finally, in 1859, Quimby settled down in Portland, Maine, where he devoted the last six years of his life to establishing a successful healing practice in which he claimed to have treated more than twelve thousand men, women, and children.

A self-educated man, Quimby wrote in a style that was confusing and at times incoherent—particularly in his discussion of mind and matter. "Men," Quimby charged, "create ideas which are matter."[41] Although his theories and practices were discussed in a number of newspaper articles and interviews that appeared before his death and in scores of letters that he exchanged with former patients, Quimby never succeeded in publishing his findings.[42] He did, however, prepare more than eight hundred pages of handwritten notes and articles that remained unpublished until 1921 and that generated considerable controversy soon after his death.[43] The Quimby manuscripts reveal a highly original, albeit undisciplined, thinker. They trace the evolution of Quimby's thinking from his initial forays into mesmerism to his eventual formulation of a nonmaterial theory of mental healing.

Writing more than twenty years before Koch's 1882 discovery of the tuberculosis bacillus, Quimby argued that "[diseases] are like fashions, and people are as apt to take a new disease as they are to fall in with any new fashion. . . . The doctor can produce a chemical change by his talk. It makes no difference what he says."[44] This view, it is worth noting, is strikingly similar to that of the American railway surgeon Warren Bell Outten, who suggested that "a physician, by virtue of mental superiority, prejudice, and suggestion could create an essentially serious condition."[45] Quimby's quasi-psychogenic conception of disease—that is, his belief that diseases were mentally induced—did not compel him to deny their somatic impact. "All effects produced on the human frame," he insisted, "are the result of a chemical change of the fluids with or without our knowledge, and all the varieties and changes are accompanied by a peculiar state of mind."[46]

Quimby's theories were not the product of wishful thinking. They were inspired by many years of practical experience.[47] Describing Quimby's method, the *Bangor Jeffersonian* reported, "His first course in the treatment of a patient is to sit down beside him, and put himself *en rapport* with him, which he does without producing the Mesmeric sleep."[48] A former patient offered a more detailed explanation. "Instead of telling me that I was not sick," Annetta Dresser recounted, "he sat beside me, and explained to me what my sickness was, how I got into the condition. . . . The general effect of these quiet sittings with him was to lighten up the mind, so that one came in time to understand the troublesome experiences and problems of the past in the light of his clear and convincing explanations."[49] Quimby himself described his treatment in the following manner:

I sit down by a sick person, and you also sit down. I feel her trouble and the state of her mind, and find her faint and weary for the want of wisdom. I tell her what she calls this feeling that troubles her; and, knowing her trouble, my words contain food that you know not of. My words are words of wisdom, and they strengthen her; while, if you speak the same words, and the sound should fall on the natural ear precisely as mine, they are only empty sounds, and the sick derive no nourishment.[50]

"To me it is perfectly plain," Quimby continued, "that if the people could see for themselves they would discard all the priests' and doctors' opinions and become law unto themselves."[51]

The Early Disciples: Warren Felt Evans
and Mary Baker Eddy

The impact of Quimby's mature doctrines was soon felt throughout United States. Beginning in the 1860s, a number of mental healing schools began to spring up throughout New England. Within three decades these schools blossomed into what many contemporaries referred to as a national craze. "The mind cure," proclaimed Julia Anderson Root, "is frequently spoken of as that 'new method,' 'the new-fangled theory,' and 'the modern craze.'"[52] The movement enlisted the support of tens of thousands of American women and men. Literally hundreds of books and pamphlets in addition to scores of periodicals proclaimed the dawning of a New Age in which mind and spirit would achieve dominion over matter and crude materialism. "No intelligent observer of the signs of the times," declared a leading proponent of metaphysical healing, "can fail to notice among philosophical minds a marked reaction against the dominant scientific materialism of the past century, and a tendency to return to a more spiritual view of human nature and the world at large."[53]

The two most prominent figures in the early days of the American mind cure movement were Warren Felt Evans and Mary Baker Eddy. Evans had visited Quimby on two separate occasions during the early 1860s. Eddy had paid him several visits throughout the 1860s and maintained a vigorous correspondence with him. Quimby's impact on Evans and Eddy was both profound and long-lasting. Indeed, it was largely through their experiences with the former clock maker that both discovered their callings.

Evans's biographer, William J. Leonard, notes that "during the twenty-five years of Dr. Evans' service as an advocate of the mental-cure system, he saw its development from the small beginnings, when Dr. Quimby and he were the only persons engaged in its practice, into almost a world-wide movement."[54] Admitted to Middlebury College in 1837, Evans remained until the following spring and then transferred to Dartmouth College, where he completed two more years of formal education before departing without his degree. Evans was married in the summer of 1840 and shortly thereafter was appointed minister of the Methodist Episcopal church at Peacham, Vermont. He remained a faithful servant to his church for the next twenty-four years.

Two events caused Evans to question his Methodist calling. The first was his exposure to the writings of Swedenborg during the mid-1850s.[55] The second was his visit to Quimby in 1863. Evans's reason for visiting Quimby remains unknown. No evidence exists suggesting that Evans had been suffering from ill health or nervousness. Indeed, the most likely explanation for Evans's trip to Portland seems to be his hope that Quimby might have something worthwhile to teach him. His hopes were more than fulfilled. "The impression I got from my father," Horatio Dresser later told Leonard, "was that Dr. Evans' Swedenborgian belief and philosophical knowledge admirably fitted him to understand Dr. Quimby's theories and methods. It was evidently a case where a word to the wise was sufficient. Hence Dr. Evans very soon concluded that he could heal in the same way."[56] Shortly thereafter Evans severed his ties with the Methodist church and embarked on a vigorous and hitherto unprecedented campaign to promote mental healing in the United States.

Evans returned to his home in Claremont, New Hampshire, and began composing what would be the first of six volumes devoted to mental healing, or what he sometimes referred to as phrenopathy.[57] During the same year that George Beard first articulated his conception of neurasthenia Evans argued that "what are called nervous diseases are among the most real ills to which man is subject."[58] But in contrast to Beard's somatic interpretation of nervous distress, Evans offered a resolutely idealistic assessment not only of nervous suffering but of all disease.

A more learned man than Quimby, Evans supplemented his personal investigations with references to Swedenborg, George Berkeley, and a host of other eminent European and American thinkers. Like Quimby, Evans rejected Cartesian dualism. "The mind being the interior of man is not," he declared, "confined to the brain, nor, as Descartes supposed, included in the Pineal gland. But it pervades and is interfused through the whole body."[59] In many respects this view bore a striking resemblance to one that had recently been articulated by a number of prominent nineteenth-century neuroscientific investigators, particularly those from Germany and Austria.[60] But in contrast to the European neuroscientists, who argued that psychological functions resulted from certain underlying organic processes, Evans claimed that organic functions resulted from underlying psychological processes. "All psychological movements," he wrote, "effect a change in the organic functions."[61]

Matter, he later wrote, "is a state of mind. And every change of the mind modifies the *appearance* that we call matter."[62] Echoing Quimby, Evans asserted that "thoughts or ideas are the most *real* things in the universe."[63] To substantiate this claim Evans cited the existence of "phantom limbs": "An amputated limb is not missed from the consciousness; the person who has suffered the mutilation *feels* it as much as he ever did, and it has the same apparent externality. He has even the sensation of pain in it. But is it external?"[64]

Evans's idealism derived in large measure from the writings of Berkeley.[65] Central to the early-eighteenth-century British philosopher's epistemology was the notion that *to be* consists in *being perceived*.[66] Berkeley espoused this idealistic doctrine in two separate works: *New Theory of Vision* (1709) and *A Treatise Concerning the Principle of Human Knowledge* (1710). Expanding on an argument that John Locke had previously proposed in the fourth edition of his famous *Essay Concerning Human Understanding*, which espoused "the importance of custom as establishing" the link between ideas and experience, Berkeley argued that "it is evident that when the mind perceives any idea, not immediately and of itself, it must be by means of some other idea."[67] Here then were the roots of what Berkeley's philosophical successors, David Hartley and David Hume, soon termed the "law of association"—a principle that held that ideas become so connected together in thought that to think of one suggests or calls up the other.[68]

That this "law" held great appeal to late-nineteenth-century American proponents of mental healing is not at all surprising. Believing that mind was solely responsible for all bodily functions, they regarded the "law of association" as not only psychologically but also physiologically significant. This law, said Evans, "is the key that unlocks many of the more mysterious phenomena of the mind, but it is one of the least familiar of the mental laws, being generally overlooked by the great majority of psychologists."[69] Anticipating Pierre Janet's conception of "fixed ideas," Evans maintained that "*fixed morbid thinking* both generated and maintained disease."[70] What was needed then was a method to overcome these so-called morbid thoughts. Deleterious, disease-causing thoughts needed to be supplanted by more healthful ideas and beliefs. "If all disease originates in some disturbed or inharmonious mental states, which ultimate themselves in corresponding bodily conditions," Evans asserted, "it becomes a question of primal importance how to induce upon a patient, as a permanent possession, the state of mind which is the opposite of that causing the disease."[71] "In all those cases," he later wrote, "the best remedy and the only specific is the opposite truth."[72]

A zealot of sorts, Evans believed "we must induce upon the patient a new mental state, and supplant the old mode of feeling and thought. We must give him in the proper sense, a new spiritual birth, or at least impregnate him with a better interior life. We must *convert* him."[73] Advocating not so much a "talking cure" as a "word cure," Evans insisted that "words, either spoken or written are absolutely necessary to the communication of thoughts from one mind to another."[74] But before this could be accomplished the patient needed to assume an impressionable and receptive state that made possible the transmission of thoughts required to "change the character and direction of his thinking."[75]

Evans attributed the agency responsible for this process to the "doctrine of sympathy," which held that "it is as natural for one mind to communicate its thoughts and feelings to another as for a flower to emit fragrance."[76] "It is well known," Evans wrote, "that, by the law of sympathy, certain diseased states both of mind and body become contagious. The convulsions of hysteria are often propagated by young women in this way. The same is true of chorea and of stammering. We insensibly imbibe the tastes, manners, habits, and even the bodily conditions of others."[77] But just as the doctrine of sympathy might give rise to certain diseases, Evans reasoned, so too might it cure them. "The doctrine of sympathy," he insisted, "is of practical value in the treatment of the sick, and can be turned to a useful account."[78] To illustrate how the doctrine functioned, he employed a technological analogy.

When a message is telegraphed from New York to London no imponderable fluid shoots along the wire but there is only the transmission of force, a vibratory wave in an elastic medium called ether. So when one mind acts upon another mind, and influences its thoughts and feelings, when the bodies they animate are separated by hundreds of leagues, the effect is produced in a similar way. There is only transmission of mental force, and the action and reaction of one spirit upon another.[79]

Evans's work was notable not for its originality but for its impact on others. Like Quimby, he put his theories into practice. Beginning with some early experiments in mental healing in New Hampshire, Evans soon established a sanitarium, the Evans Home, in Salisbury, Massachusetts. In addition to his successful healing practice Evans published several volumes and was a frequent contributor to various periodicals dedicated to the study and discussion of mental healing. His ideas spread quickly, and he soon became one of the most widely read authors on the subject.

Although Evans was the first of Quimby's followers to achieve literary prominence, he was by no means the most successful. That honor fell to Mary Baker Eddy.[80] In contrast to Evans and others proponents of what came to be known as the New Thought, Mrs. Eddy attached her mental healing doctrines to a novel religious dogma and thus extended the scope of her teachings vastly beyond the domain of mental healing. Moreover, she made considerable efforts to differentiate her doctrines from those of other mental healers. In so doing she earned the wrath of several potential allies.[81]

A chronic invalid for much of her early adult life, Mary Baker Eddy experimented with virtually every therapy available to the chronically ill of the nineteenth century. During the mid-1830s she briefly adopted the vegetarian regimen advocated by Sylvester Graham. Failing to benefit from Graham's program, she spent the better of the next two decades dabbling with mesmerism, hydropathy, and homeopathy.[82] Finding little relief from these alternatives to mainstream medicine, she consulted with Quimby in October 1862.[83] The meeting proved to be a turning point in her life. Within three weeks of her visit she published a letter in the *Portland Courier* in which she proclaimed that Dr. Quimby "speaks as never man spoke and heals as never man healed since Christ."[84] She soon returned to her home and declared herself to be on the road to perfect health.[85]

Eddy's encounters with Quimby prompted a dramatic change in her health and, perhaps more significant, contributed to a fundamental transformation of her outlook on life.

But now I can see, dimly at first and only as trees walking, the great principle which underlies Dr. Quimby's faith and works; and just in proportion to my right perception of truth is my recovery. This truth which he opposes to the error of giving intelligence to matter and placing pain where it never placed itself, is received understandingly, changes the currents of the system to their normal action, and the mechanism of the body goes undisturbed. That this is a science capable of demonstration becomes clear to the mind of those patients who reason upon the process of their cure.[86]

She continued her correspondence with Quimby until his death in 1866 and shortly thereafter began to advertise herself as a mental healer. Her first such notice appeared in an 1868 edition of the Spiritualist paper, the *Banner of Light*.[87] In addition to her healing practice, she began teaching—for a fee—Quimby's doctrines. And she commenced the arduous task of preparing a book-length treatise on the subject.

Although she sought to portray herself as an original thinker, indeed as a prophet, Eddy's writings reveal a striking resemblance to the works of both Quimby and Evans.[88] Eddy accepted Quimby's fundamental conception concerning the nature of science and health. While Evans's influence is less direct, twice in the original edition of *Science and Health* Eddy took the liberty of seizing one of his most poignant metaphors. "The electric telegraph," she proclaimed without attribution, "is a symbol of mind speaking to mind, that in progress of time will not require wires, for Spirit destroys matter, electricity, etc." "Mind, like a telegraph office," she repeated, "holds the message conveyed to the body, and to prevent any bad results we must be careful the telegram is from science instead of sense."[89]

Despite its stylistic lapses, logical flaws, and organizational shortcomings, few books have exerted a greater impact on American cultural life than *Science and Health*, first published in 1875.[90] The original edition was limited to only one thousand copies, the cost of which had been paid in advance by two of the author's students.[91] Today the Church of Christian Science boasts that more than 9 million copies are in print. Although Eddy revised her book on numerous occasions, her primary focus remained fundamentally intact. Like Quimby before her, she proclaimed that "disease is caused by mind alone."[92]

Science and Health, more than any single work, served as the first major text of the American mental healing movement. Eddy began with the proclamation that "sickness and sin have ever had their doctors, but the question is, have they become less because of them."[93] She answered her own question with a resounding no! To the contrary, she argued, physicians aggravated rather than mitigated human suffering. "Putting on the full armor of physiology, obeying to the letter, the so-called laws of health, statistics show, has not diminished sickness, nor increased longevity; diseases have multiplied and become more obstinate; their chronic forms more frequent, the acute more fatal and death more sudden, since man-made theories have taken the place of primitive Christianity."[94]

The conception of human beings as material entities, Eddy declared, had led to untold suffering: "Explaining man as a physical being evolved from matter is a Pandora's box opened on mankind, whereby hope escapes, and despair alone remains."[95] Such false opinions needed to be

countered with a vengeance. "The less thought or said of physical structure, laws of health, etc., the higher will become manhood and womanhood, the fewer diseases appear, and less harm be derived from changes
of climate, unwholesome diet, laying aside flannels, severe mental labors,
sedentary habits, heated rooms, and all the *et cetera* of physiological based on man as a structural thing, whose life is at the mercy of circumstance."[96]

Eddy's metaphysical healing doctrines rested on the premise that
disease "is caused and cured by mind alone." She rejected the prevailing medical distinction between organic diseases and diseases of the
imagination. "Mind produces what is termed organic disease, as directly
as it does hysteria, and cures it as readily." Belief in disease is what inspired bodily symptoms. "When the unconscious mental conception of
disease takes place, its symptoms and locality appear on the body the
same as in optics when the image is forced on the retina that becomes
viable to personal sense."[97]

As provocative as her theories were, Eddy's notoriety was derived
primarily from her teachings and her actual healing practices. Aware of
the opposition that her doctrines would in all likelihood elicit, she remained optimistic that her views would in time triumph. "The resistance to metaphysical science will yield slowly but surely," she declared.[98] In large part her positive outlook owed itself to her faith in her
organizational skills and her decision to situate her healing methods
within the confines of a novel religious dogma.

In 1879, while residing in Lynn, Massachusetts, she and her small
band of followers sought and received a charter as "The Church of
Christ, Scientist." Two years later she moved to Boston and founded
the Metaphysical College—a training school for practitioners of her
methods—where she was the president and sole professor.[99] Tuition at
the Metaphysical College was set at $300, an extraordinary sum for the
period and one that generated considerable controversy. It also virtually guaranteed the competition of like-minded thinkers.[100] The fee
covered the cost of twelve lessons, six of which took place in the first
week.[101] Despite the cost, Eddy had little difficulty finding students,
particularly from the ranks of her own sex.[102] In 1890 Eddy's church
consisted of 8,724 members. By 1906 it had almost 50,000 adherents,
approximately 75 percent of whom were women.[103]

That a considerably larger number of women than men were attracted to Christian Science is not surprising. Women had traditionally
been responsible for the health and care of the sick. Moreover, more

than merely filling a spiritual void in the life of Eddy's followers, Christian Science offered many American women a hitherto absent opportunity to pursue meaningful work and earn a satisfactory income. Indeed, the actions of many of these women "scientists" can plausibly be compared to the growing number of American women who were beginning to challenge the doctrine of separate spheres.[104] Women, who were excluded from virtually every meaningful career path, doubtless flocked to Eddy's church in large measure because her healing movement offered them a sense of dignity and status that many had long been denied.

The rapid growth of Christian Science had two distinct effects. On the one hand, it elicited the opposition of those who had previously chosen to overlook what they deemed to be little more than a marginal cult. On the other hand, Eddy's success inspired others who shared her antimaterialistic sentiments to follow her lead and, in effect, to compete with her.[105] By the mid-1880s Eddy's Metaphysical College was just one of four such schools in the Boston area.[106] Warren Felt Evans, Julius Dresser, and Edward J. Arens had all established competing institutions—each of which held as its fundamental idea that "disease does not come from God, that he has nothing to do with its perpetuation, but that it is one of the errors of man which can be cured by truth; the application of this truth is not by faith, but by an intelligent understanding."[107] In addition to these four major schools, a local newspaper reported that "'there are about a dozen others who practice the mind cure as a profession, and who teach classes of young and old the methods of curing.'"[108]

Midwestern Mind Cure

Interest in mental healing was not confined to New England. The mind cure movement had been spreading across the nation at a phenomenal rate.[109] In 1884 A. J. Swarts, a resident of Chicago who had earlier studied in Boston, established the Mind Cure Publishing Association and began publishing the nation's first monthly periodical dedicated exclusively to the mental healing movement, the *Mind Cure and Science of Life Magazine*.[110] Two years later Swarts followed the lead of the Bostonians and received an Illinois state charter to found the Mental Science University in Chicago. For a fee of $100 students would be instructed in the science of mental healing and receive an M.S. (mental scientist) degree. During the school's first year some thirty-seven diplomas were awarded.[111]

Unlike other proponents of mental healing who sought little more than to promote their own reputations as healers, Swarts endeavored to establish a singular, albeit eclectic, national movement. "It is not for us to discriminate between these various schools in Boston, or to give an opinion as to which one may be more correct than the others, or most successful in healing," Swarts said. "As to the one item or process of curing an afflicted person," he continued, "we endorse them all."[112] Swarts did, however, take issue with the exclusionary practices of Eddy and her followers and "strongly [disowned] the term, 'Christian Science,'" which he asserted was "pretentious and misleading."[113] Moreover, he objected to Eddy's "excessive" tuition and to her legal efforts to stifle rival healers.

Swarts's journal chronicled the early growth of mental healing in considerable detail and provided an open forum for interested men and women to articulate their concerns. Unlike Eddy's journal, which sought to promote her metaphysical doctrines to the exclusion of all others, Swarts's remained a bastion of toleration and diversity throughout its four years of existence.[114] Ultimately, however, his efforts to reconcile opposing points of view proved unsuccessful. Swarts's toleration for different schools of thought infuriated Eddy, and she repeatedly attacked him in her own journal: "A pretentious little publication called THE MIND CURE, has appeared in Chicago, and copies of the same are freely circulating in other cities. Its editor, while yet not disclaiming Spiritualism, mediumship, Mesmerism, etc., etc., still quotes enough from the pages of *Science and Health* to mislead the uninformed into the belief that he is in accord with its teaching; or, as pompously implied—the *author of them*."[115] Eddy accused Swarts of plagiarism and threatened him by referring to her legal victory in what she claimed was a similar case involving Arens, a former disciple and recent rival. Unperturbed, Swarts calmly responded to this warning in his journal and subsequently proclaimed that Evans, not Eddy, was the preeminent American mental healer.

Despite this brief foray into polemics, Swarts did not lose sight of his central aim—namely, to promote a unified and tolerant vision of mental healing on a national scale. For four years Swarts's journal was the only national forum in which proponents of mind cure, regardless of their affiliations, could express their views. Moreover, Swarts's publishing association acted as a clearinghouse for a large number of works dealing with the nascent movement. Each issue of the *Mind Cure and Science of Life Magazine* contained an extensive list of books and pamphlets published by the nation's leading exemplars of mental healing—including those of Eddy and her followers—which could be purchased through the mail. Swarts's efforts were short-lived, however. After losing money for four consecutive years, Swarts could no longer afford to publish his journal. Despite his financial failure, Swarts had accomplished a remarkable feat. He not only revealed that mental healing had a widespread, national appeal but also provided like-minded men and women with a host of previously unrecognized possibilities. His eclectic vision of mental healing served as the first essential step in establishing what over the course of the next two decades became a viable national movement wholly distinct from Christian Science.

New Thought and the Challenge to Christian Science

Prior to Swarts's efforts Christian Scientists were the only group of mental healers to command any serious scrutiny, most of which came from ministers and the press and much of which was highly critical.[116] Among the earliest such commentators was James Monroe Buckley, who in 1887 published a scathing indictment not just of Christian Science but of all schools of metaphysical healing.[117] A Methodist minister and editor of the *Christian Advocate,* Buckley maintained that the "arrogant and exclusive pretensions" of these so-called metaphysical healers were "of the nature of a 'craze.'"[118] Mental healers, he insisted, were not merely misguided and unscrupulous, they were a public menace. Moreover, Eddy and her disciples were the worst of the lot. Duped by her specious claims, thousands of credulous men, women, and children had needlessly placed themselves at risk.

The first efforts to stem the tide of Christian Science took place in the court system. Between 1887 and 1899 hundreds, if not thousands, of Christian Science healers were accused of medical malpractice. More than twenty such cases actually went to trial. Frequently acquitted on the ground that their metaphysical healing techniques, which used neither drugs nor surgery, did not constitute the practice of medicine, Christian Scientists nonetheless elicited a torrent of criticism from journalists, physicians, and ministers.[119] In 1900 William A. Purrington, an attorney, offered one of the most vituperative critiques of Christian Science to date. In a book that opened with a ghastly photograph of a child's gangrened foot that had been mistreated by a Christian Science healer, Purrington explained, "[It] has seemed worth while to collect these papers expounding the dangerous teachings of our Latter-day delusion, Christian Science, and the theory and limitations of medical legislation, if only for the sake of children and helpless adults."[120]

Such negative portrayals of Christian Science provided rival mental healers with a great opportunity. The New Thought, inspired by Julius Dresser's efforts to deny Eddy's claims of originality, acquired its cultural significance in part because of the controversy that surrounded Christian Science.[121] While sharing the same idealistic foundation as Eddy and her disciples, proponents of the New Thought were less doctrinaire in their thinking and more tolerant of both prevailing religious institutions and mainstream medical practices. Advocates of this rival mental healing movement had little desire to draw people away from either their ministers or their doctors. "New Thought is not a church, a cult, or a sect," declared one of the movement's leading exemplars, Charles Brodie Patterson. "It recognizes no limitations of any kind, creates no barriers between man and man: it asks no allegiance to creed, form, or personality, and is as much for one race as for another."[122]

Proponents of the New Thought readily conceded that their system of healing was predicated on the same set of underlying idealistic assumptions as Christian Science.[123] Their explanations for diseases virtually mimicked those of Quimby and Eddy. "From the metaphysical standpoint," a proponent of New Thought explained, "physical diseases are physical effects proceeding from mental states of unrest and discord. It is not strictly true that diseases have mental causes; but rather, diseases are mental, and they produce physical effects."[124] "Adequate study of all forms of sickness," insisted the editor of *Metaphysical Magazine,* Leander Edmund Whipple, "proves the existence of a mental origin for each case; therefore all maladies are mental rather than physical in their nature, being simply different degrees of mental distress registered in the physical system."[125] Still, the presence of these fundamental agreements did not prevent Henry Wood, among the foremost advocates of mind cure, from asserting, "[The] New Thought is no feeble imitation of its more observed neighbor, nor is its light borrowed."[126]

Wood lamented the fact that outside observers typically neglected to consider the substantial differences that distinguished these rival mental healing movements and often regarded all mental healers as "unreasonable, and sometimes fanatical."[127] To combat these perceptions he made a considerable effort to spell out in concise terms what he regarded as the critical differences between the two movements. Whereas the New Thought was "eclectic," "democratic," "open-minded," and "tolerant," Christian Science "[lodged] supreme authority in a person instead of the 'Spirit of Truth,' [proclaimed] the unreality of matter and the body, [was] an exclusive rather than a democratic and open-minded spirit, and [inculcated] the fear of 'malicious animal magnetism' instead of ignoring and overcoming it."[128] Moreover, he continued, Christian Science was "too emotional, too sentimental." Civilization was not yet ready to embrace the extreme idealism of Christian Science and its blanket rejection of materialism and all somatic therapy.[129] Men and women first needed to be weaned off their materialistic proclivities. "So long as men regard themselves primarily as material beings," Wood added, "they will rely upon material means for the healing of disease."[130]

In rejecting the agency of matter in all its forms, Eddy and her most zealous followers had needlessly put themselves and others at risk. "Many absurd and foolish things have been claimed and done," charged one critic.[131] "Some are so anxious to 'demonstrate,' that they are willing to soak themselves in a rain, unnecessarily as a testimony. Better leave that to the ducks."[132] Other critics were significantly more harsh. "What she [Mary Baker Eddy] has really 'discovered,'" charged Josephine Curtis Woodbury, "are ways and means of perceiving and prostituting the science of healing to her own ecclesiastical aggrandizement, and to the moral and physical depravity of her dupes."[133]

The greatest distinction between Christian Science and the New Thought concerned the role accorded to the patient. Eddy argued that the efficacy of mental healing depended in large part on the willingness of the patient to accept her doctrines. "A strongly material, bigoted, or opinionated man," she declared, "yields more slowly to metaphysical treatment than does a more spiritually inclined one."[134] Such faith, she implied, was a prerequisite for successful treatment. Indeed, the absence of a cure was frequently explained on this ground alone. Advocates of the New Thought rejected this argument. The mental cure, said Joseph L. Hasbroucke, "may be performed on a man who believes it to be the veriest humbug."[135]

Proponents of the New Thought adopted the theories of French hypnotist and advocate of suggestive therapeutics, Hippolyte Bernheim. Like American railroad surgeons, who had recently begun employing

Bernheim's doctrines to explain traumatic neuroses, advocates of the New Thought argued that the so-called law of suggestion provided a legitimate scientific basis not only for understanding but also for treating disease. "The metaphysical method of treating the sick person," declared W. J. Coleville, "is through mental suggestion of the right kind."[136] Coleville was just one of several exemplars of the New Thought to cite Bernheim's *Suggestive Therapeutics,* the English translation of which first appeared in 1895.[137] J. Elizabeth Hotchkiss, B. J. Fowler, Shelby Mamaugh, and several others wrote in glowing terms of the power of suggestion.[138]

Distinguishing their idealism from that of the past, proponents of the New Thought declared "the idealism of today is far more practical than the idealism of antiquity because something like a scientific basis has been prepared for it."[139] Unlike physicians, mental healers did not regard science as a means of establishing rational explanations about the natural world. To the contrary, they held a far more results-centered conception of science. Content to let their cures speak for themselves, they proclaimed that "theories, to be good and to be true must be practical."[140] Results, not their rational explanation, were what mattered most. "Any plan or system of things that will destroy or prevent disease," Julia Anderson Root said, "is so far an engine of progress. These powers we claim for metaphysical science."[141] Such a thoroughly pragmatic outlook stood at the core of the mental healing movement.

In 1893 Henry Wood published what soon became a staple in the New Thought diet, *Ideal Suggestion Through Mental Photography.* It was one of the first efforts by a proponent of the New Thought to spell out in precise terms the force by which mental healing operated. In employing the metaphor of the photograph, Wood added a novel element to the mind cure discourse. Almost a quarter of century earlier, Evans had argued that the mechanism that underlay mental healing was similar to that which might explain the telegraph. In so doing Evans had implicitly emphasized the role of the healer, not that of the patient. This emphasis on the projection of positive images, rather than on their reception, had been a central element in the systems of Quimby, Evans, and Eddy. Wood reversed this scenario. Moreover, he argued that neither the healer's personality nor his will played any significant role in mental healing. "No healer, no matter how eminent," Wood maintained, "has any inherent power to restore the health-consciousness, but he can point out the road, and, arm in arm, lovingly conduct his willing brother along its gradual ascent."[142]

Wood's 1893 work represents a midway point between the idealistic proclivities of those who came before him and the psychological orientation of those who soon followed. In *Ideal Suggestion* Wood did not explain the efficacy of mental healing by appealing to the modern science of psychology. Rather he insisted that it was "entirely based upon law, which, though belonging to the higher domain, is orderly and exact."[143] In this respect his analysis had much in common with those of other indigenous mental healers.

Wood was not the only American lay psychologist to appreciate the significance of suggestion. Thomas Jay Hudson, the former chief examiner at the U.S. Patent Office, likewise played a prominent role in popularizing the idea of psychic suggestion. Hudson's first book, *The Laws of Psychic Phenomena* (1893), sold more than one hundred thousand copies and was largely responsible for making the concepts of subjective self and suggestion household words in the United States.[144] Hudson argued that there were "six different systems of psycho-therapeutics based upon many different theories, differing widely as the poles, and each presenting indubitable evidence of being able to perform cures which in any age but the modern would have been called miraculous."[145] These included prayer and religious faith, mind cure, Christian Science, Spiritism, mesmerism, and suggestive hypnotism. These and other psychic phenomena, Hudson claimed, "could be explained as the effects of the objective mind (the ordinary mortal mind) operating by the power of suggestion upon the subjective mind, which is incapable of inductive reasoning, but which is immortal and which immediately controls the non-cerebral organs of the body."[146] Hudson hoped that his "novel" theory would supplant the doctrines of animal magnetism, Christian Science, and other fallacious explanations of hypnotism, faith healing, and kindred phenomena. He argued that although "the science of psycho-therapeutics [was] yet in its infancy . . . enough [had] been learned to simulate research."[147]

Hudson returned to the subject of suggestive therapeutics and developed his original argument in a later work, *The Law of Mental Medicine* (1904). "The aim of this book," Hudson maintained, "is primarily to assist in placing mental therapeutics on a firmly scientific basis, and incidentally to place within the reach of the humblest intellect the most effective method of healing the sick by mental processes."[148] Aware that his efforts were likely to incur the wrath of the medical profession, the former patent clerk made considerable efforts to mollify his potential critics by citing the important contributions that physicians had made to the science of mental medicine. In an effort to distance himself from Christian Scientists, faith healers, and other opponents of medical materialism, he asserted, "I have no quarrel with the medical profession, nor can I join in the indiscriminate clamor against material remedies for the cure of disease. I cannot forget that doctors of medicine were the first to discover the fundamental facts which lie at the basis of the science of mental medicine." "It is true," he added, "that the attitude of the medical profession toward all forms and theories of mental therapeutics has always been one of extreme conservatism, often savoring of unreasoning prejudice; but on the whole its influence has been salutary. If its denunciations have been bitter, it was because they have been directed chiefly against charlatanism and unscientific theories of causation."[149]

The writings of both Wood and Hudson inspired other proponents of the New Thought to emphasize the significance of suggestive therapeutics. Two recently minted journals dedicated to mental healing, the *Arena* and the *Metaphysical Magazine,* published scores of articles that focused on the power of suggestion. Mamaugh proclaimed that the "susceptibility of human beings to moral suasion and mental suggestion is an established verity."[150] He emphasized not only the psychological but also the somatic aspects of suggestive therapeutics: "By suggestion alone, despondency may be turned to hopefulness and nervous irritation largely abolished, the appetite increased and constipation very often relieved, and perverted mental impressions improved and symptoms of organic disease lessened to a considerable degree."[151] Even Wood, who had said nothing of the science of psychology in his original work, soon acknowledged the scientific foundation of suggestion. "The general psychological principles and suggestions which are active in all mental therapeutic systems, although not definitely admitted or recognized by name in Christian Science," he wrote, "are present and active in its operations."[152]

Physicians Respond

In appealing to a psychological principle rather than a divine law, proponents of the New Thought had carried their ideas and methods one step closer toward mainstream medical acceptance. More significantly, they inspired certain segments within a previously reluctant medical profession to consider the merits of their methods according to the definition of science to which physicians themselves sub-scribed.[153] During the early 1880s only a small number of physicians either cared about or concerned themselves with the practices of what many considered to be both a socially and a professionally insignificant practice.[154] "Mental science," wrote Horatio Dresser in his history of the New Thought movement, "had little influence on medical practice."[155] "Metaphysical disease and mind independent of form and motion," charged the homeopathic physician T. L. Brown, "is no part of science. Diseases without physical changes are but myths, metaphysical dreams, very large nothings never found."[156]

By the mid-1890s this situation had begun to change. A growing number of physicians were no longer so cavalier in their dismissal of what they now regarded as a legitimate threat not only to the public welfare but also to their professional livelihood. The movement, Laura Mackie declared, "is more than a passing fad; it is a great and actual danger."[157] Eliza Calvert Hall, a leading proponent of the New Thought, declared that such consideration among American physicians "shows plainly that mental healing has nearly passed the state of ridicule from people of education and culture."[158] The success of the mind cure movement, she added, was evidenced by the substantial opposition that it had evoked: "The crowning accomplishment of the ascendancy of mental healing is the strenuous efforts of the doctors to suppress such healing by law. . . . [T]he legal fight against metaphysical healing is the highest tribute that the medical profession could render it."[159]

Beginning in the late 1880s and continuing for the remainder of the century American physicians appealed to their state legislatures for restrictive licensure laws that would, among other things, put an end to lay mental healing.[160] Such behavior was nothing new. From the dawn of medicine "regular" physicians had sought to suppress alternative healing practices. Historians have explained the late-nineteenth- and early-twentieth-century efforts to revive licensure laws by offering two vastly different explanations. The first places the revival of licensure laws in the context of the nascent germ theory of disease and regards it as yet another example of both medical and scientific progress. The second claims that such laws were not driven by scientific advances but were instead an attempt by regular physicians to promote their economic and professional interests.[161] Whatever the inspiration one fact remains beyond dispute: these laws elicited a torrent of criticism from proponents of mental healing.

American advocates of mental healing appealed to the long-standing American tradition of attacking what they deemed to be a vested interest unworthy of its authoritative stature. Employing the strident rhetoric of Jacksonian democracy, B. J. Fowler, editor of the Spiritualist paper, the *Arena,* declared, "A medical hierarchy is growing up in the republic, in some respects as intolerant and despotic in its instincts as the religious hierarchy of the Dark Ages, which crushed free thought, strangled science, and rendered progress well-nigh impossible."[162] "Medical legalized monopoly," Wood added, "ruthlessly tramples upon the most sacred private domain. It is moral robbery, masquerading as humane legalism."[163]

The controversy over restrictive licensure laws reached its climax in Massachusetts. In 1898 the State Board of Registration in Medicine drafted a proposed bill that "sought to put an end to medical frauds and to require an examination of all those claiming to practice medicine."[164] The first hearing on the bill took place on February 18. On March 2 the public had a chance to respond. "Men and women," the *Boston Evening Transcript* reported, "stood several hours in a room none too well ventilated, and, until warned thrice, applauded vigorously the utterances of the speakers against the bill under consideration. . . . [N]o hearing at the State House this session has aroused such tremendous interest to those who believe themselves concerned."[165] William Lloyd Garrison was among the first to speak out against the bill. "Ostensibly an act to protect the community from malpractice," he charged, "this is really meant to secure the monopoly of treating disease to those who bear the credentials of a recognized school."[166] The most elegant critique of the proposed bill came from William James. Articulating ideas that he had previously discussed in his 1896 essay, "The Will to Believe," James declared,

Were medicine a finished science, with all practitioners in agreement about methods of treatment, a bill to make it penal to treat a patient without having passed an examination would be unobjectionable. But the present condition of medical knowledge is widely different from such a state. Both as to principles and as to practice our knowledge is deplorably imperfect. The whole face of medicine changes unexpectedly from one generation to another in consequence of widening experience.[167]

Unlike other critics of the proposed law, James questioned not the motives but the wisdom of the law's sponsors. He urged them to consider the history of their profession, which, he asserted, "is really a hideous history, comparable only to that of priest craft. Ignorance clad in authority and riding over men's bodies and souls. Let modern medicine dispel all those inherited prejudices by living the historic memories down."[168]

. James's critique was not based solely on his understanding of medical history. On the contrary, it derived in large measure from his abiding faith in science itself. Rather than suppress mental healing by a legislative enactment, he encouraged his colleagues to study such practices and learn what they could from them. "How many of my learned medical friends who today are so freely denouncing mind-cure methods as an abominable superstition," James asked, "have taken the trouble to follow up the cases of some mind cure, one by one, so as to acquaint themselves with the results? I doubt there is a single individual."[169] Earlier in the decade James had spoken out against a similar piece of legislation.[170] Both then and now his position infuriated many of his close friends in the Boston medical community, who regarded his views on the subject as being not only irresponsible but also heretical. James, of course, could not have disagreed more strongly.

In a letter to his good friend and fellow physician, James Jackson Putnam, James explained his motives for testifying against the proposed bill.

If you think that I *enjoy* that sort of thing you are mistaken. I never did anything that required so much moral effort in my life. My vocation is to treat of things in an allround manner and not to make *ex parte* pleas to influence (or to seek) a peculiar jury. *Aussi* why do the medical brethren force an offending citizen like me into such a position? Legislative licence is sheer humbug—mere abstract paper thunder under which every ignorance and abuse can still go on. . . . Bah! I am sick of the whole business, and I well know how all my colleagues at the medical school view me and my efforts. But if Zola and Col. Piquart can face the whole French army, can't I face their disapproval?—Much more easily than that of my own conscience![171]

While perhaps misplaced, James's allusion to the Dreyfus affair made clear his disdain for his medical opponents. Two days later James clarified his position.

It seems to me it is not a question of fondness or non-fondness for the mind curers [heaven knows I am not, and can't understand a word of their jargon except their precept of assuming yourself to be well and claiming health rather than sickness which I am sure is magnificent] but of the *neces-*

sity of legislative interference with the natural play of things. There *surely* can *be* not such necessity. From the general sea of medical insecurity, a law can hardly remove an appreciable quantity. . . . The profession claims a law simply on the grounds of personal dislike. It is antisemitism again. It is the justification of Armenian massacres, which we have heard of late, on the ground that the Armenians are so "disagreeable." The one use of our institutions is to force on us toleration of much that *is* disagreeable.[172]

Putnam responded that while he did not share all of James's views, he did, in fact, agree with many of his sentiments. "Sincere fanatics," Putnam told James, "are almost always, and in this case I think, certainly, of real value."[173]

Rather than suppress the mental healers by legal means, Putnam and other like-minded physicians called for an "impartial scientific" investigation of mental healing. Edes urged his fellow physicians "to look the fact squarely in the face that some persons do receive great benefit from some of these forms of treatment who have failed to do so at the hands of regular and skilled practitioners." "These cases," he continued, "should be studied and not contemptuously waved aside."[174] With respect to mind cure, Edes declared, "It is better to study it and profit by it."[175]

Inspired by Putnam and Edes's challenge, Henry H. Goddard, a doctoral student in psychology at Clark University, embarked on an extensive investigation of such practices. In 1899 Goddard published the results of his study in an article entitled "The Effects of Mind on Body as Evidenced by Faith Cures."[176] "Suggestion," he wrote, "is the bond of union between all the different methods, Divine Healing, Christian Science, Mental Science, etc. . . . [The] fundamental principle of all mental therapeutics is the law of suggestion—the law that any idea possessing the mind tends to materialize itself in the body."[177] Although certain segments within the American mental healing community were disturbed by Goddard's findings, proponents of the New Thought welcomed his conclusions. Physicians likewise gave his findings a respectable hearing. Of particular interest was Goddard's conclusion.

While we find nothing to warrant the overthrow of the science of medicine, and no power that is able adequately to take the place of a thorough knowledge of anatomy and pathology or the skill of the surgeon, we do find sufficient evidence to convince us that the proper reform in mental attitude would relieve many a sufferer of ills that the ordinary physicians cannot touch; would even delay the approach of death to many a victim beyond

the power of absolute cure, and the faithful adherence to a truer philosophy of life, will keep many a man well and give the doctor time to study his
science, and devote himself to alleviating ills that are unpreventable.[178]

Such a holding could not help but inspire more open-minded physicians to reconsider their views on the subject. Rather than call for the
suppression of the mental healers, more progressive members of the
medical establishment sought instead to consider their methods and, if
they proved effective, to use them to supplement their various somatic
therapies.

CHAPTER 5

Flirting with Psychotherapy

Somatic Intransigence and
the "Advanced Guard"

Much will be gained by recognizing at the outset, that no such
thing as a science of psychology exists, but that scientific methods
in its pursuit are readily attainable, and we may be assured that
this method will, ere long, if strictly adhered to, give us a science
of psychology.

J. D. Buck, 1880

Apathy, not antipathy, was the most common medical response to both Christian Science and the New Thought. Indeed, the
overwhelming majority of American physicians expressed little interest
in pursuing the issues raised by various proponents of lay mental healing. The refusal of most mainstream physicians to take mind cure ideas
seriously was largely attributable to their recent adoption of the somatic
paradigm. Inspired to a great extent by a broadly based epistemological
and scientific transformation that had been under way since the middle
of the seventeenth century, American and European physicians engaged
in a self-conscious and deliberate effort to follow the example of the
more rigorously physical sciences. In so doing they sought to rid medicine of its reliance on psychic or quasi-psychic entities.[1]

The ascendance of the somatic paradigm, while it signified the end of
the older psychosomatic order, did not completely abolish medical interest in psychological matters. Indeed, as the experience of the American mind cure movement reveals, rather than transform public consciousness, medical somaticism was in part responsible for generating a

backlash against what many regarded as materialism gone amok. That by 1900 the somatic paradigm had achieved superiority across the entire medical domain cannot be denied. But the unwillingness of the overwhelming majority of physicians to consider seriously nonmaterial theories of disease did not signify the death of psychological medicine. Although muted, faint echoes of the older psychosomatic tradition could still be heard.

In an odd irony, by the 1890s, when the neurological critique of asylum psychiatry had finally succeeded in convincing most American asylum superintendents of the need to consider the role of physiological factors alone in diagnosing and treating insanity, elites within the American neurological profession were just beginning to call attention to the role of mental factors in certain functional nervous disorders.[2] The disparity in emphasis was in large measure attributable to the types of patients with whom neurologists and psychiatrists came in contact.[3] For the most part neurologists worked with men and women who possessed far greater agency than those who were confined to psychiatric asylums. Thus they had little choice but to respond to their patients' demands. Treatment by a neurologist, after all, was just one of several possible options that nervous American men and women might consider. The same could not be said for the institutionalized "insane," who possessed, at best, limited capacity to influence their therapeutic regimen.

Demedicalizing the Mind

A central preoccupation of mid-nineteenth-century neuroscientific researchers involved extending the reach of the "reflex" concept to the "upper" regions of the central nervous system, including the once-sacrosanct cerebrum—thereby applying it to a broad range of psychological functions.[4] In his original discussion of the "reflex" in 1832, British physiologist Marshall Hall had divided the central nervous system into two distinct systems: one responsible for involuntary reflex functions such as respiration, circulation, and digestion; the other, for sensation, volition, and psychic functions. As Hall explained, "The cerebrum itself may be viewed as the organ of the mind,—the organ on which the *psyche*, sits, as it were, enthroned; the voluntary nerves convey the mandates of the volition to the muscles which are to be called into action. All these functions are strictly *psychical*."[5] By privileging the position of the cerebrum Hall was able to accomplish two important goals. On the one hand, he advanced the cause of physiology; on the other, he maintained a central precept of Christian morality: free will.

Many of Hall's successors challenged his narrow conception of the reflex and sought to apply the theory of reflexion to various mental functions.[6] As British physiologist William B. Carpenter asserted, "There seems no reason why [the cerebrum] should be exempted from the law of 'reflex action,' which applies to every other part of the nervous system [and to lower animals]."[7] This reversal of Hall's position had several serious consequences. As Edwin Clarke and L. S. Jacyna explain, "What had traditionally been regarded as 'mind' ceased to be a causally potent entity and became a paralleled, almost incidental series of phenomena to the mechanical reflexes of the cerebral hemispheres."[8] Cartesian dualism yielded to a novel view in which body and mind had, at long last, become integrated.[9]

Rather than banish the mind from medicine, proponents of psychophysical parallelism held that its consideration had become superfluous. John Hughlings Jackson, perhaps the most eminent neurologist of his day, summarized the parallelist position: "I do not concern myself with mental states at all, except indirectly in seeking their anatomical substrata. I do not trouble myself about the mode of connection between mind and matter. It is enough to assume parallelism. That along with excitations or discharges of nervous arrangements in the cerebrum, mental states occur, I, of course, admit; but how this is I do not inquire; indeed, so far as clinical medicine is concerned, I do not care."[10] Echoing this view, a prominent American asylum superintendent declared, "[The] expression 'disease of the mind,' should have a place in the nomenclature of modern medical science with witchcraft and demonomania. They are alike the offspring of metaphysical speculation, alike misinterpretation of phenomena."[11]

Parallelism, which rested on an analogical rather than an empirical analysis, lacked a scientifically viable foundation until 1870—the year Gustav Theodor Fritsch and Eduard Hitzig produced what appeared to be compelling empirical evidence that functional parcellation at the cortex existed.[12] The two German physicians reported their epoch-making findings in a paper entitled "On the Electrical Excitability of the Cerebrum."[13] On the basis of experiments that they conducted on dogs, Fritsch and Hitzig appeared to confirm a notion that had long since been discarded: the existence of a correspondence between particular regions of the cerebrum and specific bodily functions.[14] Moreover, the two speculated that "some psychological functions and perhaps all of them, in order to enter matter or originate from it need certain circumscribed centers of the cortex."[15]

The impact of Fritsch and Hitzig's findings was both immediate and profound. Their work prompted a torrent of literature on cerebral localization.[16] Efforts to track down and to isolate regions of the brain responsible not only for physical but also mental functions became increasingly earnest. The most conspicuous evidence in support of this endeavor came from the study of aphasia, a neurological speech disorder. Almost a full decade before Fritsch and Hitzig's experiments French philologist Paul Broca had presented "the first localization of a function in the hemisphere which met with general acceptance from orthodox scientists."[17] Within a decade of Broca's discovery of the neural speech center Fritsch, Hitzig, and Jackson were able to demonstrate that the physiological concomitants of words could be identified as cerebral motor processes, thereby "proving" what many had long speculated: a correspondence between a "higher" mental function and a specific center of the brain.[18]

The implications of this research for the study of insanity were obvious. "Although the cases thus far examined may be regarded as insufficient to establish general conclusions," John P. Gray, editor of the *American Journal of Insanity,* proclaimed, "they go to strengthen the conviction sustained by the laws of general pathology, that insanity is a physical disease of the brain, and that the mental phenomena are symptoms."[19] That microscopic investigation had yet to furnish any discernible anatomical or physiological evidence that might support this contention did little to undermine the growing belief that such lesions did, in fact, exist.[20] To claim otherwise would be to undermine the integrity of the somatic paradigm.[21]

Gray's views, although not universally embraced, were widely shared. Their apparent confirmation was not long in coming. Robert Koch's 1882 discovery of the tubercle bacillus provided the first evidence that a human disease was caused by a specific bacterium.[22] Efforts to uncover an analogous explanation for insanity and other nervous diseases provided physicians and neuroscientists with an intriguing intellectual framework. Moreover, by the early 1890s medical and cellular research had proved what had hitherto been partly speculated: "general paralysis of the insane, a form of insanity that affected a substantial percentage of male asylum patients was actually the terminal form of syphilis."[23] The discovery of the *Treponema palladum* appeared to confirm existing speculations and to provide compelling evidence that "the physical basis for all mental disease would soon be firmly established." [24] "For the first time, then," Claude Quetel observes, " 'something' had been discovered in the brains of the insane! Moreover, these anatomo-pathological lesions were not only to make general paralysis the model of organic mental diseases, they were also to swing the psychogenetic conception of madness, as defined by Pinel and Esquirol, towards an organogentic conception." [25]

The Maintenance of Psychological Medicine

In the midst of the medical revolution of the late nineteenth century the subject of mental healing had been presented in considerable detail by renowned British psychiatrist, Daniel Hack Tuke. [26] In *Of the Influences of the Mind Upon the Body in Health and Disease Designed to Elucidate the Actions of the Imagination,* Tuke explored whether "the mind's indisputable ability to heal [could] be applied and guided with skill and wisdom by the physician." [27] After more than three hundred pages in which he recounted literally hundreds of instances of mental healing, Tuke asked,

How can the foregoing facts, proving as they do, the great influence which mental states exert over the body in disease, be practically applied for therapeutic purpose? Can this unquestionable power be controlled or directed? Ought we to deliberately cause a mental shock? We have seen gout cured by the patient's window being smashed by a wagon, or his house being set afire. May we imitate these accidents to obtain the same end? [28]

Tuke's provocative questions caused little stir among his medical peers. The Anglo-American medical climate of the late 1870s and early 1880s proved inhospitable to such psychologizing. [29]

Perhaps the best evidence of American hostility to Tuke's psychological speculations can be found in the reception accorded George Beard's 1876 paper, "The Influence of the Mind in the Causation and Cure of Disease—The Potency of Definite Expectation." [30] Speaking before an audience of fellow American neurologists, Beard maintained that disease might appear and disappear without the influence of any agency other than some kind of emotion. "Mental qualities, like drugs," he explained, "could neutralize therapeutics, and they could also increase the effects of drugs." Moreover, "in disease, in ninety-nine cases out of a hundred, the emotions were supreme. The knowledge on the part of the patients that mental therapeutics was being employed in the treatment of their disease, did not discourage them; and the liability to disappointment in carrying out such therapeutics was no greater than that of attending the use of any other remedial measure." Mental therapeutics, Beard concluded, "could be applied to acute and chronic, to functional and organic diseases."[31]

The aim of his paper, Beard proclaimed, "was not to show anything new, but to introduce to the profession some special experiment, with the view of exciting a more thorough study of the subject."[32] Much to his chagrin, Beard's modest call for a systematic investigation of mental healing "aroused a furor."[33] If Beard's doctrines were to be taken seriously, venerated American neurologist William Alexander Hammond commented, "we should go back to monkery—give up our instruments, give up our medicines and enter a convent."[34] Although not all the opponents of Beard's mental healing doctrines were so strident in their rhetoric, most shared Hammond's sentiments. James Jackson Putnam, who two decades later would become one of the most prominent American medical champions of psychotherapy, asserted that he "had never seen any evidence that cure had been effected by mental influences in cases where actual disease had existed."[35] Beard's experiments, he continued, were unscientific because the emotions could not be isolated. One physician went so far as to deny the existence of mental therapeutics altogether. Such resistance to Beard's paper was not the least bit surprising. As members of a novel specialty intent on establishing its "scientific" foundation, this pioneering generation of American neurologists was unwilling to compromise its precarious professional standing by relying on a set of mental healing theories and practices that appeared to be at odds with the emerging somatic paradigm.[36]

What in the 1870s had been cause for ridicule, if not outright scorn, among American neurologists had by the first decade of the twentieth century once again become a subject of legitimate debate. Much had changed in the intervening three decades.[37] The early promise of various late-nineteenth-century neuroscientific discoveries proved difficult to realize. Neurologists had failed to demonstrate a relationship between lesions and abnormal behavior. Moreover, as Gerald Grob explains, their nosological schemes not only were rigid and vague but also relied on clinical observations rather than on more substantive biological evidence.[38] These circumstances, combined with the willingness of prominent European physicians both to investigate and to employ various mental healing techniques, did much to disabuse several prominent American neurologists and psychiatrists of their former hostility toward mental healing.

Elite American neurologists were at the fore of the campaign to legitimize the use of mental therapeutics among their professional colleagues. In an odd irony the very specialty that had compelled asylum superintendents to relinquish their once-heralded moral treatment on the ground that it was not sufficiently scientific soon embraced a mental therapy of its own.[39] That the success of the mind curists was in part responsible for this renewed willingness to consider the role of mental factors in certain functional nervous disorders few denied. "Why should we, as scientific physicians," asked Sheldon Leavitt, "allow prejudice to debar us from therapeutic resources that are apt to prove far more effective, it may be, than any in our command? Why not enter and cultivate a field now running to weeds but capable of developing the richest fruits?"[40] Leavitt's views were reiterated by a Johns Hopkins University neurologist, Lewellys F. Barker:

Educated physicians may regret the excesses of the blindly ignorant and the unscrupulously greedy, but they should not themselves err by neglecting a side of medicine which quacks have often shown themselves more capable of exercising. If the physician relies on science, experience, and training, he will surely be protected from the vagaries of psychotherapy of which those are prone who put their trust merely in introspection, instinct, or occult revelation.[41]

Rather than cite the works of Quimby, Eddy, Evans, Wood, Hudson, Whipple, Trine, and other American proponents of mind cure, American medical advocates of mental therapeutics referred instead to the writings of European physicians and scientists: Charcot, Bernheim, and Janet in France; Dubois and Dejerine in Switzerland; Breuer and Freud in Austria; Van Eeden and Van Roentergam in the Netherlands.

Somatic Intransigence

The mental healing theories and methods that crossed the Atlantic with little difficulty found acceptance by the American physicians far more arduous. The stigma of Christian Science and New

Thought was often too much to bear, and American medical proponents of mental therapeutics found themselves hard-pressed to make the case that a host of recent, medically sanctioned European experiments in hypnotism, suggestion, persuasion, and other methods were worthy of further scrutiny. Rather than stimulate professional interest in the subject, popular fascination with mental healing induced the majority of American physicians to redouble their efforts in search of both somatic explanation and somatic therapies.

Fidelity to the materialist fold was widespread. Professional unwillingness to explore the possible therapeutic uses of mental healing, claimed Lewellys Barker, was due "partly to a desire to avoid even the appearance of evil and humbug, partly to the exercise of so much zeal in those physical, chemical, and biologic studies which are flooding our science with new light that less time and attention have been devoted to psychological and psychiatric studies than they deserve."[42] Excepting railroad surgeons and a small number of neurologists and psychiatrists, the overwhelming majority of American physicians—regardless of their school or specialty—had by the final decade of the nineteenth century ceased even to consider the possibility that psychological factors might play a role in exciting, maintaining, or treating mental and nervous disorders. "Do not let us venture into deep waters of psychology," the New York neurologist Bernard Sachs warned, "unless we are in danger of being stranded by hugging too closely the shores of anatomical sciences."[43] Willing to concede that physicians were not yet "sufficiently advanced to give a rational account of the various changes underlying mental disease," Sachs nonetheless declared, "It is clearly our duty to persevere in our anatomical and experimental studies in order that we may some day reach a better solution of these many vexed problems."[44] Like Sachs, homeopathic physician T. L. Brown captured the sentiments of many in his school when he declared, "Of all things now influencing the general good of humanity, the physical causes of disease require our investigation and most earnest study."[45]

Allegiance to somatic ideology had provided late-nineteenth-century American neurologists and psychiatrists with an opportunity to push the frontiers of their respective, albeit increasingly intertwined, specialties to new heights. Much of their professional self-esteem was derived from their sense that they were playing an important part in a larger scientific enterprise.[46] Prior to his appointment at Johns Hopkins and his exposure to the most recent studies of psychopathology, Barker was himself a leading exemplar of somatic psychiatry. "The pathology of nervous diseases, with the exception of the mental forms," Barker explained, "has made rapid and encouraging progress. We have as yet, it must be admitted no pathology of mental diseases worthy of the name, nor can we expect any until our knowledge of cerebral anatomy and physiology has been much extended. Yet a beginning has been made, and we have every reason to believe that continued conscientious work will lead to important results."[47]

Moreover, when physiological and anatomical theories could not adequately explain certain disease states, a physician had little need to resort to a psychological explanation. Other somatic possibilities had not yet been exhausted. P. M. Wise, in his 1901 presidential address before the American Medico-Psychological Association, claimed,

We are being gradually drifted by clinical experience and the physiological laboratory to the conclusion that the vitalizing element of cell integrity depends more upon chemical processes than upon structure, and that we may have marked digressions from the normal without structural changes. . . . *The indications are that initial mental pathology is of a chemical nature, and leaves no traces in structure in the non-living tissues discoverable at least by present technique.*[48]

The persistence of somatic explanations was not surprising. American psychiatry and neurology had risen to prominence almost exclusively on their respective abilities to provide compelling physiological models for both mental and neurological disorders.[49]

Positing a chemical model of disease in place of a structural one enabled psychiatrists and neurologists to persist in their yet-to-be-confirmed speculations concerning the somatic etiology of all mental illness. Wise's refusal to consider the possibility that psychological factors might play a role in mental illness epitomized the intransigence of the American psychiatric community. Like ostriches with their heads stuck in the sand, most American physicians who made their careers treating nervous disorders were blind to the revolution taking place beyond the medical discourse. Given the persuasiveness of medical somaticism, American physicians who supported the professional use of mental therapeutics faced several cultural and professional obstacles. Not only did they have to distinguish their theories from those of the mind curists and other lay mental healers, but they also had to persuade their somatically inclined colleagues that psychological methods were, in fact, "scientifically" legitimate.

The Advanced Guard and the
Challenge to Somaticism

Beginning in the mid-1880s a small cohort of elite Boston-based neurologists, psychiatrists, and psychologists began to consider seriously the subjects of mental healing and psychopathology. The Boston School of Psychotherapy (or the School of Abnormal Psychology) as Eugene Taylor refers to it was a "loose-knit group of professionals who were pioneers in treating mental diseases that had no organic basis."[50] Of the Boston medical scene during the late nineteenth century, neurologist Isador Coriat wrote, "[The] interest here in psychotherapy was probably originally stimulated by William James who, as a philosopher, psychologist, and physician, was deeply interested in abnormal mental states." "During these early days," Coriat continued, "an informal psychopathological club met at irregular intervals at Dr. Prince's house."[51]

Members of this pioneering group included psychologists William James and G. Stanley Hall; neurologists James Jackson Putnam and Morton Prince; and foreign-born psychiatrists Adolf Meyer and Boris Sidis.[52] James played the most decisive role. He had almost singlehandedly defined the field of academic psychology in the United States. The first to establish a psychological laboratory in the New World and to present a synthesis of the newly emerging academic field, James inspired a generation of psychologists, neurologists, and psychiatrists. His *Principles of Psychology* (1890) was the result of a thirteen-year labor and established his reputation as one of the world's foremost psychologists. Unlike other psychologists of his generation, James argued that rather than focus on abstract entities, psychology needed to concentrate on actual experience.[53] "By appealing to experience," Ruth Leys writes, "James implicitly contravened the view that mind and body were radically distinct entities and hence were incapable of interaction."[54] Neither a materialist nor an idealist, James accorded a special role to consciousness itself, which, he argued, acted as the mediating force between experience and action.[55]

James defined science far more broadly than did many of his contemporaries. That scientific inquiry required both facts and rigorous methods with which to process them he did not deny. Where he differed from his peers, however, was in his willingness to conceive of both in their broadest possible terms. James argued that neither facts nor methods were constant. They were continually evolving. The problem, said James, was that many scientists were so blinded by received wisdom that they frequently failed to consider myriad pertinent and readily discernible clues regarding a host of matters. Such intransigence was not surprising, however. If anything, it was an endemic aspect of the human condition. "Old fogyism," James had written, "begins at a younger age than we think. I am almost afraid to say so, but I believe that in the majority of human beings it begins at about twenty-five." [56]

James's most direct contribution to the birth of American psychotherapy resulted from his discussion of habit and its relation to education. [57] He first broached the subject in the February 1887 issue of *Popular Science*. "Habit," he proclaimed, "is thus the enormous fly-wheel of society, its most precious conservative agent." [58] Making no claims of originality, James readily conceded that his views on the subject were derived from his earlier reading of Carpenter, whom he quoted at length: "It is a matter of universal experience, that every kind of training for special aptitudes is both far more effective, and leaves a more permanent impress, when exerted on the *growing* organism, than when brought to bear on the adult. The effect of such training is shown in the tendency of the organ to 'grow to' the mode in which it is habitually exercised." [59] Central to James's analysis was the proposition that by the age of thirty the character of most people "has set like plaster, and will never soften again." [60] This virtually inevitable outcome was not necessarily a limitation, however. If during their more malleable childhood years boys and girls could be encouraged to develop "good" habits and discouraged from maintaining "bad" ones, then the likelihood of a prosperous and happy adulthood could be increased dramatically.

James returned to the subject of habit in a series of public lectures that he first delivered between 1891 and 1892. [61] In *Talks to Teachers* James suggested how recent psychological findings concerning the role of habits might be of use to those responsible for the education of the young. "Education, in short," James argued, "cannot be better described than by calling it the organization of acquired habits of conduct and tendencies to behavior." While James did not dismiss the role of consciousness in education, he emphasized behavior. "Education is for behavior, and habits are the stuff of which behavior consists." "Your task," he told his audience of Cambridge schoolteachers, "is to build up a character in your pupils; and a character, as I have often said, consists in an organized set of habits of reaction." [62] Relying on theories of association psychology that had been formalized in the writings of British psychologist Alexander Bain, James stressed the link between mental perceptions and their physiological correlates: "The great thing, then, in all education is to *make our nervous system our ally instead of our enemy*. It is to fund and capitalize our acquisitions, and live at ease upon the interest of the fund. *For this we must make automatic and habitual, as early as possible, as many useful actions as we can,* and guard against the growing into ways that are likely to be disadvantageous to us, as we should guard against the plague."[63] Good habits were more than merely savings stashed away for a rainy day, they were vibrant investment capital that promised to deliver a high return.

The novelty of James's argument lay not in its epistemology but in its practical orientation. The important thing, he explained, was that "pupils, whatever else they are, are at any rate little pieces of associating machinery."[64] The teacher's task was thus to direct this process in a beneficent manner. "To break up bad associations or wrong ones, to build others in, to guide the associative tendencies into the most fruitful channels," James declared, "is the educator's principal task. But here, as with other simple principles, the difficulty lies in the application. Psychology can state the laws; concrete tact and talent alone can work them to useful results."[65]

In less than a decade James's pedagogic views found a receptive audience among several eminent Boston physicians, who began to speculate that they might be well suited for the treatment of certain types of functional nervous disorders. Among the most prominent of these was Tufts University professor of medicine, Morton Prince. More interested in questions of psychopathology than pathology, Prince approached functional nervous disorders from both a psychological and an organic perspective.[66] "The study of the pathology of these affections would be far from complete," Prince wrote, "if no account were taken of the psychical elements as a factor in the generation of the neurological process. The mental element undoubtedly plays a very important part, and particularly in maintaining the neurosis after it has been once established."[67]

Prince had not always held such views, however. Like other physicians of his generation, Prince began his medical career as a staunch proponent of the somatic paradigm. Indeed, until 1884 he specialized in diseases of the nose and throat.[68] "In spite of all its short-comings, materialism," Prince proclaimed in 1885, "is essentially the philosophy of science, and hence that which must eventually prevail." "Underneath . . . every mental act," he continued, "there flows a physical current. With every thought, sensation or emotion is associated a physical change in a material substance,—the brain."[69] Reflecting on his eventual embrace of psychological medicine, Prince explained,

I remember well how, after graduation, I had hung out my "shingle" and entered upon general practice, I expected that it would be patients with organic diseases . . . that would ring my door bell or send their calls in urgency. It was only gradually that it dawned upon me that these were but a small part of the ills for which a physician's services are needed; and I found that it was the functional disturbances of a minor and major character that to an equal extent at least with organic diseases incapacitate poor humanity from "carrying on" and which I was called upon to rectify.[70]

Prince's willingness to consider the role that mental factors played in both exciting and maintaining certain nervous diseases dated back to the early 1880s. In 1880 Prince received a firsthand education in the most recent findings emanating from France when he took his mother to Paris for a personal consultation with Charcot.[71] In addition, Prince's active participation in the medicolegal discourse concerning railway spine inspired him to consider the possible limitations of the somatic paradigm. "How can one understand," Prince asked, "how a psychical trauma, such as would be incurred in a railroad disaster, can produce not only mental perturbation but disturbances of the various physiological functions of the body, unless one has a clear conception of the relation between mental action and cerebral action?"[72]

In answering this question Prince relied almost exclusively on a physiological conception of the law of association, which, he explained, "may be stated in general terms as follows: Ideas, sensations, emotions, and volitions occurring together tend by constant repetition to become so strongly associated that the presence of one of them reproduces the others."[73] Prince's interest in associational theory had been suggested by the Baltimore surgeon John Holland Mackenzie.[74] "Having induced a violent sneeze in a lady allergic to roses by letting her sniff an artificial rose," Hale writes, "[Mackenzie] concluded that the sneeze was caused by an habitual association of ideas with bodily reactions."[75] By linking Mackenzie's findings to earlier conceptions of the unconscious articulated by Oliver Wendell Holmes and William Carpenter, Prince concluded that "*a pathological process in the nervous system, once engendered by an external agency, may afterward be awakened, on the cessation of that agency, by means merely of a physiological action or a psychological state previously associated with it.*"[76]

In an 1891 article in the *Journal of Nervous and Mental Diseases*

Prince argued that a complete pathological study of functional nervous diseases required some account of the psychic elements as a factor in the generation of the neurological process. "The mental element," he insisted, "undoubtedly plays a very important part, and particularly in maintaining the neurosis after it has been once established."[77] Citing the "well-known fact that not only may two mental states be associated together, but a mental state and a purely physiological function," Prince offered a resolutely psychogenic explanation for a host of apparently somatic symptoms:[78] "Just as mental states could become linked by association, so purely physiological functions, such as rapid heart beat, salivation, or bladder spasms could become associated with emotions, mental states, or visual images. After the association was formed, each link in the change could activate an entire pattern."[79] "The practical corollary from this theory," he concluded, "is that in a large class of neuroses we are to look for their causes, not in diseased nerves and centres, but rather in a pathological association of normal anatomical elements, and the treatment is to be directed to the breaking up of this association, and the regrouping of the nervous centres."[80]

Prince's conception of the law of association differed in one critical respect from that of the mind curists. Whereas the lay mental healers had embraced Berkeley's early-eighteenth-century formulation of the law, Prince drew instead on Bain's and James's more recently articulated physiological conception of associationism and on Carpenter's and Holmes's discussion of unconscious cerebral mechanisms.[81] In contrast to Berkeley's psychology, which was the product of a philosophical tradition, Prince's analysis was in large measure informed by a rigorous understanding of the most current physiological knowledge.[82] This physiologically rooted "law" offered Prince an eminently respectable explanation that enabled him to investigate further the psychological correlates of certain functional nervous disorders while simultaneously maintaining his fundamentally materialistic perspective.

Association theory did more than merely explain the presence of certain functional nervous symptoms; it offered a compelling theoretical basis for their treatment. Just as the theory served as the basis for James's pedagogic theories, it likewise provided Prince with a cogent rationale for a hitherto untried therapeutic regimen. Prince's "educational treatment," which he first articulated in 1898, was little more than a medical application of James's pedagogy. In "The Educational Treatment of Neurasthenia and Certain Hysterical States" Prince argued that the successful treatment of functional nervous disorders had much in common with the instruction of the young. Application of this method entailed instructing patients about the "true" nature of their symptoms; typically, this step required explaining that such symptoms were not indicative of some grave underlying organic disorder but were the product of fixed ideas, apprehensions, false beliefs, and bad habits.[83] The goal of Prince's novel therapy, much like James's pedagogy, was to suppress neurotic symptoms by the development of good habits of body and mind, which enabled the patient to return to the wear and tear of life without breaking down:

The preliminary step in the treatment is the study of the origin, history, and groupings of individual symptoms. It is surprising to find, after a searching inquiry which involves every detail concerning the origins and character of the symptoms, and the condition under which they arise, how often what seem to be a mere chaos of unrelated mental and physical phenomena will resolve itself into a series of logical events, and law and order be found to underlie the symptomatic tangle.[84]

For this therapy to succeed cooperation between doctor and patient was essential. "The attitude of the physician," Prince wrote, "should be largely that of the trainer to the athlete. He is to teach the patient how to help himself."[85] Making the patient aware of the mental nature of his symptoms and the role played by his habits and associations was only half the battle, however. On achieving this goal, the physician then had to perform the more arduous task of suppressing the symptoms by the appropriate therapeutic agents. Of the many possibilities, Prince insisted that direct suggestion was the most powerful.

Many of Prince's views were soon adopted by his Boston colleague, James Jackson Putnam. Like Prince, Putnam began his medical career as a staunch materialist.[86] During the first decade of his career as a physician he assailed mental therapeutics and the seemingly unscientific theories of functional neurosis that abounded.[87] His participation in the medicolegal discourse triggered by the rising incidence of railway spine compelled him to reconsider his somatic bias. By the mid-1880s Putnam had come to realize that "many symptoms he had once considered to be entirely physiological were in fact psychological in origin."[88] In explaining Putnam's conversion to the "psychological style," Hale writes, "Part of the impetus came from defeated expectations—the absence of somatic evidence to support overextended somatic hypotheses—and from therapeutic discouragement. A new rationale and a more sanguine outlook came from new psychological data, from the European and American rediscovery of the unconscious—the rich and subtle work of Freud's immediate predecessors, particularly Charcot and Janet."[89]

In 1899 Putnam endeavored to summarize the recent American and European investigations of both mental therapeutics and psychopathology. In a lecture entitled "Not the Disease Only, But Also the Man," the Harvard professor declared,

The splendid wave of pathological and bacteriological research that has raised the art and science of medicine to its present position of authority has set physicians trying to solve their problems in terms of pathology alone; but it is a matter for congratulation that this wave is being reinforced by another which is sweeping us toward *a better knowledge of the secrets of the mental life in health and disease.* Perhaps we may even learn thereby to interpret the teaching of pathology itself in a wider sense.[90]

Putnam encouraged his fellow physicians to embrace a larger perspective: "We all hear of the triumphs of surgery, and every doctor feels a personal pride in spreading the news of them abroad, but there are not so many who know that there are men, as yet few in number but of equal genius, who with equal devotion and study have been searching for means to change, little by little, the trend of the forces that work within the mind, and are thus silently laying the foundation of a new departure in therapeutics."[91]

Putnam's and Prince's status as elite, Harvard-educated, university-affiliated neurologists afforded them a latitude that was denied the less respectable members of their professions. Among the first American neurologists to consider seriously the possibility of exploiting recent psychological findings for therapeutic purposes and to attempt to offer a systematic analysis of the role that mental factors played in certain mental diseases, they had the freedom to entertain psychological theories and practices with little fear of professional reprisals. Indeed, by the first decade of the twentieth century neurology had risen in prominence among American medical specialties.

What Prince, Putnam, and others did for neurology, Adolf Meyer and Boris Sidis did for psychiatry. Active members in the Boston medical scene during the late 1890s, Sidis and Meyer were among the first American psychiatrists to acknowledge the contribution of psychological experimentation to psychiatric medicine. "Psychology from hovering in the clouds of metaphysical reflection," Sidis wrote, "has descended into the laboratories and is now demonstrating its truths by means of instruments and experiments."[92] Sidis, who received both a

Ph.D. and an M.D. from Harvard University, was among the first American scientists to study unconsciously motivated behavior.[93] Of special interest to him was the so-called hypnoidal state—the phase between sleep and waking, characterized by suggestibility—which he first described in 1898 and on which he relied when treating a host of patients suffering from various functional nervous disorders.[94] Shortly after the turn of the century Sidis turned his attention to the issue of multiple personality and with S. P. Goodhart published a book on the subject.[95] The importance of Sidis's contribution to the creation of a professional atmosphere supportive of what came to be known as psychotherapy cannot be underestimated. As the popular journalist H. Addington Bruce noted, Sidis and Prince shared "unquestioned preeminence among the few psychopathologists whom America has yet produced."[96]

Without question the most important American psychiatric contributor to the field of psychotherapy was the Swiss-born Adolf Meyer.[97] More than any other figure Meyer helped to shape the identity of psychiatry during the first decades of the twentieth century.[98] A student of Charcot, Hughlings Jackson, and Auguste Henri Forel, Meyer emigrated to the United States in 1892 and spent his first two and a half years working as a pathologist at the Illinois Eastern Hospital for the Insane at Kankakee, a public hospital about fifty miles south of Chicago.[99] In 1895 Meyer left his job at Kankakee for a more attractive position at the Worcester Lunatic Hospital in Massachusetts, where he remained until 1902. While at Worcester Meyer came in contact with members of the Boston school and there developed what would remain a lifelong interest in psychopathology and "functional" psychiatry, or what he would later term "psychobiology."

Reading Meyer's late-nineteenth- and early-twentieth-century work, one discovers an extraordinary synthesis of prevailing medical and psychological analyses of psychogenesis and mental therapeutics. Meyer added a voice of moderation to a debate that from its inception had been characterized by a lack of tolerance and extreme disrespect for opposing viewpoints. Meyer was an eclectic as well as a pragmatist, although not in a Jamesian sense. His conception of a "pragmatic" psychology was an extraordinarily complex matter.[100] On the one hand, like all physicians, he sought to employ a system of therapeutics that would rid his patients of pain and misery. On the other hand, he endeavored to balance this medical imperative with the demands imposed on him by prevailing "scientific" norms. For Meyer, it was not enough to satisfy the therapeutic demands of patient-consumers; physicians had a responsibility to their fellow professionals that compelled them not only to cure but also to explain their cures.

Meyer contrasted his notion of science with what he argued was an older, equally venerable understanding of the subject, but one that had failed in many instances to explain accurately the workings of the world or, more importantly, to provide an agenda for action:

To reduce the facts and events of this world to a system in which they can stand word by word as peacefully coexistent, as in an encyclopedia, with elimination of the time-component and with towering logic or noumena, was the luring dream of an earlier state of knowledge. To see things as participants of *events*, to reduce complex *events* to simpler *events*, but still events with a time-component, is the modern logic of science and also the leading feature of biological psychiatry, and we favor it especially because its schemes give us space to note essential factors and components of our observations and logic of events which were too hastily crushed in the telescoping process copied from the logic of words.[101]

For Meyer, the goal of science was neither to simplify an intrinsically complex and potentially incomprehensible natural world nor to describe its workings.[102] Echoing James, Meyer argued that for science "the most essential achievement is not the erection of a word-palace of logic or description, but the enlargement of our command of action, however modest."[103] This epistemological framework informed Meyer's understanding of mental illness.[104]

Meyer advocated a psychological approach to the study of mental illness because, *at that time,* it represented the most scientifically efficacious way of approaching the subject. Somatic explanations of mental illness had failed to yield as satisfactory a set of results as psychogenic ones. More significantly, Meyer argued, it had now "become possible to demonstrate chains of mental happenings which tend to fulfill all conditions of an experiment, *i.e.,* to single out factors, to show their natural elaboration and the development of the inevitable result; moreover, it [had] become possible to show how successful treatment depends on definite laws of modifiability of these factors."[105]

Like James, Putnam, Prince, and Sidis, Meyer believed it "is better to use the broad concepts of instincts, habits, interests, and specific experiences and capacities, than the concepts of structural analysis at the present stage of our biologic knowledge."[106]

To try and explain a hysterical fit or delusion system out of hypothetical cell alterations which we cannot reach or prove is at the present stage of histophysiology a gratuitous performance. To realize that such a reaction is *a faulty response or substitution of an insufficient or protective or evasive or mutilated attempt at adjustment* opens ways of inquiry in the direction of modifiable determining factors and all of a sudden we find ourselves in a live field, in harmony with our instincts of action, of prevention, of modification, and of an understanding, doing justice to a desire for directness instead of a neuroligizing tautology.[107]

Meyer neither argued that psychogenic theories should last for all time nor implied that lesion theory had been bad science. Both were equally legitimate on their own terms. But at this particular time one simply worked better than the other. It considered more facts more rigorously and offered a better explanation of them. In contrast to both mind curists, who could not explain their cures to the physicians' satisfaction, and physicians, whose materialistic predilections denied them the opportunity to exploit mind curists' methods, Meyer sought to offer an eminently respectable, thoroughly pragmatic, scientifically rigorous justification for the medical use of mental therapeutics.

Meyer's pragmatism was tempered by his professional allegiance, however. He was first and foremost a physician, and, unlike William James, he never doubted that physicians alone should be vested with both the care and the treatment of physical and mental disorders. A product of a different generation than James, he saw little conflict between pragmatism and professionalism. For him the two went hand in hand. Meyer's pragmatism, in fact, was inextricably bound to a professional discourse.

Meyer's ambition "was to establish a specifically American psychiatry based on the principles of James, Dewey, and other members of the Chicago school."[108] His early willingness to consider seriously the role of mental factors in psychological illness was derived in large measure not from his aspiration to challenge prevailing medical orthodoxy but from a sincere desire to perfect the practice of clinical medicine and extend the reach of professional practice. Leys points out that "Meyer practiced hypnotism briefly on his arrival in America, and although characteristically he took a conservative stand on its more popular manifestations he followed closely the debates between the rival schools."[109] In contrast to several other American medical proponents of psychotherapy who readily acknowledged the role of both Christian Science and New Thought in stimulating their thinking—though not actually influencing their work—Meyer's published writings make no mention whatsoever of the mind cure movement.[110]

Meyer argued that the theoretical advantages of working under the somatic paradigm were frequently negated by its clinical shortcomings.

Of particular concern to him was the fatalism with which physicians often approached patients whom they believed to be suffering from some indiscernible brain lesion or some equally elusive hereditary taint.[111] Having witnessed his own mother recover unexpectedly after three years of suffering through an inexplicable neurotic condition, Meyer, explains a recent commentator, "became convinced that stressful life events could precipitate 'mental breakdowns.' Such 'breakdowns' stemming from life events rather than from hereditary predisposition were reversible and did not doom the patient to insanity or crippling neuroticism."[112]

The comfort of working under the cover of fatalistic and analyzed conceptions of heredity, degeneracy, and mysterious brain diseases—and the relief from responsibility concerning a real understanding of the conditions at hand, and concerning the avoidance of preventable developments, is a powerful unconsciously cherished *protection,* very rudely disturbed by these conceptions which make the physicians partly responsible for the plain and manageable facts.[113]

To overcome this predilection, Meyer urged his colleagues to become as proficient with psychological facts as they were with anatomical ones. Meyer realized that the facts that he urged his colleagues to consider were neither readily available nor easily attained. Their compilation required considerable, detectivelike skill, and even if they could be collected, they frequently failed to offer any insight into an appropriate palliative method, let alone a cure. But when the process worked there was no denying its efficacy. Psychotherapy had a power akin to surgery, and its application required equal skill.

That mental therapeutics often succeeded when somatic therapies failed was not alone sufficient to convince Meyer of its medical utility. Phenomena that did not lend themselves to "scientific" scrutiny held little appeal for him. His advocacy of psychotherapeutics followed logically from his pragmatically established psychogenic paradigm of illness and not from some broader Jamesian notion of pragmatism. To James, the efficacy of the mind cure movement lay in the simple fact that it worked. "The plain fact remains," James wrote, "that the spread of the movement has been due to practical fruits, and the extremely practical turn of character of the American people has never been better shown than by the fact that this, their only decidedly original contribution to the systematic philosophy of life, should be so intimately knit up with the concrete therapeutics."[114] To the professionally conscious Meyer, such "pragmatism" reeked of nihilism. Mental therapeutics appealed to him not because they appealed to the masses but because they could be explained on the basis of eminently "scientific" principles—in particular, as logical extensions of a psychogenic theory of illness.

Meyer lamented the failure of his colleagues to construct a coherent and effective system of mental therapeutics. "We find," he wrote, "especially prominent therapeutic ambitions, but unfortunately too often in fields in which the object of treatment is bound to be vague and hypothetical."[115] Following the advice of Prince, Putnam, and other advocates of American psychotherapy, Meyer urged his colleagues to pay more attention to clinical observations and to prepare copious case histories when treating nervous patients. A substantial number of mental and nervous disorders were not caused by organic disturbances but by "problems of living" that the physician needed to consider when making a diagnosis. To facilitate the physician's capacity to address these issues, Meyer developed the "life-chart," which suggested that life experiences, not structural irregularities or hereditary predispositions, were often at the root of mental and nervous suffering.[116]

Skeptical of James's all-embracing pluralism but nonetheless greatly influenced by his pragmatic orientation, Meyer believed it was the duty of the scientific physician to work with all relevant psychological and historical facts and not just with those that conformed to prevailing materialistic medical theory. In so doing Meyer distinguished his conception of psychology from that of his contemporary, Cornell psychologist Edward Bradford Titchener.[117] While Meyer understood that "the formulation as to what is science depends to some extent on what [are considered] *facts*," he believed that "scientists" alone had the capacity to judge which facts were relevant and which were not.[118]

Meyer excoriated his psychiatric and neurological colleagues for their failure to take seriously the reality of psychological "experience."

Instead of analyzing the facts in an unbiased way and using the great extension of our experience with mental efforts to get square with things and with one's self in states of dreams or under dominant preoccupations, in states akin to hypnotic dissociations or a faulty development of interests and inadequacy of habits, they pass at once to a one-sided consideration of the extra-psychological components of the situation, abandon the ground of controllable observation, translate what they see into a jargon of wholly uncontrollable brain-mythology, and all that with the conviction that this is the only admissible scientific way.[119]

Meyer condemned this seemingly "scientific" approach to the study of mental illness as needlessly narrow. "Odd as it may seem," he wrote, "psychopathology has produced most fruitless debates over two of its favorite issues: The desire to understand the peculiar reaction of the mind as signs of irritation or other lesions of its organ, and the effort to use in a dogmatic way the medical formula of specific disease. Both these tendencies are legitimate and fruitful enough in their sphere, *but outside of it they become a distracting and misleading rut, away from the line of sanest development.*"[120] From such a limited perspective, he charged,

the dogma arose that what we call mental in daily life could not be scientific unless it was translated into a form of meta-neurology—a systematization of neurological inferences, usually least supported by *those who have* first-hand knowledge of the brain and its lesions. . . . Most of what is offered as neurological explanations of mental processes and especially abnormal mental processes is a tendencial [*sic*] precipitation of a mixture of truisms and assumptions into the terminology of a field in which there is today no possibility of bringing the conclusions to a test.[121]

Meyer accused his somatically inclined colleagues of engaging in tautological reasoning. Their argument went as follows: Mental illness was a disease; a disease, by definition, had a somatic etiology; therefore mental illness must have a somatic etiology. Such reasoning, he argued, was not only logically fallacious but also scientifically naive—especially when one considered the myriad other more plausible, factually based, empirically verifiable explanations for a host of mental symptoms. "Why then should we have to insist so on the 'physical disease,' if it is a mere formula of some vague obstacles, while the functional difficulties give a plain and controllable set of facts to work with?" "The maintenance of the disease-concept," he added, "had a great advantage for orderly thinking, but like the neo-vitalistic modes of presentation of biological facts, it would be most detrimental if it should be considered as more than a formula of available facts or a starting point of more fundamental work. Under all circumstances we must beware, however, of any *a priori* definitions which might rule out strings of facts because they are mental."[122]

Meyer insisted that a theory of psychogenesis better explained certain forms of mental illness, not because it was more logical, more rational, more precise, or even more capable of yielding promising therapeutic results than were materialistic theories, but because at that time it was more readily amenable to scientific scrutiny—which to Meyer implied actual experimentation. "The main point," Meyer wrote, "is that we shall use system in the examination of psychic symptoms as well as we do the physical symptoms, and that a knowledge of the abnormal workings of the patient's mind is the foundation of a knowledge of the nature of the disease (i.e., pathology), and of therapeutics."[123]

Meyer believed that physicians had a choice. They could accept a medical theory that presupposed the existence of lesions that no microscope had discovered and hereditary formulas that offered little hope for prevention, therapy, or cure, or they could construct a hypothesis based on discernible, albeit difficult to attain, psychological evidence that appeared to offer promising therapeutic results. Meyer recommended the latter course. He realized, however, that the sirens of materialism were difficult to silence. The syphilitic model of insanity continued to exert a powerful grip on the medical imagination. "The most serious cause for relapses into opposition to psychogenic interpretations," he asserted, "is the blind acceptance of any anatomical finding as definite evidence of an autonomous disease, after the paradigma [*sic*] of general paralysis."[124]

In a series of articles that appeared just before and shortly after the turn of the century in the *American Journal of Insanity,* the *Journal of Nervous and Mental Disorders,* the *Psychological Bulletin,* the *American Journal of Psychology,* and several other prominent professional journals, Meyer laid out his position as the leading exemplar of a distinctly American functional psychology, or psychobiology. "The fundamental principle on which the psychiatry of today is built," Meyer told his psychiatric colleagues, "is undoubtedly this biological conception of man. From the purely materialistic conception of the middle of this century this biological view has developed which does better justice to our entire experience, not solving ultimate problems, to be sure, but furnishing a rational working basis."[125] Meyer realized, however, that a theory that did "better justice" to a set of experiences need not endure forever. Always willing to substitute new knowledge for old and to consider new facts so long as they lent themselves to systematic investigation, Meyer was temperamentally ill-suited to sanctify received wisdom, especially when viewed in the context of the dramatic discoveries brought forth by the novel science of psychology. "[The] customary pathological laboratory," he declared, "is not sufficient to meet the needs of the study of so-called mental disease."[126]

Although he applauded the contributions of John Gray, Meyer challenged Gray's extreme materialism.[127] While Gray had "achieved the practical aim to harmonize theory," Meyer explained, "he went from one extreme—the tendency to systematic ignoring of the somatic factors in the lay public—to another extreme, the disregard of the mental factors."[128] Meyer did not question the necessity of establishing a working hypothesis to explain physical or mental disorders in the absence of discernible empirical evidence. That a particular hypothesis might likewise serve the interests of both the medical profession and the mentally disabled was, moreover, nothing to scoff at. He realized that such speculations played a vital role in scientific inquiry. But dogmatic adherence to what was, after all, only a hypothesis was another matter entirely.

Lesion theory, Meyer argued, epitomized the problems endemic to what he deemed to an oxymoronic notion of scientific orthodoxy. It was one thing to respect tradition, quite another to be bound to it. "So numerous were the anatomical and histological discoveries," Meyer maintained, "that they absorbed all the attention and what was not known yet nevertheless put down in terms of some kind of 'lesion' and the *knowledge of the lesion* was the pathology." But, "the mere *assumption* of a hypothetical lesion is no solution and not even necessarily the most stimulating hypothesis."[129] That another "more stimulating" hypothesis could better explain the presence of mental and nervous disorders was indisputable. Ample evidence existed that lent credibility to the notion of psychogenesis. Rather than assume the presence of some hypothetical lesion in order to explain mental illness, Meyer urged his colleagues to consider a host of facts that had hitherto fallen outside of the clinical domain. Such facts included, among other things, a patient's prior experiences. As examples of psychogenesis, Meyer described several cases of men and women whose mental and nervous sufferings were apparently attributable to prior lifetime experiences.

One example of Meyer's style of analysis can be found in the case of an apparently hysterical young woman who as a child, Meyer explained, had been "taken advantage of by a neighbor's boy at six. She did not dare tell any one for shame, and without knowing what it all meant, she imagined things about it, that she had become different from others."[130] Over the course of the next several years, certain painful experiences elicited a great variety of hysterical symptoms that, if one neglected to consider the prior childhood trauma, would appear to be without any reasonable foundation and, given prevailing medical wisdom, most likely would be attributed to some indiscernible bodily irregularity. According to Meyer, there was no reason to hypothesize the presence of some elusive lesion or hereditary taint, for the cause of the woman's ailment could be readily determined by analyzing the facts of her life.

For every step there are adequate causes; usually causes that would not have upset you or me, but which upset the patient. Now what makes the difference between her and you and me? Do we not, to explain it usefully and practically, have to express it in the very facts of the history. Every step is like an experiment telling us the story, and giving us the concrete facts to be minded; while to speak merely of "hysteria" or later of "dementia praecox" gives us no clue as to what to prevent, and what sore spots to protect and what weak sides to strengthen, but only a general characterization of the possible mischief and the probable absence of a palpable lesion, and the fact that the disorder consists of a faulty hanging together of the mental reactions or adjustments, shown and promoted by previous maladjustments.[131]

Meyer rejected lesion theory not because it failed to provide a compelling rationale for the presence of mental and nervous disorders—of that there was little dispute—but because he believed there was a more compelling, factually contingent explanation that could better serve the interests of doctors and patients. "I started out from the realization," he wrote, "that in some diseases we are continually promising ourselves lesions, and over that we neglect facts which are even now at hand and ready to be sized up and the very things we must learn to handle."[132]

Psychotherapy had a clear and singular meaning for Meyer. It entailed "the regulation of action and is complete only when action is reached."[133] Echoing the sentiments expressed by both William James and Morton Prince in the 1890s, Meyer argued that "habit-training is the backbone of psychotherapy; suggestion is merely a step to the end and of use only to the one who knows that the end can and *must* be *attained*. Action with flesh and bone is the only safe criterion of efficient mental activity; and actions and attitude and their adaptation is the issue in psychotherapy."[134] Meyer eagerly embraced the efforts of his medical colleagues to perfect psychological theories of causation and psychological therapies for treating functional disorders. "This attempt at a medical psychology," he wrote, "gets most of its material from the needs of clinical analysis of symptoms. It is full of hypothetical constructions, but on the whole, on the ground of well-founded analogies. It is a consistent elaboration of neurological hypotheses."[135]

Enduring Somaticism: 1906–1908

The efforts of James, Putnam, Prince, Sidis, Meyer, and like-minded physicians and psychologists to redress not only the epistemological but also the practical shortcomings of the somatic paradigm were only partially successful. Even among the small number of American physicians who conceded that psychotherapy had been used effectively in Europe, there remained a pervasive belief that it could not be used successfully with "high-strung, intelligent American people."[136] Although the visits of Pierre Janet in 1904 and 1906 and the translation of Paul Dubois's *Psychic Treatment of Nervous Disorder* in 1906 by William Alanson White and Smith Ely Jelliffe had a marked impact on certain elites within the American medical community, neither of these events induced a dramatic shift among the rank and file.[137]

In an effort to clarify the various controversies raised by the subject of psychotherapy, Boston neurologist Edward Wylis Taylor addressed an audience composed of neurologists and psychiatrists from Boston, New York, and Philadelphia in November 1907.[138] Recounting a number of gatherings he recently held with several Boston-area physicians, Taylor concluded that many in the profession had little awareness of what was meant by psychotherapy and that large numbers were "highly skeptical" of the possible practical utility of mental methods of treatment.[139] Particularly significant was the attitude of conservative physicians whose distaste for mental therapeutics was largely attributable to their disdain for alternative healers. To win them over, Taylor insisted, it was imperative that the medical embrace of psychotherapy not appear as "a confession of defeat at the hands of the great body of irregular practitioners."[140] On the contrary, it required following the same course as with other novel medical procedures. To that end, Taylor called on his like-minded colleagues "to publish cases illustrative of definite methods; to state facts simply and without recourse to overmuch speculation; and finally, to maintain an attitude of conservatism in the interpretation of results, such as would be demanded in physical science."[141]

Promoting psychotherapy among the broader public was a considerably more delicate matter. If done imprudently it threatened not only to aggravate an already chaotic public situation but also to derail the internal medical campaign by further antagonizing conservative members of the profession. To avoid such an outcome Taylor opposed the idea of offering popular lectures on the subject.[142] Events of this nature, he argued, left too much room for misinterpretation. A better avenue for promoting the movement was through periodicals—so long as physicians themselves did the writing. If the medical profession took it upon itself to direct the popular discourse, physicians would have little reason to fear any possible public misconception. "There is no reason," Taylor insisted, "why ascertained facts in medicine should not be given the same publicity as any other matter of knowledge."[143] He praised the recent efforts of Drs. George L. Walton and Frederick Peterson. The former had written a series on "worry" for the November and December 1907 issues of *Lippincott's Monthly Magazine,* and the latter had published an article on "overwork" for the November 9, 1907, issue of *Collier's Weekly.*

Taylor objected to the efforts of other medical proponents of psychotherapy to ally themselves with nonmedical personnel. Efforts to work with nonphysicians, regardless of their qualifications, would likely antagonize conservative physicians and thereby compromise the capacity of the medical profession to shape the course of American psychotherapy. What was needed "is the cooperation of all regular practitioners toward a common end." "Our essential aim," he concluded, "should be to develop a permanent interest in the psychotherapeutic movement within the ranks of the profession, and to do nothing which can in any way retard this effort."[144]

Taylor's paper provoked a lively discussion, and as Taylor noted in his remarks that followed the discussion, the audience's reaction reinforced his original contention concerning the medical profession's antagonism toward and ignorance of psychotherapy.[145] Conservatives responded to his presentation by claiming that psychotherapy was neither so novel nor so deserving of attention as Taylor had maintained. Charles Dana suggested that Taylor "had dwelt with more emphasis than was just, upon the neglect of psychotherapy." Bernard Sachs agreed: "Do not let us waste too much time and energy on what people are now pleased to call psychotherapy." "Psychotherapy," Francis Dercum insisted, "does not convey a new idea despite its clothing of a new phraseology. . . . [I]t is literally as old as the human race, the term alone, high-sounding and impressive is new, that is all." John K. Mitchell, the son of S. Weir Mitchell and an accomplished physician in his own right, noted that those who frequently advocated the medical use of mental healing often failed to consider the significance of one of its most prominent, albeit elusive, features, the *"personality* of the physician,—a gift, this, which cannot be taught or learned."[146]

Taylor's allies did not remain silent in the face of this mounting criticism. Joseph Collins, a prominent New York neurologist, was among the first to speak out in favor of Taylor's analysis. Arguing that psychotherapy held an important place in the treatment of a certain class of patients, Collins spoke of the need for a rational and teachable method of psychotherapy: "The trouble is that no method of psychotherapy has yet been formulated and unless such formulation has resulted it cannot be taught systematically." To which William Alanson White rejoined, "Surely if we can practice psychotherapy, and if we know what we are doing when we practice it, we can tell other people how to do the same thing."[147]

The most vigorous arguments in support of psychotherapy came from Jelliffe, Putnam, and Prince. One of the co-translators of Dubois's influential book on persuasion, Jelliffe provided a splendid response to those who criticized psychotherapy on the ground that it was old. "So is the knowledge of opium and of belladonna," he asserted. "Both were used probably before man could read or write, but that does not imply that we are not better acquainted with the more intimate structure of these drugs today and cannot use them to greater advantage at the present time than our forefathers did, not withstanding the ages that they have known." Prince followed up on this comment: "Psychotherapy may be 'as old as the hills,' but the educational treatment, as such, was not old but modern. In making allusion to the antiquity of psychotherapy, it was evident that many of the speakers had a very slight conception of its principles and less of its methods and technique."[148]

In the midst of this commotion Putnam interjected that he thought it worthwhile to say a few words about the Emmanuel movement. Although he neither endorsed nor criticized every detail of the movement, Putnam expressed his belief that certain functional nervous disorders had "religious as well as medical bearings and that if an individual minister felt a qualification and desire to tackle this problem he should be helped to do so in the way which would be predictive of the best results." "No one," he continued, "can foretell exactly how far this present movement will reach or what form it will eventually assume, but it would be unwise for physicians to adopt an attitude of complete aloofness."[149]

Putnam's comments elicited little response. Although news of this "movement" had recently begun to spread to other cities, few physicians outside the Boston area had any reason to believe that the Emmanuel movement might threaten them in any way. The controversy concerning the future of psychotherapy in the United States, most believed, would remain an internal medical matter. What Taylor's speech and the response it generated reveal is that even as late as November 1907, only a tiny minority of American physicians appreciated the significance that psychotherapy would soon have not only for the medical profession itself but for American culture as well.

CHAPTER 6

Embracing Psychotherapy

*The Emmanuel Movement and the
American Medical Profession*

In November 1906 James Jackson Putnam penned a brief
letter to his good friend and colleague, Richard C. Cabot. "The Neurasthenic Class, which your suggestion first put into my mind," Putnam
wrote, "is going to be provisionally launched tomorrow evening in the
Vestry of the Emmanuel Church, where Dr. Worcester and I are to explain the plan and I am to make a brief address. . . . May we not hope
at least to excite an interest, making practical some of the fundamental
principles of psychology and philosophy and mental hygiene? I feel sure
that many persons would be much interested to be told in simple language and in reference to practical learning, what the scientific people
are doing." [1] Within two years Putnam's hopes were dashed. In a public letter to the *Boston Sunday Herald* the Harvard Medical School professor renounced his ties to what had become a full-blown national
movement and conceded that his early support had been seriously misplaced: "I have spent many sleepless nights the last year worrying over
injury I may have done in allowing my name to stand sponsor for a
state of affairs that I deeply feel is of harm to the public." [2]

Although not unprecedented, the willingness of a prominent American physician to air his views in public was by no means common. The
decision of Putnam and other critics of what came to be known as the
Emmanuel movement to express their concerns in such a glaringly visible manner was fueled in large measure by the realization that they
were losing their capacity to direct the course of psychotherapy in the
United States. Putnam's changing sentiments were just one small gust

in a much larger storm that had swept the topic of psychotherapy into the homes of virtually every literate American.[3]

Whereas more than thirty years of vigorous internal professional debates had failed to generate a consensus among American neurologists and psychiatrists regarding the scientific legitimacy and clinical efficacy of mental therapeutics, in two short years the Emmanuel movement had forced the American medical community to confront squarely and publicly a subject that it had long avoided.[4] More than any other single factor the Emmanuel movement not only raised the American public's awareness of psychotherapy but also compelled the American medical profession to enter a field that it had long neglected.

What came to be known as the Emmanuel movement was initially conceived as a local cooperative venture between Boston physicians and Episcopalian ministers. It began as an experiment in public health that aimed to provide impoverished victims of neurasthenia and other functional nervous disorders with a "fusion of religious faith and scientific knowledge."[5] The movement's name stemmed from its affiliation with one of Boston's most venerated institutions, the Emmanuel Church, which was located on Newbury Street near the Public Garden. By 1909 a host of similar ventures had been launched across the nation, in Brooklyn, Buffalo, Detroit, Philadelphia, Baltimore, Seattle, and elsewhere. No longer confined to the Episcopalian church, the psychotherapy movement's appeal transcended denominational boundaries. Baptists, Presbyterians, Congregationalists, Unitarians, and Universalists all enlisted in the cause.

Although the program's medical and clerical champions had realized early on that this unprecedented medical-pastoral venture might arouse the ire of their more intransigent colleagues, they failed to anticipate not only the popular allure of their program but also the almost ubiquitous professional opposition that their efforts would soon elicit. Shortly after the program's inauguration Canadian-born journalist H. Addington Bruce declared, "Signs are multiplying that the medical profession, which has hitherto been conspicuous for its opposition to the mental healers, is beginning to show a serious interest in their claims."[6] In a telling statement, journalist Ray Stannard Baker added, "Though there is a union of ministers and doctors in the work of the Emmanuel Movement, yet back of it all lies a real struggle of the two professions to attain a greater influence over the lives of men."[7]

Whereas the frequently overlapping Euro-American medical-cultural discourses regarding neurasthenia, railway spine, hysteria, and mind cure were all vital prerequisites for the establishment of so-called scientific psychotherapy in the United States, neither alone nor taken together were they capable of generating widespread American medical interest in the topic. Like the mind cure movement, the Emmanuel movement both tapped into and stimulated an already existing demand for mental therapeutics. Where it distinguished itself from its less respectable rivals was in its capacity to exert a profound impact on the American medical profession.

Both the popular coverage of and public enthusiasm for the Emmanuel movement triggered an almost instinctual prudence from more conservative members of the medical and clerical establishments. Such nonsense, they claimed, bore a stark resemblance to the ideas and methods espoused by the more ordinary mind cure quacks. Attacking psychotherapy as being no different from Christian Science, New Thought, or any of the other healing cults, the movement's professional critics waged a vigorous campaign against what they deemed an equally insidious cult arising from within their own ranks.[8] In response to this rising tide of professional opposition, several physicians who initially supported the movement withdrew their backing. Others, who under more ordinary circumstances might not have given the psychotherapeutic efforts of a few Boston ministers and physicians a second thought, began a vigorous professional and popular campaign to discredit the movement and to usurp its function. The movement's defenders responded in kind. As a result what had formerly been an endogenous, if not actually an esoteric, neurological, psychiatric, and religious discourse became grist for the public mill.

The Emmanuel movement distinguished itself from prior American efforts to legitimate mental healing by the social standing of its promoters and by the coverage it received. In many respects the former fueled the latter. Prior to 1910 the *Readers' Guide to Periodical Literature* does not cite a single article on either Freud or psychoanalysis; it does, however, list thirty-one articles on the Emmanuel movement.[9] In contrast to both Christian Science and New Thought, each of which had been painted in relatively unflattering colors, the Emmanuel program's fusion of "science" and established religion was initially depicted in highly favorable terms. One article boasted that "this union of religion with sound science . . . is the most tremendous alliance yet made for the benefit of suffering humanity."[10]

This positive assessment derived from the eminence of the program's founders. Both were pillars of the cultural establishment. Protestant, male, and educated in the finest European universities, Elwood Worcester and Samuel McComb faced few, if any, of the obstacles that impeded the efforts of their less respectable rivals. These facts alone distinguished the Emmanuel movement from virtually all other contemporary religious healing movements. Worcester, chief rector of the Emmanuel Church, possessed credentials that rivaled, if not surpassed, those of virtually all American academic psychologists: in addition to holding degrees from Columbia University and the General Theological Seminary, he had also earned a Ph.D. in philosophy at Leipzig, where he had studied with Max Heinz and Wilhelm Wundt.[11] Worcester's recently arrived assistant, Samuel McComb, could boast of virtually identical qualifications.[12]

Before coming to Boston in 1904 Worcester had spent several years in Pennsylvania, where he taught classes in psychology at Lehigh University and later served as minister to the St. Stephen's Episcopalian Church in Philadelphia. At St. Stephen's Worcester came in contact with Philadelphia's famed neurologist and writer, S. Weir Mitchell.[13] Worcester and Mitchell were more than mere acquaintances. Later in life Worcester recounted that Mitchell had been his "most interesting parishioner and . . . most intimate friend."[14] Indeed, despite Mitchell's later condemnation of the program, Worcester credited him with having first suggested the idea of establishing a clerical-medical alliance to promote psychotherapy.[15]

One day, as we were walking up Walnut Street, Dr. Mitchell stopped and said: "Rector, if you and I should get together and establish a work on the basis of sound religion and sound science, we could put [mentioning a person he detested] out of business." I left Philadelphia soon after this occasion, and I do not know if Dr. Mitchell ever thought of these words again. They remained in my mind, however, and they were destined to play an important part in my subsequent life.[16]

Several years passed before Worcester had the chance to put Mitchell's suggestion into practice.

Soon after his arrival in Boston Worcester met Joseph Hersey Pratt, a young internist at Boston's Massachusetts General Hospital who had recently devised a home treatment program for the city's impoverished victims of tuberculosis.[17] Lacking the financial resources to institute his plan, Pratt turned to Worcester's Emmanuel Church for financial support. Worcester graciously acceded to the request. The inspiration for Pratt's program derived from a December 1904 encounter in Asheville, North Carolina, with Dr. Charles L. Minor. An expert on tuberculosis, Minor had developed a home treatment program not for the poor but for the wealthy, who despite their means refused to avail themselves of expensive sanitariums. Pratt's program, although similar, was not an exact replica of Minor's. In contrast to Minor's personally directed home treatment program, Pratt's plan centered on a weekly meeting of the Emmanuel Church Tuberculosis Class, during which Pratt "focused on bolstering his patients' faith, and encouraging their adherence to the arduous regimen of enforced bed-rest considered so essential to the cure."[18]

To Worcester, Pratt's project demonstrated "what faith and devotion, through the employment of the best methods of science, could accomplish."[19] Pratt "was like a father surrounded by his children. Kind, merry, highly skillful and optimistic, he inspired all his patients by his confidence and hope."[20] Worcester declared in a widely read article, "The success of Pratt's program showed me that the physician and the clergyman can work together with excellent results."[21] Later in life he wrote, "[The] success of our Tuberculosis Class moved me to undertake another service to a larger group of unhappy, unstable men and women, to persons suffering from physical and nervous affections . . . and to the victims of injurious habits such as alcoholism and other drug addictions."[22]

Worcester's inspiration to begin a psychotherapy class was not based exclusively on Pratt's program, however. His earlier experiences with both the "higher criticism" and the "new psychology," he claimed, were equally significant. Worcester cited with equal frequency the biblical scholarship of Ernest Renan, Adolf von Harnack, and Theodore Keim and the psychological investigations of Gustav Theodor Fechner, Wilhelm Wundt, and William James. From the former, Worcester concluded that "something valuable had been lost from the Christian religion, and that Christianity had not always been so unsuccessful in its appeal to human nature as it [now was]."[23] From the latter, Worcester became aware of the subconscious mind, the law of suggestion, and the scientific method. "Above all," Worcester added, "I learned from psychology the advantage of a scientific method in dealing with myself and with other men."[24]

From the start Worcester and McComb had little trouble enlisting the aid of prominent neurologists and psychiatrists. Two pillars of the Harvard medical community, Putnam and Cabot, provided much needed backing at a critical stage in the program's development. They were joined by Drs. Isador Coriat, James G. Mumford, Joseph H. Pratt, and Joel E. Goldthwait. Perhaps even more significant was the attitude of Bishop William Lawrence. Lawrence had the authority to squelch

Worcester's program if he feared that it might impair the church's pres-
tige.[25] Never alluding to the movement in public and referring all re-
quests for information directly to the ministers, the bishop maintained
an attitude of "benevolent neutrality."[26] Despite the later opposition
of several prominent physicians, ministers, and psychologists, the historian John Gardner Greene notes that at no time were Worcester or
McComb "opposed by the one man whose opposition could have done
decisive harm to their cause."[27]

The Program Begins

The Emmanuel program commenced with a series of
public lectures in November 1906. Putnam, Cabot, Worcester, and
McComb spoke on a host of topics ranging from recent psychological
investigations to Jesus' healing ministry. Worcester concluded the lectures with the announcement that he and McComb, accompanied by
two psychiatrists, would set aside some time the following morning to
meet with anyone who desired to discuss their "moral problems or psychical disorders." Worcester expected a modest turnout but was confronted with an entirely different situation, which he later described in
vivid detail:

I found one hundred and ninety-eight men and women, suffering from
some of the worst diseases known to man, old chronic maladies, rheuma-
tism, paralysis, indigestion, conditions which lay totally outside of our
province. *Thus, from the very beginning, our carefully prepared scheme was
taken out of our hands and committed to the people.* Our physicians were in
despair, but they stuck to their guns and manfully distinguished some cases
which seemed promising and furnished us with a number of diagnoses.[28]

In a few short weeks Worcester and McComb had more than two hundred patients on their hands.[29] Over the next several months the two
ministers and the program's medical consultants formalized the process
by which patients were selected to participate in the program. Candi-
dates for psychological treatment were required to bring a letter from
their physicians. Those lacking such letters were referred for examination to one of the physicians of the parish who agreed to examine, free
of charge, all who applied for admission to the health class.[30]

In its final form Worcester's program consisted of three mutually
reinforcing elements: a medical clinic where physicians provided free

weekly examinations; a weekly health class at which eminent physicians, clergymen, and psychologists lectured on a variety of issues relating to physical, mental, and spiritual health; and private sessions during which the minister employed psychotherapy. The health class was modeled after Pratt's "successful" tuberculosis class. "The idea," Putnam said, "is to have a series of conferences where questions will be asked and answered, and talks given by suitable persons." [31] Meeting each Wednesday evening from November through May, the class typically attracted between 250 and 500 individuals. Its aim was to promote physical, mental, and spiritual health. All segments of the population were represented, but the overwhelming number were women.[32] Each class began with a prayer, after which Worcester, McComb, or a guest speaker would deliver a lecture on some relevant spiritual, medical, or psychological issue. At the close of the lecture the congregation was invited to an upper room for a social hour and refreshments.[33]

Although the Emmanuel class received considerable coverage in the press, it aroused little controversy. The same could not be said for the private psychotherapy sessions with the minister. An early proponent of the movement described the sessions as "a sermonette preached to a congregation of one at the moment of extreme suggestibility."[34] One of Worcester's early disciples explained, "After the discussion and the prescription of good books the patient is seated in the comfortable morris chair before the fire, which I take care by this time to have burning low—is taught by rhythmic breathing and by visual imagery to relax the muscles, and is led into the silence of the mind by tranquilizing suggestion. Then in terms of the spirit, the power of the mind over the body is impressed upon the patient's consciousness, and soothing suggestions are given for the relief of specific ills."[35] This therapy derived its force from the minister's spiritual and moral authority. Treatment usually lasted from fifteen minutes to an hour depending on the difficulties encountered.[36]

The Movement Spreads

Not long after the program was established a number of prominent clergymen began visiting the Boston church to learn firsthand of the medical-clerical venture. By the autumn of 1908 *Good Housekeeping* reported the initiation of church-sponsored clinics throughout the East Coast and Midwest.[37] Among the most prominent were those

of Bishop Samuel Fallows of Chicago and the Reverends Robert Mac-
Donald of Brooklyn, Loring W. Batten of New York, and Albert Shields
of San Francisco.[38] Fallows's reputation prompted others throughout
the region to take the movement seriously and helped to inspire what
soon became a vibrant national debate concerning both the nature and
the control of psychotherapy in the United States. Longtime foes of
Christian Science, Fallows and his wife had coauthored *Science of Health
from the Viewpoint of the Newest Christian Thought* (1903) shortly after
the turn of the century. This work stressed the compatibility of orthodox Christianity with "the belief in the supremacy of the inner and immortal self over the entire external world."[39]

Although more harmonious with mainstream Protestant denomina-
tions than Christian Science, "Christian Metaphysics" suffered from the
same shortcomings as its less respectable rivals. Each neglected to consider the most recent "advances" in neurology, psychiatry, and academic
psychology. It took Fallows little time to see the virtue of Worcester's
more inclusive program. Soon after he learned of the work being done
in Boston he commenced with plans to institute a similar venture in his
home city of Chicago.[40] By the spring of 1908 the *Brooklyn Eagle* reported that "the parlors of St. Paul's Church have been crowded with
people seeking help and light upon the movement. Remarkable results
have already followed the efforts put forth."[41] Fallows proved to be one
the movement's most prominent supporters. He devoted virtually all of
his time and energy to the work. He lectured throughout the region,
published a number of articles espousing not Christian Metaphysics but
"Christian Psychology," and wrote a book-length work on the subject,
Health and Happiness; or Religious Therapeutics (1908).[42]

Whereas the first ministers to embrace Worcester's program were fellow Episcopalians, not all of his clerical supporters came from the ranks
of his denomination. Indeed, one of Worcester's earliest and most vocal
champions was the Reverend Dr. Robert MacDonald of the Washington Avenue Baptist Church in Brooklyn, New York. The author of *Mind,
Religion, and Health* (1908), MacDonald proved to be one of Worcester's most able lieutenants.[43] On February 16, 1908, the Baptist minister delivered the first of what would be several published sermons devoted to the Emmanuel movement to an overflowing audience at the
Washington Avenue Baptist Church. The reception to MacDonald's
sermons was for the most part overwhelmingly positive. Robert E. Peele
of Ebenezer, South Carolina, wrote to say that he was "in thorough
sympathy with the Emmanuel Movement." W. E. J. Gratz of Elizabeth,

New Jersey, reported that "for a great many years, [he had] been look-
ing for just what this Emmanuel movement is giving us—a clear rational, scientific basis for the presentation of a sadly neglected truth." Not
everyone was convinced by MacDonald's lectures, however. I. D. Grover
of Brooklyn, New York, charged that "all this talk of 'hypnotic touch,'
'subconsciousness,' 'thought producing diseases as readily as germs,' etc.,
smacks too much of Christian Science and Spiritualism and their ilk."[44]

In the Public Eye

From its inception the Emmanuel program operated in
the public light and under considerable professional scrutiny. Such attention was a mixed blessing. On the one hand, it extolled Worcester's
many achievements and inspired others to become familiar with his efforts; on the other, it frequently exaggerated and in several instances
grossly distorted the true nature of the program.[45] To combat scores
of distortions and misconceptions concerning their program, Worcester
and McComb commenced what would become a multiyear effort not
only to explain but also to promote the work being done at the Emmanuel Church. The two men provided the nation's booming periodical press with scores of articles discussing various aspects of their work,
distributed a brief series of pamphlets that offered a more detailed description of their efforts, and published the best-selling book, *Religion
and Medicine*. In addition to these literary ventures, Worcester and Mc-
Comb embarked on an extensive lecture tour that took them to several
American and European cities.

Both men denied that these highly visible endeavors stemmed from
any aim to launch a national movement. The decision to publicize their
work, Worcester later insisted, derived from little more than a desire
to set the record straight; it had, he said, been thrust upon them by
"the sensational press [which] saw in our doings an unending source of
weird stories and caricature. They were determined to find something
wild and fanatical in our work and meetings and, when they could not
discover it, they would invent it."[46] Although there is some merit to
Worcester's claim, the actions of the two ministers suggest that their
motives were not nearly so humble as they would later maintain. Evidence exists suggesting that from the start both Worcester and McComb
had high hopes for their program. In a personal letter to Putnam,

Cabot expressed "dismay . . . over hearing Dr. McComb, that first evening, prophesy a vast extension of the church healing movement."[47]

As early as March 1907, when the program was not yet four
months old, McComb declared, "I propose to set forth as clearly as I
can the fundamental principles on which the Emmanuel Church *movement* is based."[48] More notable than the minister's words was the
medium in which they appeared. They were featured in the "Happiness and Health" department of the popular women's monthly magazine, *Good Housekeeping*.[49] The following month, the magazine's editors proudly boasted that "*Good Housekeeping* [had] been chosen by
Rev. Drs. Worcester and McComb as the periodical through which the
good news shall be spread, accordingly it will assist clergymen, physicians and others in establishing centers and introducing the work in
their churches or districts."[50] The *Good Housekeeping* series continued
for almost two years.

A plethora of articles detailed all phases of the "movement." Readers
received biographical information regarding the movement's founders
and details concerning many of the formal aspects of the program. In
addition to these informational pieces, the magazine offered its readers
an opportunity to express their concerns. The editors received and responded to scores of letters from their almost exclusively female audience. Advice was offered for a vast range of problems such as "house-
keeper's anxiety," "fear of failure," "business after business hours,"
"sleeplessness," and "artistic temperament." Perhaps most significantly,
child-rearing practices were discussed in considerable detail. In addition to articles written by Worcester, McComb, and other clergymen,
the magazine included pieces by the movement's medical champions:
Coriat, Cabot, Barker, and Putnam.

The *Good Housekeeping* articles typically relied on anecdotal information rather than statistical and factual analysis that might lend further credence to the claims of the author. This perspective was especially
common when discussing the actual results of the movement. *Good
Housekeeping*'s readers learned of the case of Mrs. A. who, after a few
short weeks of treatment, testified that she had "journeyed homeward
feeling that [she] had never been nearer heaven ever before in [her]
life." Readers also received news of the formerly reckless Miss B. who,
as a result of her encounter with Dr. Worcester, had been transformed
into a "bright, clever, and entertaining" young woman. And it was
not just women who benefited from the program. The magazine reported that after a few short weeks of treatment, Mr. Packard, who had

come "to Dr. McComb the embodiment of utter hopelessness and despair . . . might have posed as a 'happiness advertisement.'"[51]

Good Housekeeping's literary franchise on the Emmanuel movement lasted throughout most of 1907.[52] Excepting a brief piece that McComb had prepared for *Harper's Bazaar,* the only other national magazine to discuss the "movement" prior to 1908 was *World's Work.* In its December 1907 issue Rollin Lynde Hart featured the Emmanuel program in an article provocatively entitled "'Christian Science' Without Mystery." Hart's piece was notable in two respects. Whereas the *Good Housekeeping* series had been conducted under the aegis of the program's medical and clerical champions, Hart had no personal affiliation with the plan. Moreover, in contrast to *Good Housekeeping, World's Work* appealed to a predominantly male audience. Hart proved to be the first of several lay commentators who would seek to distinguish Worcester's program from Christian Science. "Unlike Christian Science," Hart declared, the Emmanuel plan was "both Christian and scientific; Christian in that it affirms the reality of sin, scientific in that it heals by methods endorsed by the leading neurologists and psychologists of our epoch." After discussing the movement's underlying philosophy and plan of action, Hart asked, "Doesn't all this sound reasonable?"[53] He then chronicled the experiences of five patients—a clergyman, a businessman, an elderly man, a young woman, and a female schoolteacher—who as a result of their treatment by Worcester and McComb had overcome a wide array of nervous afflictions.

Soon after the publication of Hart's article, a number of other national magazines published articles on the "movement." Within a span of several months articles concerning the movement appeared in *Century, North American Review, Current Literature, Popular Science Monthly, Outlook, American Magazine, Independent, Review of Reviews,* and a host of other national periodicals. Like the articles that appeared in *Good Housekeeping,* those who appreciated these magazines made great use of anecdotal information. But in contrast to the *Good Housekeeping* series, the articles in the more masculine periodicals were often supplemented with a variety of facts and statistics. In a piece that he prepared for *Outlook,* Cabot, a pioneer in the statistical analysis of treatment outcomes, provided a cursory statistical assessment of the program's first year.[54] From a sample of 178 men and women who had been diagnosed at the Emmanuel clinic, Cabot reported that 82 were suffering from neurasthenia, 24 from insanity, 22 from alcoholism, 18 from fears or fixed ideas, 10 from sexual neuroses, 5 from hysteria, and

17 from a number of other miscellaneous disorders. From this sample Cabot reported that there were 123 known results, 61 percent of which were positive. Moreover, he detected no evidence that their course of treatment by the ministers had any detrimental effects on the patients. "The seventy-five cases in which undoubted benefit has resulted," Cabot therefore concluded, "should be put down with clear gain, and nothing to offset it."[55]

Cabot's *Outlook* piece seemed to provide compelling statistical justification for the program. The following month McComb supplemented Cabot's findings in an article that he prepared for *Century*. McComb boasted that the Emmanuel program's brand of psychotherapy had been applied to a wide array of functional disorders. The list of ailments that had been cured was extensive. It included

all functional disturbances of the digestive apparatus; congestive, neuralgic, and anemic headaches, certain forms of paralysis, simulated epilepsy, neurasthenia, hypochondria, psychasthenia, hysterical pains, functional insomnia, melancholia, nervous irritability, hallucinations, morbid fears, fixed ideas (including a long list of troubles dignified with Greek names, such as monophobia, claustrophobia, agoraphobia, and so forth), incipient insanities, stage fright, worry, stammering, abuse of tobacco, alcoholism, morphinism, cocainism, kleptomania, suicidal tendencies—in a word, the vast and complicated field of what is technically called the functional neuroses and the psycho neuroses.[56]

More impressive than the contents of McComb's list was the impression it created. Psychotherapy was depicted as being something that bordered on the miraculous.

In addition to the ongoing magazine campaign, the distant travels of Worcester and McComb proved to be of particular importance in spreading the Emmanuel idea.[57] After a year of practical experience the two ministers became convinced that the time had come to reach out and share their findings with other congregations throughout the United States and abroad.[58] "Doctor McComb and I," Worcester recounted, "were constantly called on to preach and lecture on weekdays in distant cities and to carry on public debates with physicians, psychologists, clergymen and laymen in the Church Congress, colleges, medical meetings, and other places where questions were freely asked and criticism freely administered."[59] The 1908 edition of the *Emmanuel Year Book* states, "From all parts of the country came invitations to address medical societies, ministerial meetings, clubs, and popular gathering of various kinds."[60]

Early in 1908 the Archbishop of Canterbury invited Worcester to discuss his work before a committee composed of members of the Pan-Anglican assembly. Unable to accept the invitation, Worcester requested that McComb attend in his place. The assistant minister proved to be a more than adequate substitute. Although he did not win the committee's formal endorsement for the Boston program, he succeeded in having the members acknowledge the potential virtues of a clerical-medical alliance.[61] The *New York Times* reporter Allan L. Benson recounted McComb's speech before the full assembly of the London conference. He wrote that on hearing a bell that signaled McComb's allotted thirty minutes had come to an end, McComb attempted to stop talking, but "the audience wouldn't let him. The whole assembly rose to its feet and from every quarter there were cries of 'Go On! Go On!'"[62] McComb also spoke in various London churches and addressed several meetings of the city's physicians and ministers. As was the case in the United States, these lectures and meetings received considerable coverage in the city's press and shortly before McComb departed for Boston a similar movement, known as the Church and Medical Union, began in London.[63]

In the summer of 1908 Worcester and McComb supplemented their magazine campaign and lecture tours with an intensive three-week course of lectures on religious therapeutics that attracted considerable attention. More than 140 people enrolled, including the Reverend Samuel S. Marquis, dean of St. Paul's Episcopal Church in Detroit. Students received intensive instruction in the most recent psychological studies and psychotherapeutic knowledge from Worcester, Coriat, and other practitioners of church-sponsored psychotherapy. Many returned to their home parishes eager to put to use their newly acquired knowledge to institute their own church-sponsored psychotherapy programs. Moreover, to facilitate the growth of their movement Worcester and McComb arranged for the publication of a series of pamphlets detailing the many different aspects of the movement. Although the proposed series was to include nine separate articles, the completed version contained only seven. The cost of each was set at twenty-five cents, though many were distributed free of charge. The Emmanuel Church published the initial pieces in-house. The remaining ones were published by Moffat, Yard and Company of New York.[64]

As significant as they were in promoting the Emmanuel message, the pamphlets were quickly superseded by the publication of *Religion and Medicine* in August 1908. Written jointly by Worcester, McComb, and Coriat, this work was one of only five books listed under the subject heading "Psychotherapy" in the *Index Catalogue of the Library of the Surgeon-General's Office*.[65] Promoted by its publisher as a book "which sets forth in clear and non-technical language the principles, and the methods by which these principles have been applied, that underlie the notable experiment in practical Christianity known as the *Emmanuel Movement, Religion and Medicine* was heralded by the editors of *Current Literature* as "some of the most illuminating pages yet written on the subconscious mind."[66] The book was reviewed in virtually every major newspaper and medical and religious periodical and soon became the single most important text of so-called scientific psychotherapy in the United States. A reviewer for the *New York Times* declared, "The book is marked throughout with admirable modesty and moderation."[67] In his review H. Addington Bruce wrote, "No more needed book on the general subject of psychotherapy has lately come forth, and none more likely to exert beneficent influence wherever read."[68] In addition to receiving laudatory reviews, *Religion and Medicine* sold almost two hundred thousand copies.[69]

Religion and Medicine provided a more detailed discussion of the movement than had ever appeared previously; it allowed Worcester, McComb, and Coriat to speak in their own voices. Unlike the numerous newspaper and magazine articles that had discussed the movement during the prior eighteen months, it offered an unsullied expression of the work being done in Boston. Moreover, it served as a text for others seeking to imitate the Boston venture. What its coauthors failed to realize was that their four-hundred-plus page book would also provide a highly visible target for those seeking to derail the psychotherapy movement. Although the book's title was bound to evoke Eddy's earlier work *Science and Health,* the authors insisted, "Our movement bears no relation to Christian Science, either by way of protest or of imitation, but it would be what it is had the latter never existed."[70] Anticipating those who might question their motives, they stressed the lack of adequate treatment for functional nervous disorders—especially for the poor—in the United States.

Echoing the views of the mind curists, Worcester readily acknowledged his views on the limits of medical materialism: "One reason why American physicians are slow to avail themselves of psychical influence in combating disease is that they have been educated in a too narrowly materialistic school of science which assumes that only material objects possess reality and which thinks that the mind can be safely ignored."[71] This assertion was by no means radical, however. Similar statements had been made by Putnam, Prince, Sidis, Meyer, and several prominent American physicians who frequently chastised their professional brethren for their ignorance of scientific psychology. Indeed, the most provocative feature of *Religion and Medicine* had little to do with its critique of medical materialism or its discussion of the unconscious. Rather, it pertained to the authors' statements concerning the ultimate effects of the movement. "What we have done," Worcester maintained, "other men and other churches can do as well or better, and it is with the earnest hope that other qualified persons may be induced to help us and to relieve us of the pressure of patients from distant cities that we issue this tentative and imperfect statement."[72]

Medical Opposition: The Quest for Control

Even before the publication of *Religion and Medicine* a number of prominent physicians had begun to express reservations about Worcester's movement. Medical opposition reflected a combination of ideological concerns and professional self-interest. Frequently the latter took precedence over the former. Physicians who attacked the movement typically expressed great concern for their roles as medical professionals. Willing to acknowledge the efficacy of certain types of mental healing, the movement's medical critics sought to restrict the practice of psychotherapy to licensed physicians.

In a January 1908 address before the New York Neurological Society, Charles Dana spoke directly to the issue of control. He urged his more intransigent, somatically inclined colleagues to take seriously the growing public interest in religious psychotherapeutics: "There is already a wave of public interest in the matter, which we at least must watch if we take no definite attitude toward it. It seems as if a certain large group of minor psychoses are to be taken in hand by the clergy, cooperating with medical men, and it is seriously proposed to have psychotherapeutics as part of the religious work of our churches. Already centers of this work exist in Boston, Chicago, and this city."[73] Rejecting the claims of those who argued that the "best attitude to take towards the [Emmanuel] movement was one of aloofness, believing that it will die out," Dana argued instead that a decided position should be taken against it. "We can reasonably assert that the care of the sick is safest in the hands of those trained for the purpose. But if we say this," Dana asked, "will we not have to assert also that medical men are using the forces of therapeutics, and using them more skillfully and effectively than clergymen, or nonmedical therapeutics can do?"[74]

The first direct medical assault on the Emmanuel movement took place on February 28, 1908. Addressing the section in Neurology and Psychiatry of the Medico-Chirurgical Faculty of Maryland, Clarence B. Farrar, an associate in psychiatry at Johns Hopkins University and future editor of the *American Journal of Psychiatry,* delivered a vitriolic critique of Worcester's program.[75] It was no surprise, Farrar claimed, that the Emmanuel movement arose in Boston, "the land of witchcraft and transcendentalism."[76] Farrar argued that the Emmanuel movement represented a retreat to the benighted past during which the priest-physician administered to sick and suffering souls.[77] Worcester and his followers, he declared, failed to recognize the long-known fact that "perturbations of the soul (mental diseases) are, in reality, diseases of the nervous system, and more particularly of the brain, and that, therefore, their treatment was the proper work of the physician and not of the priest."[78] Farrar's criticism of the movement was not merely an expression of his somatic bias. It likewise reflected his desire to secure for the medical profession the exclusive right to administer psychotherapy. The ministers' motives, he claimed, were anything but disinterested. On the contrary, the Emmanuel movement was a deliberate effort to restore the church's diminishing authority. "Knowing, however, that an intelligent public would no longer unquestionably bow to theologic authority in these matters, and realizing that the old theocracy was inevitably crumbling," Farrar charged, "the brilliant maneuver with which we are now familiar was executed. It was nothing else but a bold and triumphant gasconade. A truce was sounded and science was bidden to parley."[79]

The following month, Philadelphia neurologist Charles K. Mills picked up where Farrar left off. Speaking before the Philadelphia County Medical Society, Mills addressed the rising passion for psychotherapy generated by Worcester's recent visit to the city of brotherly love. "A wave of increasing interest in psychic medicine," he warned, "appears to be passing over our country. An old, old story is being repeated by new raconteurs; an old, old subject is being presented in a garb not entirely new, but with new trimmings and adornments."[80] To safeguard the public interest, Mills insisted "that psychotherapy like medicinal or mechanical or surgical or climatic, or any other sort of therapy *belongs to the physicians* and not to the clergyman, however sincere the latter may be in his idea that it his duty to invade the province of his medical brother."[81] Despite his unwitting influence on Worcester, S. Weir Mitchell expressed a similar view. In an address before the American Neurological Association he declared, "The so-called suggestion used in induced hypnotic states is utterly outside the true domain of the clergyman and if needed should be and remain part of the therapeutic agencies in the hands of physicians alone."[82] The practice of psychotherapy, he continued, was not something to be taken lightly: "I have treated a large number of neurasthenics and need hardly assure you that there are many cases which are simple and which intrusive psychotherapy would severely injure."[83]

Mitchell's paper generated a lively discussion.[84] One the one hand, Francis X. Dercum, Bernard Sachs, and Phillip Coombs Knapp defended Mitchell's argument and in so doing affirmed their allegiance to the somatic paradigm and to exclusive medical control. "The word, psychotherapy," Dercum charged, "offers no advantage over the old term of treatment by suggestion." "Dr. Mitchell's conclusions," Bernard Sachs declared, "might stand forth as the sane sentiment of this Association, in opposition to the psychotherapy idea." "In their craze for matters psychical," Philip Coombs Knapp added, many medical proponents of psychotherapy had "neglected fundamental principles of the art of medicine. The whole tendency of this present move in favor of psychoanalysis and psychotherapy has been to neglect, as Dubois cheerfully neglects, the physical basis which is so often at the bottom of the nervous disorders."[85]

On the other hand, James Jackson Putnam, Adolf Meyer, and Charles Dana argued that while the practice of psychotherapy might not be the panacea that many of its proponents claimed it to be, physicians nonetheless had a professional responsibility to take the subject seriously. In perhaps the most provocative commentary on the subject Dana asserted,

We as neurologists are confronted with the fact that an enormous number of mentally sick people are running around and getting their psychotherapeutics from the wrong well. They go to the seven different kinds of cures which Dr. Mitchell has spoken of, and a great many of them are injured by them. We do not believe that this is the best way for these people to be treated. We feel that there ought to be some definite forms of psychotherapeutics. What are we going to do with the large number who won't come to us and will go to anyone else who will raise his psychic standard? We must find out the good behind these false methods and organize it into some wise scientific measure which can prescribe. Until we do this there will be a continual succession of new cults, Christian Science, Osteopathy, etc., to the discredit of medicine and more especially psychiatrists and neurology.[86]

Dana was certainly not alone in making such a charge. An increasing number of physicians were beginning to embrace his view that American physicians needed to investigate more vigorously the claims of the mind curists and other nonmedical mental healers.

The promotional efforts of Worcester, McComb, and their followers did more than merely hasten the willingness of formerly intransigent physicians to consider seriously the subject of psychotherapy. They also generated a backlash among certain physicians who had originally supported Worcester's venture. Of these, the most notable was James Jackson Putnam. By the summer of 1908 Putnam himself began to express serious reservations about the direction of Worcester's movement. While vacationing in New York he sent Worcester an eighteen-page, handwritten letter in which he expressed his fear that Worcester and McComb might have originally misled him and the other physicians who had endorsed their initial, humble-sounding venture back in the autumn of 1906. This fear was fueled in large measure by the publication earlier that summer of *Religion and Medicine*.

In discussing that important matter I make at once the assumption that the movement was not ever designed to remain under your personal leadership or that of your church. In everyone's estimation this fact counts much in forming a judgment of its value and significance. If my present opinion seems to you radically different from those which you had good reason to think I entertained two years ago, I can only say that I have thought about the matter since then, to a degree and in a way that I had not, at that time, and furthermore, that I did not then conceive,—could not easily have conceived, what since has taken place.[87]

While still a staunch believer in the efficacy of psychotherapy, Putnam argued that he no longer supported its application by nonmedically trained professionals.

Individual physicians may fail to appreciate their splendid opportunity, individual clergymen may have a certain special moral fitness for doing part of the doctor's work. But these conditions are incidental and local; they constitute an obvious reason physicians should be made to feel the full weight of the clergymen's criticisms and suggestions *but not sufficient reason for an attempt to supersede physicians or rather the medical profession, or to lower its standing in the eyes of the community.* Yet this is what the Christian Science movement has avowedly tried to do, and what the Church-based healing movement is doing without wishing it.[88]

Despite Putnam's eloquent statement regarding the Emmanuel movement's unwitting effect on the medical profession, Worcester persisted in promoting his venture and thereby soon brought the full wrath of the medical profession on himself. Earlier that summer, Worcester had accepted an extraordinarily lucrative offer—$5,000—from Edward Bok, editor of *Ladies Home Journal,* to produce a series of articles for the popular women's monthly. Although he initially declined the offer, Worcester soon reconsidered. "I estimated," he later wrote, "that I could write an article a day and I knew that I should never earn that much money again in my natural life. So I accepted."[89] After considerable editing Worcester's first article appeared in November 1908, and the series continued until the following March.[90]

Putnam's growing apprehensions concerning the direction of Worcester's movement generated the first serious blow to Worcester's leadership role in the American psychotherapy movement—his exclusion from W. B. Parker's newly minted journal, *Psychotherapy: A Course of Readings in Sound Psychology, Sound Medicine, and Sound Religion.*[91] In an effort both to promote psychotherapy and to counteract the growing number of charges against it, leading academic, medical, and clerical figures engaged in a short-lived collaborative project that aimed not only to demystify but also to legitimate the practice by trained professionals.[92] In the fall of 1908 the first issue of *Psychotherapy* became publicly available. The intention of what ultimately became a three-volume, twelve-issue collection containing close to ninety articles was "to present in attractive and intelligible form and in a conservative manner the results of the best thought [and] the latest investigations, of the scientific and medical world, in this field."[93]

As originally conceived, the articles in *Psychotherapy* were to focus on one of five overlapping categories: general or descriptive, physiological, psychological, religious, and historical. Contributors included a host of eminent physicians and professors in both Europe and America as well as members of the American religious establishment who advocated the use of psychotherapy.[94] Conspicuously absent, however, were Worcester and McComb. Parker's refusal to include any work from the original clerical sponsors of the Emmanuel movement derived from a conflict with Worcester that had been fueled in large measure by James Jackson Putnam's changing sentiments concerning the rector's ambition. The Harvard neurologist had become increasingly frustrated with Worcester's promotional efforts on behalf of the Emmanuel movement, and during the summer of 1908 he threatened to withdraw his support from Parker's venture if it took the form of an "Emmanuel Church Course."

Realizing that Putnam's support was critical to the legitimacy and hence the success of *Psychotherapy*, Parker assured him that the course was in no way connected to the Emmanuel movement: "It is in no sense a church undertaking but essentially an educational undertaking. It is comparable most closely, I think, to the course offered to the old Chautauqua Reading Circles and like them aims primarily to inform and instruct."[95] But given the undeniable contribution of the church healing movement to American psychotherapy, Parker continued, he felt obliged to include representatives of the movement in *Psychotherapy*. The course, he declared, "cannot ignore the large part that has been played by the church movements—it would be not only incomplete but unscientific if it attempted to deal with the subject [of psychotherapy] without giving adequate attention to these aspects."[96]

Although as late as August 1908 Parker expressed his hope that Worcester might contribute to the project, he made it a point to inform Putnam, "I should not consider this a very prominent part" of the course.[97] Worcester refused to accept such a diminished role, however, and he and Parker soon found themselves at odds. In a personal letter to Putnam dated September 19, 1908, Parker spoke explicitly of his conflict with the minister:

You are doubtless aware that I have had a somewhat unwelcome experience owing to Dr. Worcester's attempt to dominate this Course of Readings and to make it subordinate to his Emmanuel movement. This I very naturally refused to do, and have had to sacrifice whatever advantage there may have been in Dr. Worcester's cooperation, but I think he is wholly at fault in his attempt to have it appear that Psychotherapeutics in America is his creation.[98]

The exclusion of Worcester from the course did not signify a refusal on Parker's part to acknowledge the church's importance to American psychotherapy. Articles by the Reverends Loring Batten, Lyman Powell, Samuel Fallows, and Albert B. Shields more than compensated for Worcester's absence.

The New York and Boston Controversies

What had been largely a private matter between Parker, Putnam, and Worcester soon became a highly visible public controversy. In the autumn of 1908 Loring W. Batten, Episcopal rector of St. Mark'sin-the-Bouwerie, announced his intention to establish a "Healing Mission" along the lines of Worcester's Emmanuel class.[99] News of Batten's intentions spread quickly. *Good Housekeeping* reported that "one of the latest and most important accessions to the list of the Emmanuel clinics is that of St. Mark's (Episcopal) church in New York City."[100] Interest in Batten's proposal increased when seven of the city's Episcopal ministers announced that Worcester himself, along with McComb and Coriat, had accepted their invitation to deliver a series of lectures beginning on Thanksgiving morning. The publicity generated by the news of their forthcoming visit not only helped to entrench the movement in New York City but also provoked a backlash from conservative physicians and ministers that would ultimately doom it.

The weeks preceding Worcester's visit to New York were marked with controversy fomented in large measure by a letter from New York neurologist Joseph Collins to the *New York Times*. On the same day during which a front-page headline proclaimed "Christian Scientist Held," a headline on page six reported, "Dr. Joseph Collins Attacks Prospectus of Rev. Dr. Batten of St. Mark's." "What is there about the ministerial profession," Collins asked, "that gives them a peep into the human mind and its diseases, or the human body and its diseases that is not vouchsafed to the physicians? On their investiture with orders, are they likewise given a divine potency to open the Pandora chest of the pathologist? Is it not possible that the average man or woman may by years of laborious study prepare himself or herself to recognize disease and learn how most expeditiously and safely to overcome it, quite as well as the man who had no experience with disease and therapeusis save his own arrogance?"[101]

Nine months before, in an article in the *American Journal of Medical Science*, Collins had expressed what can only be considered grudging admiration for his nonmedical rivals: "I am merely emphasizing the fact that no source of knowledge is too mean or contemptible for us to disdain it, and, that it does not detract from the dignity of our calling to admit the instructive value of these sources."[102] More significantly, he had declared, "I am opposed to the claim that it requires special skill to treat nervous disorders successfully [i.e., beyond those belonging to a general practitioner], and I contend that the general practitioner should study the proper manner of treating them, with the same care he studies infant feeding or the treatment of typhoid fever."[103] Why the change of position? The answer to this question, I suspect, concerns the threat of competition from nonmedically trained "psychotherapists." The growing allure of the Emmanuel movement compelled Collins to reconsider his former views regarding who was best suited to practice psychotherapy. Soon several other prominent physicians and neurologists would join him in publicly condemning Worcester's movement.

Collins's November 7 letter to the *New York Times* proved to be just the first shot in an extended volley of criticism leveled against the Emmanuel movement. During the next several days the *Times* reported considerable dissension among the city's neurologists. Both A. W. Catalin and Moses Allan Starr, as well as Dickinson S. Miller, the Columbia University professor of philosophy, enthusiastically endorsed Worcester's burgeoning movement.[104] "I do not believe," Starr declared, "that the admitted miracles of Lourdes and of St. Anne de Beaupre are supernatural. But since the human mind in its weakness demands some supernatural theory to account for these miracles, why is it not legitimate for the Protestant Church as well as the Catholic to adopt means calculated to produce the ends desired; especially as this means cannot be termed in any sense evil?"[105] Collins immediately shot back: "My letter to the *New York Times* was a protest against the assumption on the part of Elwood Worcester, D.D., Ph.D., and his followers that there is any justification for their engaging in the practice of medicine; against the arrogation to themselves of a power or capacity to deal with disease therapeutically that is beyond the acquisition of a man or woman who devotes his or her life to the study of disease; against the pretense of Worcesterism that its practices are scientific, and against the unseemliness of directing the finger of scorn and the voice of contumely against its parent, Christian Science."[106]

Collins did not have the last word, however. In yet another letter to the *Times,* Dickinson Miller argued that Worcester's claims were anything but extraordinary and that Collins's critique bordered on the disingenuous. "Dr. Worcester says that suggestion will relieve many functional disorders," Miller wrote. "This is exactly what the medical profession at large would say. He says that he has not yet found a case where it will relieve organic disorders. Here also he is supported by the majority of the medical profession."[107] Miller's public endorsement of the clerical uses of suggestion provoked a scathing indictment from Henry Rutgers Marshall, a former president of the American Psychological Association. Marshall challenged Miller's contention that ministers could safely administer suggestive therapeutics. Comparing psychotherapy to surgery, Marshall argued that "the operation should not be indulged in carelessly, nor without facing the fact that as life may be saved at the expense of bodily mutilation, so freedom from vicious habit and pain and worry may be gained at the expense of the weakening of personality."[108] Miller responded by asserting that there was little empirical basis to Marshall's argument. He then proceeded to savage Marshall's analysis:

It is a pity that legend should begin to depict Dr. Worcester as a kind of clerical Svengali, tampering through his uncanny arts with the personalities of his trustful patients. This Dr. Worcester is a creature of the imagination quite as much as Svengali himself. Dr. Marshall speaks of "the radical form of suggestion urged on us by the psychotherapist." I do not know to whom he refers. The methods of mental treatment or "psychotherapy" are many: explanation, encouragement, work-cure, psychic education, suggestion, and others. With all of these, ideas of the philosophy of life may be associated. With all of them, therefore, religion may be associated. Into all of them reason may enter. It is the sanest appeal that is best.[109]

In the midst of the highly visible public discussion of psychotherapy two of the city's most prominent medical journals entered the debate. On November 14 both the *New York Medical Record* and the *New York Medical Journal* included editorials on the movement. "While it [the medical-clerical venture] was confined to the Emmanuel Church people in Boston," the *Medical Record* quipped, "it was generally regarded as a sort of Neo-Eddyism, one more of the many queer fads with which the citizens of that town are wont to amuse themselves, and little more was thought of it."[110] Such eccentricities could easily be overlooked. But now that Worcester's program had spread to other cities responsible physicians could no longer remain silent—lest they wish to set a dangerous precedent. The editorial concluded by asserting that "when men speak with the confidence, shown by the authors of *Religion and Medicine,* of matters concerning which their words show them to have only uncertain knowledge, it is but a step to the rejection of all advice and suggestion from the physician."[111] In direct contrast to the *Medical Record* editorial, the *New York Medical Journal* declared, "As regards our own impression, we do not see in the movement anything subversive of the prerogatives of medical men in their daily work; the ecclesiastic, as represented by Dr. Worcester and Dr. Batten, seem to us to stand ready to cooperate with the medical profession, and not in the least disposed to antagonize it."[112]

New York City's highly publicized controversy concerning Worcester's forthcoming visit and Batten's "Healing Mission" soon spread to other cities. A similar episode erupted in Boston later that month when a local reporter asked James Jackson Putnam to respond to the *Medical*

Record's editorial. Putnam did so in writing, and the *Boston Herald* published his letter on the front page beneath the towering headline, "Convinced that the 'Emmanuel Movement' Is a Mistake." "[While] I have a high respect for the characters and purposes of its founders," Putnam wrote, "I am convinced that movement is a clear mistake. It is clear that clergymen, without adequate preparation, are assuming responsibilities of a kind that physicians are not considered qualified to assume until after years of study and of training. The question is whether the best interests of the community are really being served by this movement, and in my opinion this is not the case."[113]

Worcester and McComb did not remain silent. "The men who have taken up the work," they declared, "are able and experienced, and they are working under the direction of equally able and conscientious physicians. The immense response which our movement has met with, not only in this country, but also in others of the civilized world, proves how great is the need of help that we are offering."[114] In the Sunday issue of the *Herald* Putnam offered a lengthy reply. "When Dr. Worcester originally consulted me, just two years ago," Putnam explained, "I was at first much interested in his plan. I did not then realize what the outcome was to be. When I did realize it I expressed my criticism to Dr. Worcester, as I have done from time to time ever since—on two occasions at considerable length."[115] Of particular concern to Putnam was the direction of the movement. "The only real question," he explained, "seems to be one of future policy."[116] And on this critical point Putnam sided with the medical critics. The movement needed to be checked.

Just as the leading New York medical journals had expressed their concerns during the New York controversy, the *Boston Medical and Surgical Journal* entered the fray. Conceding that the medical profession could do more to promote the instruction of psychotherapy in the nation's medical schools, a November 26 editorial proclaimed that "it is not for a moment to be conceived that the great field of mental therapeutics is to be turned over to the churches, nor is it conceivable that representative medical men will indefinitely stand between the public and the minister to pass on patients which it is their manifest duty to treat themselves."[117] But the field of mental therapeutics had never "belonged" to physicians. It was not theirs to turn over to the churches, or to anyone else for that matter. If anything, the opposite was true. Lay proponents of mental healing were not stealing patients away from physicians. On the contrary, physicians were seeking to lure potential patients away from the lay mental healers.

By publicly assailing the movement, medical critics of Worcester's program hoped to establish themselves as the only legitimate source of mental healing in America and seize control of a market that they had long neglected. "The only knowledge which is of value in the field of abnormal psychology and mental therapeutics," the *Boston Medical and Surgical Journal* asserted, "has been gained from the laborious investigations of psychologists and physicians. . . . The field is foreign to the ordinary clerical mind and is not a matter which in any large way concerns the churches. It is, however, essentially a medical problem, and one which the profession is quite capable of handling in the future as it has in the past."[118] But saying that psychotherapy was "essentially a medical problem" did not make it so. Moreover, the assertion that physicians had handled the subject in the past was an egregious distortion that contradicted three decades of somatic intransigence and widespread unwillingness to take seriously the complaints of men and women afflicted with functional nervous disorders.

The New York and Boston controversies were more than mere local events. They were portents of what was to come. Newspapers throughout the region covered the dispute. The *New Jersey Herald* reported, "In the face of the volleys of criticism and denunciation which have been leveled by prominent Boston neurologists at the so-called 'Emmanuel Movement' for the cure of functional nervous diseases, certain of its sponsors now admit that the charge that dangers lurk in 'its spread to other churches' and in the administration of methods by 'untrained and unqualified men' may have a valid foundation."[119] On December 31 an editorial writer for the *Boston Medical and Surgical Journal* opined, "While we may regret the fact that the medical profession as yet has not completely aroused itself to its privileges and responsibilities, we entirely disagree with the statement that physicians are not concerned with the need which the Emmanuel movement seeks to meet."[120] A growing number of American physicians agreed. "What personally I feel," John Jenks Thomas asserted, "is that all methods of treatment of disease are with greater safety left in the hands of medical men and that by cooperation with clergymen in the future, as in the past, the often perplexing moral and religious questions that may arise in these curious functional nervous disorder can be best met."[121] "By whom should the treatment be carried out?" Robert T. Edes asked. "Obviously by the physicians."[122]

In an attempt to meet this mounting criticism and to defend the Emmanuel movement four Boston physicians, Richard C. Cabot, Joseph H. Pratt, Joel E. Goldthwait, and James G. Mumford, jointly wrote a letter dated January 15, 1909, in which they argued for reforming rather than destroying Worcester's movement.[123] But their effort proved to be too little and too late. With their defense in tatters, proponents of the Emmanuel movement found themselves increasingly under siege. Physicians, ministers, and academic psychologists all joined arms in the attacks.

Echoing the views expressed by previous medical critics, New York alienist Allan McClane Hamilton charged, "The *motif* of the Emmanuel movement . . . simply consists in the fact that there are a certain number of clergymen who become amateur doctors, their particular religion not forming the basis for any therapeutic plan, and they meddle with things of which they naturally know but little and injure themselves in their own calling at the same time."[124] An editorial in the *Old Dominion Journal of Medicine and Surgery* agreed: "[Great] masses of our people are now being blindly led by the promises of these movements to dizzy psychic heights, and this has so encouraged the originator and teachers that they have developed expansive delusions of the most ridiculous variety." Just as Christian Science was fading, the editorial continued, "another cult is arising, more insidious, more fascinating, more intellectual, holding out with one hand the *apparent* sanction of an established church and with the other holding in reserve the caduceus of the medical profession, to be used when necessary."[125]

In early May several prominent neurologists convened in New Haven, Connecticut, for a three-day symposium on psychotherapeutics.[126] The symposium was chaired by the associate editor of *Psychotherapy*, Frederick H. Gerrish, and included James Jackson Putnam, Morton Prince, Edward W. Taylor, Ernest Jones, and several other neurological exemplars of psychotherapy.[127] Echoing the views expressed by many of Worcester's medical critics, Gerrish opened the conference by declaring, "[Most] physicians and some neurologists have little appreciation of this branch of the healing art."[128] Ernest Jones, whose militant advocacy of psychoanalysis made him a maverick among the participants, agreed that physicians had to meet the challenge posed by both lay and religious mental healers. "The sooner we honestly face the shameful but undeniable fact that unqualified empirics can relieve distressing affections in cases that have defied medical skill, can produce results where we fail," Jones asserted, "the sooner will this flagrant lack in our system of education be remedied, and the better will it be for the dignity and honor of the medical profession." Until physicians learned to exploit the methods of their nonmedical rivals, Jones concluded, "our profession must submit to being the prey of the charlatan and the mock of the sufferer."[129] Four months later Freud himself offered a similar analysis. In an interview with a Boston reporter the Viennese neurologist declared, "When I think that there are many physicians who have been studying modern techniques of psychotherapy for decades and who yet practice it only with the greatest caution, this undertaking of a few without medical training, or with superficial medical training, seems to me at the very least a questionable good."[130] Freud's views were forcefully reiterated by John K. Mitchell: "Most earnestly should we insist that the *treatment* of a patient, whether it be surgical, medical, or psychic, should for the safety of the public, be in the hands of the doctor."[131]

Clerical Opposition

Physicians were not alone in condemning the Emmanuel movement. Leading religious figures from the Protestant establishment also assailed Worcester's popular venture. "We can imagine nothing so fatal to *real religion*," declared the Episcopal minister J. Edgar Johnson, "as the encouragement of the notion that people are invited to accept our religion for the sake of their health." Acknowledging the impressive credentials of those who founded the Emmanuel movement, Johnson nonetheless feared "the hasty adoption of Christian Therapeutics by those who are ill prepared for the venture."[132] The Boston minister Chauncey Hawkins attacked the movement on other grounds: "I believe that out of this movement there is coming a shallow type of ethics, the same as originated through the multitude of healing movements, among which Christian Science, Mental Healing, and the Emmanuel Movement are classed."[133] Hawkins's views were reiterated by George L. Parker, a minister from Salem, Massachusetts: "I protest against any theory that reduces the Gospel to a mere curing system, anything that makes it a mere religious watering-place, a sort of spiritual Baden-Baden or French Lick Springs. . . . Psychotherapy has too much the atmosphere of a drawing-room end-of-the-century fad. It is interesting for nervous dilettantes and those who have not much else to interest or employ them."[134] James Monroe Buckley, Methodist minister and editor of the *Christian Advocate,* provided an equally critical assessment of the Emmanuel movement: "For Dr. Worcester, his motives, his ardor, his indefatigable labors, I have nothing but admiration. But the foregoing facts and considerations, and others for which there is not room here, compel me to believe that for parishes or congregations to sustain a clinic as a part of their regular work presided over by the pastor, would be detrimental both to the church and the medical profession."[135]

In contrast to the views expressed by Hawkins, Taylor, and Buckley, the Congregational minister George A. Gordon's opposition to the Emmanuel movement derived from a subtle, albeit compelling, analysis of the role of professionalism and expertise. Expressing sentiments similar to those that Putnam had earlier conveyed in his September 1908 letter to Worcester, Gordon argued that the Emmanuel movement led the sick "to underestimate the service of the expert; it turns them away from the true source of hope—knowledge, experience, scientifically qualified men; it raises in them false expectations, feeds superstitious feeling, revives the popular belief in miracle, and blinds the community to the inviolable order of human life."[136] In recognizing the vital role of professionalism itself, Gordon offered not so much an attack of the Emmanuel movement as a defense of expertise. One of the more insightful responses to Gordon's article came from the minister of the Union Church in Haverhill, Massachusetts, George Henry Hubbard. Given the role of specialization among American physicians, Hubbard questioned the very meaning of medical expertise. If we are speaking of medical practice, Hubbard wrote, "the most skillful surgeon may be a layman in medicine and the medical practitioner a layman in surgery. The osteopath is a layman in the use of drugs and the drug doctor a layman in osteopathy. As for psychotherapy, the average physician of any school is as truly a layman as is the average minister or lawyer or tradesman."[137]

Hubbard did not deny the existence of experts. What he questioned, however, was whether all physicians—regardless of their specialty—were entitled to pronounce themselves experts on every single question regarding sickness and health. Moreover, Hubbard asked, "If we agree who are the laymen and who are the experts, are we are ready for the next step? Does it follow that the expert is the only person fit to practice a given art?"[138] But such thoughtful questions were the exception rather than the norm. In the debate to shape the future of American psychotherapy virtually none of the participants ever seriously addressed this critical issue.

The most eloquent clerical critic of the Emmanuel movement proved to be the dean of the Yale Divinity School, the Reverend Charles R. Brown:

Let the young physicians be more fully instructed in the medical schools in the principles of psychology as well as in the facts of physiology. The mood and the need of our age imperatively demand it. By that thorough study the physicians themselves will be made competent to render service along those lines, and they will also be the more inclined to invite the cooperation of the minister of religion. Let the minister of religion forsake any secondary ambitions they may have to become amateur dabblers in medicine; let them strive to be more fully competent in aiding the people "to live in the vision and service of the greatest ideals of the race." [139]

In large measure the mounting clerical antagonism to Worcester's program proved to be even more damaging than the medical opposition, and it would not be long before the two ministers ceased their efforts to promote their work.

Psychological Opposition

American academic psychologists were no less divided on the issues raised by the popular American psychotherapy movement than were physicians or ministers. Whereas Dickinson Miller and James R. Angell were outspoken champions of the movement, others were considerably less supportive. Among the most hostile psychological critics of the Emmanuel movement were Lightner Witmer, Henry Rutgers Marshall, and Hugo Münsterberg. Witmer, the director of the Psychological Clinic at the University of Pennsylvania, had earned a reputation as an expert on mental retardation. On December 15, 1908, he presented the first of three articles that criticized the American psychotherapy movement. [140] "Whatever Dr. Worcester's practice may be in his own church clinic," Witmer declared, "the principles of psychotherapy to which he and his associates adhere, are based upon neither sound medicine, sound psychology, nor to our lay mind, upon sound religion." [141]

More representative of the professional psychological criticism were the views expressed by Henry Rutgers Marshall and Hugo Münsterberg. Marshall argued that religion and medicine, despite their invaluable service to the community, were best kept separate. The skills and temperament required in each realm were frequently ill suited for the other.

The effective physician must be a man of keen insight, sound judgment, unwarped by emotionalism, and wise; yet at times even "worldly wise."

It cannot be maintained that clergy are as a rule recruited from those in whom these characteristics are markedly displayed, nor that their training and occupation tend to emphasize these qualities. We cannot but group together the Christian Science healer and the Emmanuel movement leaders as men who lightly take upon themselves work which the most serious experts in medicine study with the deepest care and handle with the greatest caution.[142]

Although Münsterberg shared Marshall's opposition to the Emmanuel movement, he recognized its important contribution to the medical profession. "The ministers first saw what the physicians ought to have seen before," Münsterberg declared, "but the physicians will see it more fully and more correctly."[143] In the preface to his popular 1909 book, *Psychotherapy,* Münsterberg wrote, "[The] aim of this book is not to fight the Emmanuel Church movement, or even Christian Science or any other psychotherapeutic tendency outside the field of scientific medicine. I see the element of truth in all of them, but they ought to be symptoms of transition. Scientific medicine should take hold of psychotherapeutics now or a most deplorable disorganization will set in, the symptoms of which no one ought to overlook today."[144]

Final Defense

In an article in the April 1909 issue of the *Harvard Theological Review*, Putnam declared that the movement was "still on trial." The critical issue was "whether the community should endorse a new form of medical specialty, represented by persons without adequate training for their task."[145] His answer, which he had already made clear during the recent Boston controversy, was that it should not. In the face of such overwhelming medical, clerical, and psychological criticism Worcester and McComb made one final effort to defend their movement. In the spring of 1909 the two men published *The Christian Religion as a Healing Power.*[146] Conceding that the popularity of their work had placed their movement in jeopardy, Worcester and McComb attempted to respond directly to the criticism leveled against them by their medical, clerical, and lay opponents. They insisted that it was a lack of familiarity with their work that had bred the scorn of the medical community, and they chastised their medical critics for failing to acquire a firsthand education concerning the true nature of their program. "[When] physicians, professing to speak in the name of science, attack a work that is open to inspection without attempting to acquaint themselves with its aims, limitations, or practice," the rector charged, "they bring scientific method into contempt, and show how slight a part science plays in the training of the average medical practitioner." [147] And McComb wrote, "Physicians, no matter how famous, who have made no use of the moral and religious motive are not in a position to deny its efficacy; and if they were truly scientific, they would not do so." [148]

The ministers' criticism of the movement's clerical opponents was even less charitable. Ministerial opposition to the work, Worcester declared, "has come in every instance from men who have reached a time of life when opinions are crystallized and it is too difficult to accept anything new. Their real quarrel is not with us or our work, but with the new spirit that is passing over the world of thought which they are unable to grasp." [149] "The doctrinaire theologian," McComb added, "objects to the therapeutic use of Christianity on the grounds that such use is a degradation of the lofty purposes which this religion was designed to subserve. . . . We contend, on the other hand, that the Christian religion is never more in its element, never shines with a greater glory, than when it is seen entering the dark places of our experience to cast out the demons of fear, worry, passion, despair, remorse, over-strained grief, and disgust of life, and to make the soul and body a fit temple for the holy spirit." [150] In addition to defending the movement against "doctrinaire theologians," McComb responded directly to those who accused the movement of being hedonistic in character and who warned that if widely copied would "cheapen religion by putting the emphasis as to the meaning of life upon personal comfort and absence of pain rather upon character, pain or no pain." [151]

By the end of the first decade of the twentieth century few American physicians were willing to challenge McComb's assertion regarding both the necessity and the efficacy of mental therapeutics. Whereas just a decade before only a tiny minority had even flirted with the possibility of systematically employing mental therapeutics, on the eve of Freud's historic visit to United States in September 1909 a substantial plurality, if not an outright majority, of American physicians were now willing to defend vigorously their exclusive right to employ a method that many in the profession had previously maligned and a substantially greater number had simply ignored.

The failure of *The Christian Religion as a Healing Power* to silence their critics convinced Worcester and McComb that any additional efforts on their behalf to salvage their movement would be futile. After publishing a few brief articles on their work in early 1910 the two ministers abandoned efforts to defend their movement. Seeking to avoid any future controversy, Worcester and McComb deliberately chose to suppress a work that was to have been a companion to *Religion and Medicine* after it had already been set in type.[152] Moreover, by the summer of 1910 magazine references to the Emmanuel movement ceased abruptly.[153] According to the *Readers' Guide* the last popular reference to the Emmanuel movement was May 1910.[154] No longer in the public spotlight, the movement "disappeared completely from current discussion."[155]

In rare moments of candor certain physicians readily conceded that the Emmanuel movement had acted as a vital catalyst in inspiring the medical profession to take the subjects of psychology, psychopathology, and psychotherapeutics more seriously. "For renewed interest in these subjects," John C. Fisher asserted, "we have to thank the Emmanuel movement."[156] A Massachusetts physician, Homer Gage, agreed. Although not without its shortcomings, the Emmanuel movement, Gage argued, warranted praise for adding clarity to the medical debate on psychotherapy. By inspiring the doctor and psychologist to renew their study of the nature, limitations, and practical application of psychotherapy it had recalled "the practicing physicians from too cold a materialism; and [prevented] the dehumanized scientist from taking the place of the doctor of the old school."[157] As H. Addington Bruce proclaimed, more than any other single factor, the Emmanuel movement had "aroused the medical profession to a belated recognition of the importance of scientific study and utilization of the mental factor in medicine."[158]

CHAPTER 7

Conclusion

The Emmanuel movement did far more than introduce the vocabulary of psychotherapy to the American public. It compelled a hitherto reluctant American medical profession to stake an important jurisdictional claim.[1] Taken alone, each was a considerable feat; taken together, they were revolutionary. By offering the imprimatur of respectable science to psychotherapy American physicians contributed to a radical transformation in the role that mental therapeutics would play in mainstream American culture. No longer confined to the margins, psychotherapy acquired a central position that it has continued to occupy for almost a full century.

The willingness of physicians to enter the previously much-maligned market of mental therapeutics reflected a novel professional calculus. Whereas during the 1880s American physicians specializing in the treatment of functional nervous disorders rightly feared that employing practices similar to those of Mary Baker Eddy and her ilk might compromise their precarious professional standing, by the first decade of the twentieth century such a concern, while not irrelevant, no longer factored so prominently in their calculations.[2] More secure in their professional standing, early-twentieth-century American physicians concluded that the benefits of entering the mental healing market outweighed the risks.

In contrast to earlier generations of American physicians who had initially embraced such diverse practices as phrenology, hypnotism, and spiritualism only to abandon them at the first sign of popular enthusiasm, medical proponents of scientific psychotherapy were drawn to the practice in large measure because of that enthusiasm.[3] That factors internal to the practice of medicine contributed to this response cannot be denied. Both the renewed awareness of the doctor-patient rapport that arose as a result of the various efforts to treat neurasthenic patients and the increasing familiarity with European neurological and psychiatric discourse were crucial variables in this process. They were far from the most important, however. More significant was the impact of various nonmedical factors—particularly the growing awareness of the psychic dimensions of traumatic neuroses inspired by the railway spine controversy, the begrudging recognition of the therapeutic successes achieved by various lay mental healers, and finally the overwhelming public enthusiasm for the Emmanuel movement.

By offering a professionally sanctioned and scientifically respectable alternative to the various lay mental healing therapies that predominated in the popular cultural landscape, American physicians hoped to secure a dominant position in a market they had long neglected. In the long term they failed. Medical enthusiasm for psychotherapy did little to dampen interest in alternative therapies let alone to diminish the allure of Christian Science and other analogous healing movements. The market was simply too unwieldy to be dominated by a single player, however powerful that player might be. In the short term, however, medical proponents of psychotherapy achieved a stunning, though perhaps unwitting, effect. They created a viable cultural space for a new type of psychotherapy.

It was in this highly charged medical-cultural context that psychoanalysis was first introduced to the American public.[4] In September 1909 Freud delivered a series of lectures at Clark University in Worcester, Massachusetts. His talks received ample coverage not only in the scholarly but also in the popular press.[5] As with prior mental healing movements, proponents of psychoanalytic theory—in particular, of dream interpretation—were paraded across the nation's newspapers and magazines as exemplars of the latest "scientific" advances. America's reading public was confronted with a variety of articles on the subject, many written by eminent psychologists themselves.[6] Freud's ideas generated considerable public curiosity. His provocative analyses of dreams, slips of the tongue, the unconscious, and infantile sexuality not only made for good copy but also stimulated a lively professional debate among physicians and psychologists. What they did not do, however, was substantially alter the course of American psychotherapy.

Indeed, more significant than the content of Freud's ideas was the context in which they were received. The fundamentally positive reception of psychoanalysis in the United States during the second decade of the twentieth century can be attributed to a host of factors that had little to do with the substance of Freud's theories. The allure of psychoanalysis derived in large measure from the unprecedented combination of popular and professional enthusiasm for mental therapeutics that existed at the time of its introduction in the United States. Had Freud delivered his lectures just three years earlier, in, say, 1906, chances are great that they would have received little fanfare. But by standing on the modest shoulders of Worcester and McComb, Freud received far more than an honorary degree from Clark University, perhaps even far more than he desired. His ideas—modified though they may have been—rapidly spread across an entire continent.[7]

Other scholars have made important contributions to evaluating the cogency of those ideas and to exploring their subsequent dissemination in the United States. That such tasks extend vastly beyond the scope of this project is hardly worth mentioning. What does warrant brief consideration here, however, are the ramifications of this voluminous and still expanding body of scholarship. The impact of such a surfeit of literature has grossly distorted our understanding not only of the history of psychotherapy but also of the history of psychiatry in the United States. The contribution of psychoanalysis to these respective realms, while certainly significant, is not nearly so profound as the sheer volume of scholarship on the subject suggests.

When Freud first set foot on American soil, psychotherapy was already integrally woven into the fabric of American culture and American medicine. True enough, psychoanalysis added new textures and new hues. What it did not do, however, was to alter the underlying pattern. At least not immediately, perhaps not at all.[8] The American melting pot had done to psychoanalysis what it had done to millions of foreign-born men, women, and children. It allowed it an opportunity to reinvent itself—but at the price of assimilation. In America the aim of psychoanalysis would no longer be to transform misery into common everyday unhappiness; it would be the pursuit of happiness itself, a goal that had been first propounded in the nation's founding document. Moreover, Freud's harsh determinism would give way to an upbeat American environmentalism. In these respects, and in several others, early-twentieth-century American psychoanalysis, for better or worse, owed an important though often unstated debt to American culture itself.

Whereas the history of psychoanalysis in America (and for that matter everywhere else) has been amply documented, the histories of other psychotherapies have remained largely unexamined, if not actually drowned out altogether by the profusion of what, for want of a better term, I shall call Freud studies. I do not mean to suggest that psychoanalysis has not warranted the attention it has received, though I must confess I have certainly entertained this notion. My point is more modest—namely, that despite having achieved hegemonic status among an elite cadre of American physicians and other custodians of culture, psychoanalysis neither supplanted the eclectic blend of psychotherapies that preceded it nor prevented alternative psychotherapies from emerging in the future. If anything, it had the opposite effect. That is to say, psychoanalysis not only added greater legitimacy to the much broader market in mental therapeutics but also helped to spawn a host of competing psychotherapies (to say nothing of psychoanalyses) that had little, if any, allegiance either to Freud himself or to the medical profession. As Nathan Hale points out, "By the 1970s guides were published to what had become a 'psychotherapy jungle,' with at least 130 recognizable varieties of 'psychosocial' therapies."[9] The story of these other psychotherapies begs to be written.

It is not only the study of non-Freudian psychotherapies that has suffered as a result of this preoccupation with the history of psychoanalysis. Even more significant has been the almost wholesale neglect of psychiatry's somatic side, which has only recently begun to arouse the interest of professional historians.[10] Such work is long overdue. The fascinating stories of barbiturate-induced narcosis; the surgical removal of teeth, tonsils, stomachs, and other organs; malarial fever therapy, metrazol shock therapy, electroshock therapy, insulin coma therapy; and lobotomy and psychopharmacology, although known to experts in the field, have received little, if any, scrutiny in the less specialized historical and popular literature on the field. While scholars too numerous to count continue to wage a now-tiresome debate over the significance, legitimacy, salience, *whatever* of psychoanalysis, an extraordinary historical record relating to the somatic side of twentieth-century psychiatry still waits to be mined. There is little left to excavate from Freud's city. It's time to move on and dig again.

Notes

Chapter 1

1. While only psychiatrists (i.e., M.D.'s) have the authority to prescribe drugs, both clinical psychologists (Ph.D.'s and Psy.D.'s) and social workers (M.S.W.'s)—provided they are licensed by their respective state boards—are legally entitled to practice "psychotherapy" and, perhaps more importantly, to receive compensation from insurance companies.

2. It was not until the January 1904 issue of *Index Medicus* that "psychotherapy" first appeared in the subject index, and another two years would pass before the word appeared as a separate subject heading. *Index Medicus*, 2d ser., 2 (1904). On page 37, a reference appears to a French article written by the Swiss neurologist Paul Dubois. Barbara Sicherman claims psychotherapy's first appearance in *Index Medicus* takes place in 1906. See Sicherman, "The New Psychiatry: Medical and Behavioral Science, 1895–1921," in *American Psychoanalysis: Origins and Development*, ed. Jacques M. Quen and Eric T. Carlson (New York: Brunner, Mazel, 1978). While Sicherman is correct in terms of the listings under the category, "Therapeutics, Materia Medica," which appears at the beginning of each monthly issue, she neglects to consider the subject Index that appears in the year-end issue of each volume. "Suggestion," which first appears in the February 1886 issue of *Index Medicus*, 1st ser., 8 (1886) is replaced by "Psychotherapy" in the April 1906 issue.

3. This point is not universally accepted. Francis Gosling has argued that "throughout the years from 1870 to 1910 physicians of all types displayed increasing recognition that psychological treatment alone could have just as great an effect on neurasthenic patients as physical remedies." There are two flaws in this assertion. The first concerns the time frame. Prior to 1900 there is little evi-

dence suggesting that American physicians *self-consciously* sought to employ psychological treatment. The second flaw is more substantive. At no time, either before or after 1900, did any American physician of note ever advocate the application of "psychotherapy" to the exclusion of all somatic therapies. See Francis G. Gosling, *Before Freud: Neurasthenia and the American Medical Community, 1870–1910* (Urbana: University of Illinois Press, 1987).

4. David W. Wells, *Psychology Applied to Medicine* (Philadelphia: F.A. Davis, 1907), 123.

5. John Hughlings Jackson, *Selected Writings of John Hughlings Jackson,* 2 vols., ed. J. Taylor, G. Holmes, and F.M.R. Walsh (London: Hodder and Stoughton, 1932), 1:452.

6. George Beard, *Practical Treatise on Nervous Exhaustion (Neurasthenia): Its Symptoms, Nature, Sequences, and Treatment* (New York: William Wood, 1880), 114.

7. S. Weir Mitchell, "The Treatment by Rest, Seclusion, et., in Relation to Psychotherapy," *Journal of the American Medical Association* 50 (1908): 2037.

8. Claude Quetel, *History of Syphilis,* trans. Judith Braddock and Brian Pike (Baltimore: Johns Hopkins University Press, 1990); Allan M. Brandt, *No Magic Bullet: A Social History of Venereal Disease in the United States since 1880* (New York: Oxford University Press, 1985); Daphne A. Roe, *A Plague of Corn: The Social History of Pellagra* (Ithaca: Cornell University Press, 1973); Elizabeth W. Etheridge, *The Butterfly Caste: A Social History of Pellagra in the South* (Westport, Conn.: Greenwood, 1972); and Otto Marx, "What Is the History of Psychiatry?" *American Journal of Orthopsychiatry* 40 (1970): 598.

9. For a summary of American medical attitudes regarding mental therapeutics, see Edward Wylis Taylor, "The Attitude of the Medical Profession Toward the Psychotherapeutic Movement," *Boston Medical and Surgical Journal* 157 (26 December 1907): 843–850.

10. Hugo Münsterberg, *Psychotherapy* (New York: Moffat, Yard, 1909), 360.

11. Richard C. Cabot, "The American Type of Psychotherapy," in *Psychotherapy: A Course Reading in Sound Psychology, Sound Medicine, and Sound Religion* 1 (1908): 1.

12. Robert C. Fuller, *Americans and the Unconscious* (New York: Oxford University Press, 1986), 97.

13. John C. Burnham, "Psychology and Counseling: Convergence into a Profession," in *The Professions in American History,* ed. and introd. Nathan O. Hatch (Notre Dame: University of Notre Dame Press, 1988), 183.

14. Nathan G. Hale, Jr., *Freud and the Americans: The Beginnings of Psychoanalysis in the United States, 1876–1917* (New York: Oxford University Press, 1970), 72.

15. George Frederick Drinka, *The Birth of Neurosis* (New York: Simon and Schuster, 1984), 287; For other examples of this type of analysis, see James Hoopes, *Consciousness in New England: From Puritanism and Ideas to Psychoanalysis and Semiotic* (Baltimore: Johns Hopkins University Press, 1989), 237–238. Building on Hale's work, Castel et al. contend, "At the end of the last century, however, the somatic style in mental medicine fell into crisis and neurologists were thereby prevented from capitalizing fully on their gains. The results of research on brain lesions proved disturbing, and disease classifications

based on the structure of the nervous system were widely viewed as abstract and arbitrary, incapable of providing an adequate account of complex mental pathology." Robert Castel, Françoise Castel, and Anne Lovell, *The Psychiatric Society*, trans. Arthur Goldhammer (New York: Columbia University Press, 1982), 26. Regarding the applicability of Kuhn's theory to the history of psychiatry, Dowbiggin observes, "Psychiatry as a profession may be in a perpetual state of Kuhnian crisis by virtue of its inherent cognitive and empirical difficulties. As a result, psychiatric knowledge has a fluid character that—combined with the fact that it never ceases to be free of 'social' considerations—virtually guarantees that it will be a shifting blend of cultural attitudes, social values, political beliefs, and professional imperatives." See Ian Dowbiggin, "French Psychiatry, Hereditarianism, and Professional Legitimacy, 1840–1900," *Research in Law, Deviance and Social Control* 7 (1985): 135–165. See also Dowbiggin's *Inheriting Madness: Professionalization and Psychiatric Knowledge in Nineteenth-Century France* (Berkeley: University of California Press, 1991), 166.

16. Thomas S. Kuhn, *The Structure of Scientific Revolutions*, 2d ed. (Chicago: University of Chicago Press, 1970); For an excellent analysis of Kuhn's impact, see David Hollinger, "T. S. Kuhn's Theory of Science and Its Implications for History," in *In the American Province: Studies in the History and Historiography of Ideas* (Bloomington: Indiana University Press), 105–129.

17. Charles E. Rosenberg, "Body and Mind in Nineteenth-Century Medicine: Some Clinical Origins of the Neurosis Construct," *Bulletin of the History of Medicine* 63 (1989): 189.

18. Gerald N. Grob, "Rediscovering Asylums: The Unhistorical History of the Asylum," in *The Therapeutic Revolution: Essays in the Social History of American Medicine*, ed. Morris J. Vogel and Charles E. Rosenberg, 135–157 (Philadelphia: University of Pennsylvania Press, 1979); Richard Harrison Shyrock, "The Medical History of the American People," in *Medicine in America: Historical Essays* (Baltimore: Johns Hopkins University Press, 1966), 5.

19. Edward Shorter, *From Paralysis to Fatigue: A History of Psychosomatic Illness in the Modern Era* (New York: Free Press, 1992), 233–253.

20. Gerald N. Grob, *Mental Illness and American Society, 1875–1940* (Princeton: Princeton University Press, 1983), 112.

21. John Hughlings Jackson, *Selected Writings of John Hughlings Jackson*, 2:212; quoted in Michael J. Clark, "The Rejection of Psychological Approaches to Mental Disorders in Late Nineteenth-Century British Psychiatry," in *Madhouses, Mad-Doctors, and Madmen: The Social History of Psychiatry in the Victorian Era*, ed. Andrew Scull (Philadelphia: University of Pennsylvania Press, 1981), 271–312; also see Rosenberg, "Body and Mind," 193–194.

22. Lester S. King, *Transformations in American Medicine: From Benjamin Rush to William Osler* (Baltimore: Johns Hopkins University Press, 1991), 174. On the American reception of germ theory, see Grob, *Mental Illness*, 122; James H. Cassedy, *Medicine and American Growth, 1800–1860* (Madison: University of Wisconsin Press, 1986), 83; and John Duffy, *The Sanitarians: A History of American Public Health* (Urbana: University of Illinois Press, 1990), 196.

23. See Grob, *Mental Illness*, 108; J. Sanbourne Bockoven, *Moral Treatment in American Psychiatry* (New York: Springer, 1963); John C. Burnham, "Psychiatry, Psychology, and the Progressive Movement," in *The Professions in*

American History, ed. Nathan O. Hatch, 188–189 (Notre Dame: Notre Dame University Press, 1988); and Wells, *Psychology Applied to Medicine,* vii.

24. Walter Bromberg, *The Mind of Man: The Story of Man's Conquest of Mental Illness* (New York: Harper & Brothers, 1937), 198–199.

25. Few issues have elicited greater controversy in the history of psychiatry than the significance of moral therapy. Virtually all historians of psychiatry agree that the late eighteenth century and early nineteenth century was a time of unprecedented medical awareness of mental illness. This consensus rapidly disintegrates, however, when efforts are made to assess the significance of this previously absent medical concern. Although the erection of asylums throughout Europe and North America, the imposition of the so-called moral treatment, and the oversight of medical doctors are universally regarded as hallmarks in the foundation of modern psychiatry, the cultural and historical ramifications of these developments are hotly contested by historians, sociologists, and myriad other scholars. "Traditional" historians tend to take nineteenth-century "reformers" at their word and thereby regard this period as among the most progressive episodes in the history of mental medicine. By way of contrast, "revisionists" argue that "this very humanization of madness and crime created new forms of repression" leading ultimately to a drastic regimen of social control over a host of marginal members of society—many of whom had long been left alone. For a representative, though by no means exhaustive, sample of "traditionalist" interpretations of moral therapy, see Bromberg, *The Mind of Man;* Albert Deutsch, *The Mentally Ill in America: A History of Their Care and Treatment from Colonial Times* (Garden City: Doubleday, Doran, 1937); Gregory Zilboorg, in collaboration with George W. Henry, *A History of Medical Psychology* (New York: W. W. Norton, 1941); Franz G. Alexander and Sheldon T. Selesnick, *The History of Psychiatry: An Evaluation of Psychiatric Thought and Practice from Prehistoric Times to the Present* (New York: Harper and Row, 1966); and Norman Dain, *Concepts of Insanity in the United States, 1789–1865* (New Brunswick: Rutgers University Press, 1964). For some revisionist interpretations, see Michel Foucault, *Madness and Civilization: A History of Insanity in the Age of Reason,* trans. Richard Howard (New York: Vintage Books, 1973); Christopher Lasch, "Origins of the Asylum," in *The World of Nations: Reflections on American History, Politics, and Culture* (New York: Alfred A. Knopf, 1973), 6; David Rothman, *The Discovery of the Asylum: Social Order and Disorder in the New Republic* (Boston: Little, Brown, 1971); idem, "Social Control: The Uses and Abuses of the Concept in the History of Incarceration," in *Social Control and the State,* ed. Stanley Cohen and Andrew Scull, 106–117 (New York: St. Martin's Press, 1981); Andrew Scull, *Most Solitary of Afflictions: Madness and Society in Britain, 1700–1900* (New Haven: Yale University Press, 1993); idem, "The Discovery of the Asylum Revisited," in *Madhouses, Mad-Doctors, and Madmen,* 144–165; idem, "Moral Treatment Reconsidered," in *Social Order/Mental Disorder: Anglo-American Psychiatry in Perspective* (Berkeley: University of California Press, 1989), 80–94; idem, "A Failure to Communicate?" in *Rewriting the History of Madness: Studies in Foucault's* Histoire de Folie, ed. Andrew Still and Irving Velody (London: Routledge, 1992); idem, "Madness and Segregative Control: The Rise of the Insane Asylum," *Social Problems* 24 (1977): 338–351.

26. Norman Dain and Eric T. Carlson, "Milieu Therapy in the Nineteenth Century: Patient Care at the Friend's Asylum, Frankford, Pennsylvania, 1817–1861," *Journal of Nervous and Mental Disease* 131 (October 1960): 277–290; Oskar Diethelm, "An Historical View of Somatic Treatment in Psychiatry," *American Journal of Psychiatry* 95 (1939): 1165–1179; Bockoven, *Moral Treatment*, 10–19, 69–80.

27. Proponents of moral therapy, explains Roy Porter, "were not interested in a 'talking cure,' or in 'working through' problems. Theirs was a psychiatry which operated not through peeling off layers of consciousness or recovering the repressed, nor even through a 'meeting of the mind,' but by making people want to be good." Roy Porter, *Mind Forg'd in Manacles: A History of Madness in England from the Restoration to the Regency* (Cambridge: Harvard University Press, 1987), 226.

28. Prior to 1910 the *Readers' Guide to Periodical Literature* does not list a single article on either Freud or psychoanalysis.

29. John C. Burnham explains, "One can easily account for the rise of psychotherapy and the rise of behaviorism in terms of the internal histories of psychiatry and psychology. But the fact that these movements coincided in time with the Progressive social reform movement, and the fact that social control was an aim of reformers in politics and science, can be accounted for only by treating the developments in psychiatry and psychology and in all other middle-class endeavors as part and parcel of the Progressive movement itself." John C. Burnham, "Psychiatry, Psychology, and the Progressive Movement," in *Paths into American Culture: Psychology, Medicine, and Morals* (Philadelphia: Temple University Press, 1988), 192; see also Drinka, *The Birth of Neurosis;* George Gifford, ed., *Psychoanalysis, Psychotherapy and the New England Medical Scene, 1894–1944* (New York: Science History, 1978); Eugene Taylor, *William James on Exceptional Mental States: The 1896 Lowell Lectures* (New York: Charles Scribner's Sons, 1984).

30. For examples of works that make this mistake, see Alfred Booth Kuttner, "Nerves," in *Civilization in the United States,* ed. Harold Stearns (New York: Harcourt, Brace, 1922), 427–442. See also Henry Alden Bunker, Jr., "From Beard to Freud: A Brief History of the Concept of Neurasthenia," *Medical Review of Reviews 36* (1930): 108–114; Philip Wiener, "G. M. Beard and Freud on 'American Nervousness,'" *Journal of the History of Ideas 17* (1956): 269–274; and Kenneth Levin, "S. Weir Mitchell: Investigation and Insights in Neurasthenia and Hysteria," *Transactions and Studies of the College of Physicians of Philadelphia* 38 (1970): 168–173.

31. *Index Catalogue of the Library of the Surgeon-General's Office* 11, 2d ser. (1906): 603–607.

Chapter 2

1. Josef Breuer and Sigmund Freud, *Studies on Hysteria*, trans. James Strachey (New York: Basic Books, 1955).

2. The secondary literature on shell shock and war neuroses is extensive. Good places to start are Elaine Showalter, *The Female Malady: Women, Madness, and English Culture, 1830–1980* (New York: Penguin Books, 1985), 167–194; Wolfgang Schivelbusch, *Railway Journey: The Industrialization of Time and Space in the 19th Century* (Berkeley: University of California Press, 1989), 150–158; Judith Lewis Herman, *Trauma and Recovery: The Aftermath of Violence—From Domestic Abuse to Political Terror* (New York: Basic Books, 1992), 20–28; Martin Stone, "Shell Shock and the Psychologists," in *The Anatomy of Madness,* ed. William F. Bynum, Roy Porter, and Michael Shepard (Cambridge: Cambridge University Press, 1985); and Allan Young, *The Harmony of Illusions: Inventing Post-Traumatic Stress Disorder* (Princeton: Princeton University Press, 1995).

3. Lawrence M. Friedman, *A History of American Law,* 2d ed. (New York: Touchstone Books, 1985), 471.

4. Exact figures for train accidents and injuries prior to 1889 are impossible to determine. The newly established Interstate Commerce Commission did not begin compiling such statistics until 1889.

5. Walter Licht, *Working for the Railroad: The Organization of Work in the Nineteenth Century* (Princeton: Princeton University Press, 1983), 191. The corresponding figures for Great Britain differed significantly: one trainman in every 329 was killed and one in 30 was injured.

6. See Robert B. Shaw, *A History of Railroad Accidents, Safety Precautions and Operating Practices* (n.p.: Vail-Ballou Press, 1978).

7. Although there are literally scores of books and articles devoted to the history and cultural significance of neurasthenia, there are only a small number of English-language works that consider the subject of railway spine. See Eric Caplan, "Trains, Brains, and Sprains: Railway Spine and the Origins of Psychoneuroses," *Bulletin of the History of Medicine* 69 (1995): 387–419; Ralph Harrington, "The Neuroses of the Railway," *History Today* 44 (1994): 15–21; idem, "The 'Railway Spine' Diagnosis and Victorian Response to PTSD," *Journal of Psychosomatic Research* 40 (1996): 11–14; Allard Dembe, *Occupation and Disease: How Social Factors Affect the Conception of Work-related Disorders* (New Haven: Yale University Press, 1996), 107–119; Young, *Harmony of Illusions,* 1–28; Ian Hacking, *Rewriting the Soul: Multiple Personality and the Sciences of Memory* (Princeton: Princeton University Press, 1995), 184, 192–193; Thomas Keller, "Railway Spine Revisited: Traumatic Neurosis or Neurotrauma," *Journal of the History of Medicine and Allied Sciences* 50 (1995): 507–524; Schivelbusch, *Railway Journey,* 134–170; Drinka, *The Birth of Neurosis,* 109–122; Michael R. Trimble, *Post-Traumatic Neurosis: From Railway Spine to Whiplash* (New York: John Wiley and Sons, 1981); Gosling, *Before Freud,* 91–92; Hoopes, *Consciousness in New England,* 243–244; Edward M. Brown, "Regulating Damage Claims for Emotional Injuries before the First World War," *Behavioral Sciences and the Law* 8 (1990): 421–434; and Hale, *Freud and the Americans,* 87–88. Together these works provide a fairly accurate, albeit general, discussion of the neurological discourse on the subject of railway spine. None goes substantially beyond this discourse, however. Drinka and Schivelbusch offer some interesting cultural speculations. Trimble provides a more rigorous discussion of some of the primary medical texts on the subject.

Gosling concentrates on the role of neurasthenia, and Hoopes explores the distinctions between functional and structural notions of disease that informed the debate.

8. Morton Prince, "The Present Method of Giving Expert Tension in Medico-Legal Cases, as Illustrated by One in which Large Damages were Awarded, Based on Contradictory Medical Evidence," *Boston Medical and Surgical Journal* 122 (1890): 77.

9. Shobal Vail Clevenger, *Spinal Concussion: Surgically Considered as a Cause of Spinal Injury, and Neurologically Restricted to a Certain Symptom Group, for which Is Suggested the Designation Erichsen's Disease, as One Form of the Traumatic Neuroses* (Philadelphia: F. A. Davis, 1889), 207.

10. Charles D. Dana, "The Traumatic Neuroses: Being a Description of the Chronic Nervous Disorders that Follow Injury and Shock," in *A System of Legal Medicine,* vol. 2, ed. Allan McClane Hamilton and Lawrence Godkin (New York: E. B. Treat, 1894), 299.

11. John G. Johnson, "Concussion of the Spine in Railway Injuries," *Medico-Legal Journal* 1 (1883–1884): 515 (italics added). See Landon Carter Gray's comments following William J. Herdman, "Traumatic Neurasthenia (Railway Spine, Spinal Concussion), What Is It, and How Can It be Recognized?" *International Journal of Railway Surgery* 2 (1898): 221.

12. Erichsen was certainly not the only physician of his day to focus on the particular medical issues raised by railway injuries. Two fellow countrymen and surgeons, William Camps and Thomas Buzzard, had also published brief essays on the subject of railway accidents. "The extent of the injuries which may be caused by a railway accident," Camps proclaimed, "are not, in my judgment, very easily or adequately to be realized or appreciated. The actual destruction of life and limb of which we read with so much that excites in us the emotion of horror, forms but a part of the suffering really undergone by the unfortunate victims. There is something in the crash, the shock, and the violence of a railway collision, which would seem to produce effects upon the *nervous system* quite beyond those of any ordinary injury." William Campe, *Railway Accidents or Collisions: Their Effects upon the Nervous System* (London: H. K. Lewis, 1866). Also see Thomas Buzzard, "On Cases of Injury from Railway Accidents," *Lancet* (1866): 23, 186.

13. John Eric Erichsen, *On Railway and Other Injuries of the Nervous System* (London: Walton and Maberly, 1866), v.

14. John Eric Erichsen, *On Concussion of the Spine, Nervous Shock, and Other Obscure Injuries to the Nervous System in Their Clinical and Medico-Legal Aspects* (New York: William Wood, 1883), 158–159.

15. See next chapter; see also George Beard, "Neurasthenia, or Nervous Exhaustion," *Boston Medical and Surgical Journal* 3 (1869): 217–219. For a discussion of Beard's contribution, see Charles Rosenberg, "The Place of George Beard in Nineteenth-Century Psychiatry," in *No Other Gods: On Science and American Social Thought* (Baltimore: Johns Hopkins University Press, 1976), 98–108; and Barbara Sicherman, "The Use of Diagnosis: Doctors, Patients, and Neurasthenia," *Journal of the History of Medicine and Allied Sciences* 32 (1977): 33–54.

16. Erichsen, *On Railway and Other Injuries,* 9.

17. Ibid., 96–100. This is a paraphrase.

18. Trimble neglects to consult Erichsen's pioneering 1866 series of lectures in which he first expresses his ideas and treats the topic of hysteria in a radically different manner than he did in his revised and expanded 1875 edition.

19. As Mark Micale explains, prior to Charcot's work of the 1880s, "the great majority of physicians, including many of the most 'progressive' doctors of the day, held that hysteria, in some undefined but definite way, was, as it always had been, intimately caught up with the female generative system." Mark S. Micale, "Charcot and the Idea of Hysteria in the Male: Gender, Mental Science, and Medical Diagnostics in Late Nineteenth-Century France," *Medical History* 34 (1990): 370. In his dissertation, Micale provides an excellent summary of the treatment of male hysteria prior to Charcot's reassessment of the issue in the 1880s: "Diagnostic Discrimination: Jean-Martin Charcot and the Nineteenth-Century Idea of Masculine Hysterical Neurosis" (Ph.D. dissertation, Yale University, 1987). For an excellent general treatment of the history of hysteria, see Ilza Veith, *Hysteria: The History of a Disease* (Chicago: University of Chicago Press, 1965); see also Sander L. Gilman, ed., *Hysteria Beyond Freud* (Berkeley: University of California Press, 1993).

20. Historians have provided compelling and persuasive evidence that gender issues played a substantial, perhaps even the dominant, role in late-nineteenth-century psychiatric theories and practices. Class also factored into the analysis concerning mental distress, but there is widespread consensus that issues of class failed to occupy as prominent a position as those of gender. The discourses germane to both neurasthenia and hysteria, the two most popular, if not actually the most prolific, nervous disorders of the late nineteenth century are among the most gender-centered issues of the age. Indeed, as both Janet Oppenheim and Elaine Showalter argue, it was not until the First World War that Anglo-American physicians widely embraced the notion that men as well as women might experience hysteria. See Janet Oppenheim, *Shattered Nerves: Doctors, Patients and Depression in Victorian England* (New York: Oxford University Press, 1991), and Showalter, *Female Malady.*

21. Erichsen, *On Railway and Other Injuries,* 70–71.

22. Ibid., 127.

23. Carroll Smith-Rosenberg, "The Hysterical Woman: Sex Roles and Role Conflict in Nineteenth-Century America," in *Disorderly Conduct: Visions of Gender in Victorian America* (New York: Alfred A. Knopf, 1985), 205. Smith-Rosenberg's statements regarding hysterics apply equally well to victims suffering from a host of apparently nonsomatic disorders. See Robert A. Aronowitz, "From Myalgic Encephalitis to Yuppie Flu: A History of Chronic Fatigue Syndromes," in *Framing Disease: Studies in Cultural History,* ed. Charles E. Rosenberg and Janet Golden (New Brunswick: Rutgers University Press, 1992), 155–181.

24. As quoted by Herbert W. Page, *Injuries of the Spine and Spinal Cord Without Apparent Mechanical Lesion and Nervous Shock in their Surgical and Medico-Legal Aspect* (London: J. & A. Churchill, 1883), 193.

25. D. R. Wallace, "Spinal Concussion and John Eric Erichsen's Book," *Railway Surgeon* 1 (1894–1895): 249.

26. R. M. Hodges, "So-Called Concussion of the Spinal Cord," *Boston Medical and Surgical Journal* 104 (1881): 338. Schivelbusch incorrectly dates this article at 1883: *Railway Journey*, 144 n.24.

27. Johnson, "Concussion of the Spine," 504.

28. D. R. Wallace, "A Reply to Dr. Swearingen," *The Railway Surgeon: Official Journal of the National Association of Railway Surgeons* 1 (1894–1895): 259.

29. "Railway Accidents and Railway Evidence," *British Medical Journal* 2 (December 1, 1866): 612.

30. John Eric Erichsen, "Mr. Erichsen's work 'Railway and Other Injuries of the Nervous System,'" *British Medical Journal* 2 (1866): 679.

31. Ibid., 670.

32. Hodges, "So-Called Concussion," 388.

33. Ibid., 361.

34. His 1881 prize-winning essay was entitled "Injuries to the Back without Apparent Mechanical Lesions, in their Surgical and Medico-Legal Aspects."

35. Page, *Injuries of the Spine*.

36. Thomas Furneaux Jordan, "Shock after Surgical Operation," *British Medical Journal* 1 (1867): 136. For biographical details, see "Thomas Furneaux Jordan," *Plarr's Lives of the Fellows of the Royal College of Surgeons of England* (Bristol: John Wright & Sons, 1930), 1:635–637. For a history of surgical shock, see Peter English, *Shock, Physiological Surgery, and George Washington Crile: Medical Innovation in the Progressive Era* (Westport, Conn.: Greenwood, 1980). Of particular significance is English's first chapter, "Surgical Shock Before Crile: A Disorder of the Nervous System," 3–20.

37. Trimble, *Post-Traumatic Neurosis*, 27.

38. Page, *Injuries of the Spine*, 147.

39. James Paget, "Nervous Mimicry," in *Clinical Lectures and Essays* (London: Longmans, Green, 1875): 2:172–252. Reprinted from *Lancet* 2 (1873): 511–513, 547–549, 619–621, 727–729, 773–775, 833–835.

40. Page, *Injuries of the Spine*, 204 (italics added).

41. Brown, "Regulating Damage Claims," 425–426.

42. Page, *Injuries of the Spine*, 205.

43. James Jackson Putnam, "Recent Investigation into the Pathology of So-Called Concussion of the Spine," *Boston Medical and Surgical Journal* 108 (1883): 217.

44. Dana, "The Traumatic Neuroses," 300.

45. Putnam, "Recent Investigation," 217.

46. Ibid., 219.

47. G. L. Walton, "Possible Cerebral Origins of Symptoms Usually Classed Under 'Railway Spine,'" *Boston Medical and Surgical Journal* 109 (1883): 337. Historian Jan Goldstein makes the important point that while "Charcot shared the view that hysteria was not a variety of full-fledged insanity—indeed, this was the generally accepted view of the psychiatrists of his day— . . . for him its lesser severity did not constitute a detraction." Jan Ellen Goldstein, *Console and Classify: The French Psychiatric Profession in the Nineteenth Century* (New York: Cambridge University Press, 1987), 331–332.

48. Mark Micale, "Hysteria Male/Hysteria Female: Reflection on Comparative Gender Construction in Nineteenth-Century France and Britain," in *Science and Sensibility: Gender and Scientific Inquiry, 1780–1945,* ed. Marina Benjamin (Oxford: Basil Blackwell, 1991), 363–411; Oppenheim, *Shattered Nerves,* 293–319; Shorter, *From Paralysis to Fatigue,* 191–192.

49. My discussion on Charcot is derived from the following sources: Henri Ellenberger, *The Discovery of the Unconscious: The History and Evolution of Dynamic Psychiatry* (New York: Basic Books, 1970), 89–109; Frank J. Sulloway, *Freud, Biologist of the Mind: Beyond the Psychoanalytic Legend* (New York: Basic Books, 1979), 28–49; Ernest Jones, *The Life and Work of Sigmund Freud* (New York: Basic Books, 1953), 1:221–267; Peter Gay, *Freud: A Life for Our Time* (New York: W. W. Norton, 1988), 46–53; Edward Shorter, *From Paralysis,* 167–196; Kenneth Levin, "Freud's Paper 'On Male Hysteria' and the Conflict Between Anatomical and Physiological Models," *Bulletin of the History of Medicine* 48 (1974): 377–397; idem, *Freud's Early Psychology of the Neuroses: A Historical Perspective* (Pittsburgh: University of Pittsburgh Press, 1978); Trimble, *Post-Traumatic Neurosis,* 34–56; Mark S. Micale, "Charcot and the Idea of Hysteria in the Male: Gender, Mental Science, and Medical Diagnostics in Late Nineteenth-Century France," *Medical History* 34 (1990): 363–411; idem, *Diagnostic Discrimination: Jean-Martin Charcot and the Nineteenth-Century Idea of Masculine Hysterical Neurosis* (Ann Arbor: University Microfilms, 1987); Leon Chertok, "On Objectivity in the History of Psychotherapy," *Journal of Nervous and Mental Diseases* 153 (1971): 73–78; idem, "Hysteria, Hypnosis, Psychopathology," *Journal of Nervous and Mental Diseases* 161 (1975): 367–378; and Ola Anderson, *Studies in the Prehistory of Psychoanalysis: The Etiology of Psychoneuroses and Some Related Themes in Sigmund Freud's Scientific Writings and Letters, 1866–1896* (n.p.: Scandinavian University Books, 1962).

50. Micale, "Diagnostic Discrimination," 387. Micale adds, "Charcot's inspiration for the trauma came from a rather specialized medico-legal debate, originating outside France, over what was then called 'railway spine'" (79); Chertok adds, "In point of fact Charcot drew part of his inspiration from the Anglo-Saxon investigations (by Putnam, Page, etc.) on male hysteria resulting from railway accidents." "Hysteria," 369.

51. For a British perspective, see Lorraine J. Daston, "British Responses to Psycho-Physiology, 1860–1900," *Isis* 69 (1978): 192–208.

52. Shorter, *From Paralysis,* 176. Even Freud, who would later minimize the significance of somatic factors in psychic events, acknowledged the presence of organicity in his and Breuer's now-famous volume of 1895, *Studies on Hysteria.* As the editor points out, "Freud was devoting all of his energies to explaining mental phenomena in physiological and chemical terms. . . . It was not until 1905 [in his book on jokes, chapter 5] that he first explicitly repudiated all intention of using the term 'cathexis' in any but a psychological sense and all attempts at equating nerve-tracts or neurons with paths of mental association." In a note, the editor adds, "The insecurity of the neurological position which Freud was still trying to maintain in 1895 is emphasized by the correction he felt obliged to make thirty years later in the very last sentence of the book. In

1895 he used the word, '*Nervensystem*' ('nervous system'); in 1925 he replaced it by '*Seelenleben*' ('mental life')." Freud and Breuer, *Studies on Hysteria*, xxiv.

53. Page himself had been aware of Charcot's early work on hysteria, but he seemed to have been oblivious to the physiological significance the French neurologist attached to the disease. Moreover, at the time when Page had first read Charcot, Charcot had neither written a single word on the topic of male hysteria nor begun his investigation of hypnotism. In the single reference that Page made to the French master's work, he cited Charcot's assertion concerning the elusive nature of certain hysterical symptoms and the fact that many patients were themselves "quite surprised when [their] existence is revealed to them" (*Lectures on Nervous Diseases*, 1877). Like the numerous citations he provided from other medical authorities, the passage that Page quotes from Charcot's work was used primarily to reinforce Page's central argument concerning the specious nature of Erichsen's doctrines.

54. Jean-Martin Charcot, *Lectures of Localization in Diseases of the Brain* translated by E. P. Fowler (New York: William Wood, 1878), preface.

55. The source of Charcot's interest in hypnotism is commonly believed to be an 1875 article, "The Somnambulistic Provocation," by Charles Richet, in which Richet argues that hypnosis involves physiological changes in the nervous system and is itself a form of neurosis (Charles Richet, "Du somnabulisme provoqué," *Journal de l'anatomie et de le physiologie normales et pathologiques de l'homme et des animaux* 2 [1875]: 348–377). See Levin, "Freud's Paper," 50. For a brief summary of Charcot's views on hypnotism, see Jerome M. Schneck, "Jean-Martin Charcot and the History of Experimental Hypnosis," *Journal of the History of Medicine and Allied Sciences* 16 (1961): 297–300. Schneck contrasts Charcot's interest in the experimental uses of hypnosis with Bernheim's focus on its potential therapeutic value. For a discussion of the popular perception of hypnosis in France, see Robert G. Hillman, "A Scientific Study of Mystery: The Role of the Medical and Popular Press in the Nancy-Salpêtrière Controversy on Hypnotism," *Bulletin of the History of Medicine* 39 (1965): 163–182. Hillman asserts that the controversy between Charcot and Bernheim made "hypnotism a subject of general knowledge" (173).

56. Sulloway contends that the study of hypnotism was "a bold step in his medical career, since in France, as elsewhere, the whole subject had been in considerable scientific disrepute for almost a century [ever since the debates over mesmerism in the 1780s]. Four years later, in 1882, Charcot delivered a paper on hypnotism at the *Academie des Sciences* in which he personally endorsed the phenomenon of hypnotism." The paper, Sulloway continues, brought about a "complete reversal within France of the negative attitude in official science toward mesmerism or 'animal magnetism'—a subject that the *Academie des Sciences* itself had twice formally condemned" (30).

57. See Levin, "Freud's Paper," 384–385. Freud, who had recently visited with Charcot, charged that Charcot's school "speaks therefore, of the physical or physiological phenomena of hypnosis." As quoted in Levin; Sigmund Freud, "Preface to the Translation of Bernheim's *Suggestion*," *Complete Psychological Works* 1:77.

58. Shorter, *From Paralysis*, 176.

59. In his dissertation Micale provides an excellent summary of the treatment of male hysteria prior to Charcot's reassessment of the issue in the 1880s. For an excellent general treatment of the history of hysteria, see Veith, *Hysteria*.

60. Micale, "Charcot," 370.

61. Ibid., 370.

62. Micale, "Diagnostic Discrimination," 85.

63. Micale, "Charcot," 385. In his dissertation Micale asserts, "Charcot's inspiration for the trauma came from a rather specialized medico-legal debate, originating outside France, over what was then called 'railway spine'" (79).

64. J.-M. Charcot, *Clinical Lectures on Certain Diseases of the Nervous System*, trans. E. P. Hurt (Detroit: George S. Davis, 1888), 99.

65. Ibid., 99.

66. Ibid., 100.

67. My analysis here follows from Micale, "Charcot," 387–390.

68. Charcot (1888). Charcot cites the work of Putnam, Walton, Page, Oppenheim, and Thomsen in support of his doctrines.

69. Quotation from Micale, "Charcot," 394, citing Charcot's *Leçons du Mardi* 2, lesson 15, 352.

70. For an extensive discussion of hysterical symptoms, see Daniel Hack Tuke's *Dictionary of Psychological Medicine* (Philadelphia: P. Blakiston, Son, 1892), 618–627. In his discussion of male hysteria, Tuke noted, "The difficulty of diagnosis is much increased by the frequent occurrence of purely fraudulent imitation of such cases" (625).

71. Micale makes the point that Charcot's neurological conception of hysteria was a blow to gynecologists, alienists, and obstetricians. See "Diagnostic Discrimination."

72. As quoted in Trimble, *Post-Traumatic Neurosis*, 45 (italics in original).

73. Anderson, *Studies in the Prehistory of Psychoanalysis*, 59.

74. Micale provides an excellent discussion of this resistance in his dissertation. He devotes the final section of his work to what he terms a "speculative" analysis of the "internal resistance" to the concept of masculine hysteria.

75. For a provocative treatment of the British reaction to female hysteria, see Showalter, *Female Malady*, 145–167.

76. Philip Coombs Knapp, "Nervous Affections Following Railway and Allied Injuries," in *Text Book on Nervous Disease by American Authors*, ed. Francis X. Dercum (New York: Lea Brothers, 1895), 159.

77. Landon Carter Gray, discussion following Dercum's paper, "Two Cases of 'Railway-Spine' with Autopsy," *Transactions of the American Neurological Association* 21 (1896): 43.

78. Philip Coombs Knapp, "Nervous Affections Following Railway Injury ('Concussion of the Spine,' 'Railway Spine,' and 'Railway Brain')," *Boston Medical and Surgical Journal* 119 (1888): 422. He cites Westphal's "Three Cases of Railway Spine Thought to be due to Minute Hemorrhages."

79. For a discussion of Oppenheim's views, see Clevenger, *Spinal Concussion*, 77–117, and "Recent View on 'Railway Spine,'" *Boston Medical and Surgical Journal* 115 (1886): 286–287.

80. H. Oppenheim, *Diseases of the Nervous System,* trans. Edward E. Mayer (Philadelphia: J. B. Lippincott, 1900), 741. Emphasis in original.

81. For a succinct biographical summary of Knapp's professional accomplishments, see *Dictionary of American Medical Biography: Lives of Eminent Physicians of the United States and Canada, from the Earliest Times,* ed. Howard A. Kelly and Walter L. Burrage (Boston: Milford House, 1971), 708-709.

82. Knapp, "Nervous Affections" (1888), 421.

83. Knapp, "Nervous Affections" (1895), 136.

84. Landon Carter Gray, "Traumatic Neurasthenia," *International Clinics* 2 (1893): 144-150.

85. F. X. Dercum, "The Back in Railway Spine," *American Journal of Medical Sciences* 102 (1891): 264.

86. Edward Spitzka, "Spinal Injuries as a Basis of Litigation," *American Journal of Neurology and Psychiatry* (1883): 540-543.

87. Charles Dana, "Concussion of the Spine and Its Relation to Neurasthenia and Hysteria," *Medical Record* 26 (1884): 617.

88. I do not mean to suggest that scientific issues can ever be fully divorced from social and cultural circumstances. But the degree of their attachment is not always constant. While there is a good deal to be said for work that emphasizes the often-symbiotic relationship between science and culture, it is platitudinous and often incorrect to make too much of the supposed false dichotomy between the two realms. While some "science" is no doubt very much a part of the underlying culture that produces it, not all "science" is necessarily so.

89. Brown, "Regulating Damage Claims," 424.

90. Clevenger, *Spinal Concussion,* 207.

91. Brown, "Regulating Damage Claims," 428-430.

92. Harold N. Moyer, "The So-Called Traumatic Neurosis," *Railway Surgeon* 8 (1901-1902): 151.

93. Thomas G. Morton, "Some Medico-Legal Experiences in Railway Cases," *Journal of the American Medical Association* 21 (1893): 522.

94. John Punton, discussion following D. S. Fairchild's "Some Points in the Examination and Diagnosis of Traumatic Nerve Affections," *Railway Surgeon* 7 (1900-1901): 158.

95. Hugh Burford, "The Railway Surgeon as Medico-Legal Expert," *International Journal of Surgery* 11 (1898): 148.

96. D. R. Wallace "A Reply to Dr. Swearingen," *Railway Surgeon* 1 (1894-1895): 259.

97. Gary Y. Schwartz, "Tort Law and the Economy in Nineteenth-Century America: A Reinterpretation," *Yale Law Journal* 90 (July 1981): 1764.

98. Schwartz reports that "[in] California appellate opinions, one can detect two hundred forty-eight jury verdicts for plaintiffs, only twenty-six for defendants. In suits against railroads, the breakdown in verdicts is one hundred eleven to twelve. In New Hampshire after 1850, there were one hundred and forty-seven jury verdicts for plaintiffs, but only twenty-two for defendants. During the entire nineteenth century, in suits against towns for highway accidents, the jury verdict ratio was forty-one to nine; in all tort suits against the railroads, it was seventy-one to four." "Tort Law," 1764. See Richard A. Posner, "A Theory of Negligence," *Journal of Legal Studies* 1 (January 1972): 92; Friedman, *History of American Law,* 2d ed., 471. "Uppermost in the minds of both judges and lawyers of the time," Malone explains, "was a seething, although somewhat

covert, dissatisfaction over the part they felt the jury was destined to play in these cases against corporate defendants." Web Malone, "The Formative Era of Contributory Negligence," in *Tort Law in American History*, ed. and introd. Kermit L. Hall (New York: Garland, 1987): 300.

99. "Possibly," speculates Schwartz, "upper-class judges felt no sympathy for injured blue-collar workers." Schwartz, "Tort Law," n. 399, 1771; Friedman, *History of American Law*, 470; See Morton J. Horwitz, *The Transformation of American Law, 1870–1960: The Crisis of Legal Orthodoxy* (New York: Oxford University Press, 1992), 57–59, 113–116, 123–143. Not all legal historians share this interpretation, however. After reviewing more than 1,500 appellate cases from 1875 to 1905, Posner writes, "I discern no systematic bias in the law of negligence as it was applied between 1875 and 1905 in favor of industrial growth and expansion, except insofar as the efficient use of resources may be thought to foster, or perhaps to be the equivalent of, economic development. The common law seems to have been fairly evenhanded in its treatment of the claims of victims and injurers." "Theory of Negligence," 73.

100. See J. Barculo, *Haring* v. *New York and Erie R.R.*, 13 Barb. 2, 15 (N.Y. 1853).

101. The distinction that nineteenth-century American judges made between injured workers and injured passengers is a subject that demands more serious intention than I can offer in this brief summary. Posner explains this distinction by arguing, "[The] rule that common carriers owed a higher duty to their passengers signifies that passengers expect (and are willing to pay for) a high level of safety—because the railroad has a comparative advantage in accident prevention (indeed, passengers are normally helpless to avert an accident) and because a collision or derailment (like a plane crash today) is likely to kill or seriously injure them." "Theory of Negligence," 38; Schwartz adds: "Because the high speeds of the new railroads created 'hazards to life and limb,' and because railroads were 'entrusted [with] the lives and safety' of their passengers the New Hampshire Supreme Court held railroads liable to passengers for 'even the smallest neglect.'" "Tort Law," 1743. Also see Licht, *Working for the Railroad*, 197.

102. "The railway does not owe a like duty to its passengers, to its servants, to persons who are rightfully upon public highways which adjoin or cross its lines, to persons who come upon its line or premises as mere licensees, and to persons who trespass upon its line or premises." Christopher Stuart Patterson, *Railway Accident Law: The Liability of Railways for Injuries to the Person* (Philadelphia: T. and J. W. Johnson and Co., 1886), 2–3.

103. R.R.R. v. Derby, 14 Howard 468, as quoted in Patterson, *Railway Accident Law*, 232; contrast this view to Patterson's claim that "railways do not warrant to their servants the safe condition of their line, nor the security of their appliances and machinery, and they guarantee only that due care shall be used in constructing and in keeping in repair, and in operating the line, appliances and machinery" (300).

104. Henry Hollingsworth Smith, "Concussion of the Spine," *Journal of the American Medical Association* 13 (1888): 181.

105. For discussion of fraudulent cases, see Hodges, "So-Called Concussion," 387; Morton, "Some Medico-Legal Experiences," 520–525; C. J.

Cullingworth, "Fraudulent Damage Claims in Railroad Accidents," *The Medico-Legal Journal* 1 (1883–1884): 175–178; Pearce Bailey, "Simulation of Nervous Disorder Following Accidents," *Railway Surgery* 3 (1896–1897): 439–442; Herbert Judd, "The Medico-Legal Aspect of Concussion of the Spine," *Journal of the American Medical Association* 13 (1889): 188–194; L. Bremer, "A Contribution to the Study of Traumatic Neuroses (Railway Spine)," *Alienist and Neurologist* 10 (1889): 437–455.

106. James Syme, "On Compensation For Railway Injuries," *Lancet* (January 5, 1867): 2.

107. Judd, "The Medico-Legal Aspect," 188.

108. Erichsen, *On Railway and Other Injuries*, 97.

109. R. Harvey Reed, "The National Association of Railway Surgeons—Its Objects and Benefits," *Fort Wayne Journal of Medical Science* (later *Journal of the National Association of Railway Surgeons*) 1 (January 1889): 6.

110. For a complete list of the membership, see *Fort Wayne Journal of Medical Science* 2 (1889–1890): 442–446. There is a wide, albeit not well-organized, body of periodical literature that discusses the National Association of Railway Surgeons. Some of the more valuable sources are *Medico-Legal Journal*, 1–20; *Railway Age; Railway Surgeon: Official Journal of the National Association of Railway Surgeons* 1–9; and *International Journal of Surgery* 11 (1898). These volumes contain articles that focus on a host of issues and are the best source of information on railway spine from the perspective of the railroad industry itself.

111. B.A. Watson, "The Practical Relation of the So-Called 'Railway Spine' and the Malingerer," *Railway Age* 16 (1891): 214.

112. Milton Jay, discussion following Webb J. Kelly, "Not a Case of 'Railway Spine,'" *Journal of the American Medical Association* 24 (1895): 446–448.

113. Reed, "National Association of Railway Surgeons," 6.

114. Ibid., 8.

115. See William A. Hammond, "Certain Railway Injuries to the Spine in their Medico-Legal Relations," *Fort Wayne Journal of the Medical Sciences* 2 (1889–1890): 409–424; F. X. Dercum, "Railway Shock and Its Treatment," *Fort Wayne Journal of the Medical Sciences* 2 (1889–1890): 229–249; Pearce Bailey, "Simulation of Nervous Disorder Following Accidents," *Railway Surgery* 3 (1896–1897): 439–442; Pearce Bailey, "The Injuries Called Spinal: Their Relations to Railway Accidents," *Railway Surgery* 4 (1897–1898): 483–489; idem, "The Medico-Legal Relations of Traumatic Hysteria," *Railway Surgery* 5 (1898–1899): 555–559, 578–580.

116. For a succinct summary of Bell's accomplishments, see *Dictionary of American Biography*, 1:153–154.

117. Bell's speech was quoted in the *Boston Medical and Surgical Journal*, *Railway Surgeon*, and *Journal of the American Medical Association*, just to name a few.

118. Clark Bell, "Railway Spine," *Medico-Legal Journal* 12 (1894–1895): 133.

119. Ibid., 135.

120. Ibid., 137.

121. John E. Parsons, Esq., "Mental Distress as an Element of Damage

in Cases to Recover for Personal Injuries," in Allan McClane Hamilton and Lawrence Godkin, *A System of Legal Medicine* (New York: E. B. Treat, 1894), 2:385.

122. J. H. Greene, "Hypnotic Suggestion in Its Relation to the Traumatic Neuroses," *Railway Age* 17 (1892): 814.

123. Ibid.

124. For a succinct summary of Bernheim's views on suggestion and the controversy between him and Charcot, see Ellenberger, *Discovery of the Unconscious,* 85–89.

125. W. B. Outten, discussion following John Punton's "The Treatment of Functional Nervous Affection Due to Trauma," *Railway Surgeon* 4 (1897–1898): 31.

126. Outten, "Railway Injuries: Their Clinical and Medico-Legal Features," in *Medical Jurisprudence: Forensic Medicine and Toxicology,* ed. R. A. Witthaus and Tracy C. Becker (New York: William Wood, 1894), 591.

127. Ibid., 572 (emphasis added).

128. Ibid., 573.

129. Ibid., 591.

130. Quotation from R. M. Swearingen's "A Review of Dr. Wallace and the Railway Surgeons on Spinal Concussion," *Railway Surgeon* 1 (1894–1895): 254.

131. Outten, "Railway Injuries," 625.

132. David S. Booth, "The Neuropath and Railway Neuroses," *Railway Surgeon* 9 (1902–1903): 63.

133. R. S. Harnden, discussion following William Herdman's "Traumatic Neurasthenia (Railway Spine, Spinal Concussion): What Is It, and How Can It Be Recognized," *International Journal of Surgery* 11 (1898): 221.

134. George Ross, discussion following Booth, "Neuropath," 66.

135. See Silas Weir Mitchell, *Wear and Tear or Hints for the Overworked* (Philadelphia: J. B. Lippincott, 1872); idem, "Rest in Nervous Disease: Its Use and Abuse," in *A Series of American Clinical Lectures,* ed. E. C. Seguin (New York: G. P. Putnam's Sons, 1876); idem, *Fat and Blood: An Essay on the Treatment of Certain Forms of Neurasthenia and Hysteria,* 4th ed. (Philadelphia: J. B. Lippincott, 1888); and idem, "The Evolution of the Rest Treatment," *Journal of Nervous and Mental Disease* 31 (1904): 368–373.

136. For a historical perspective on the rest cure, see Smith-Rosenberg, "Hysterical Woman," 195–216; Charles E. Rosenberg and Carroll Smith-Rosenberg, "The Female Animal: Medical and Biological Views of Women and Her Role in Nineteenth-Century America," *Journal of American History* 60 (1973): 332–356; Ann Douglas Wood, "'The Fashionable Diseases': Women's Complaints and Their Treatment in Nineteenth-Century America," in *Clio's Consciousness Raised: New Perspectives in the History of Women,* ed. Mary S. Hartman and Lois Banner (New York: Octagon Books, 1976), 1–22; Suzanne Poirier, "The Weir Mitchell Rest Cure: Doctors and Patients," *Women's Studies* 10 (1983): 15–40; Susan E. Cayleff, "'Prisoners of Their Own Feebleness': Women, Nerves, and Western Medicine—A Historical Overview," *Social Science and Medicine* 26 (1988): 1199–1208; John S. Haller, Jr., "Neurasthenia: Medical Profession and Urban 'Blahs,'" *New York State Journal of Medicine*

473 (1970): 2489–2496; idem, "Neurasthenia: The Medical Profession and the 'New Woman' of the Late Nineteenth Century," *New York State Journal of Medicine* 474 (1971): 473–482; John S. Haller, Jr., and Robin M. Haller, *The Physician and Sexuality in Victorian America* (Urbana: University of Illinois Press, 1974): 2–43; T. Jackson Lears, *No Place of Grace: Anti-Modernism and the Transformation of American Culture, 1880–1920* (New York: Pantheon Books, 1981); and Tom Lutz, *American Nervousness, 1903: An Anecdotal History* (Ithaca: Cornell University Press, 1991).

137. John Punton, "The Functional Treatment of Nervous Affection Due to Trauma," *Railway Surgeon* 4 (1897–1898): 27.

138. Ibid., 28.

139. Outten, discussion following Booth, "Neuropath," 66.

140. John Eric Erichsen, letter to the editor, *Texas Sanitarian* 3 (1894): 448–449.

Chapter 3

1. Shorter, *From Paralysis*, 201–232.

2. Despite Beard's contribution to American neurology, his life work has failed to arouse the interest of any potential biographer. Several insightful articles contain interesting bits and scraps about his life. A good place to start is with Charles Dana, "Dr. George M. Beard: A Sketch of His Life and Character, with Some Personal Reminiscences," *Archives of Neurology and Psychiatry* 10 (1923): 427–435. For more recent examples, see Charles E. Rosenberg, "George M. Beard and American Nervousness," in *No Other Gods: On Science and American Social Thought* (Baltimore: Johns Hopkins University Press, 1976), 98–108; Barbara Sicherman, "The Use of Diagnosis," 33–54; Eric T. Carlson, "George Beard and Neurasthenia," in *Essays on the History of Psychiatry,* ed. Edwin R. Wallace IV and Lucius C. Pressley (Columbia: W. S. Hall Psychiatric Institute, 1980), 50–57.

3. E. H. Van Deusen, "Observation on a Form of Nervous Prostration (Neurasthenia) Culminating in Insanity," *American Journal of Insanity* 25 (1868–1869): 445–461. Van Deusen's role in the discovery of neurasthenia was frequently overlooked by Beard's neurological colleagues. This neglect generated considerable frustration among members of the AMSAII. C. H. Hughs, writing in an 1880 issue of the *Alienist and Neurologist* made it a point to credit Van Deusen's "original" paper: "In this instance, as in many others, the medical superintendents of the hospitals for the insane, in this country, have anticipated the profession outside of them in important contributions of clinical medicine." "Notes on Neurasthenia," *Alienist and Neurologist* 1 (1880): 439.

4. Van Deusen, "Observation," 445.

5. Ibid., 445.

6. George M. Beard, "Neurasthenia, or Nervous Exhaustion," *Boston Medical and Surgical Journal* 3 (1869): 218.

7. W. A. McClain, "The Psychology of Neurasthenia," *Medical Record* 48 (1895): 81–83.

8. See Nathan G. Hale, Jr., *James Jackson Putnam and Psychoanalysis* (Cambridge, Mass.: Harvard University Press, 1971), and Bonnie Ellen Blustein, *Preserve Your Love for Science: Life of William Alexander Hamilton, American Neurologist* (Cambridge: Cambridge University Press, 1991); also see Rosenberg, "George Beard," 98.

9. McClain, "Psychology of Neurasthenia," 81–83.

10. See George Cheyne, *The English Malady: or, A Treatise of Nervous Diseases of All Kinds* (London: Wisk, Ewing, and Smith, 1733).

11. Edward Cowles, "The Mechanism of Insanity," *American Journal of Insanity* 48 (1890–1891): 55.

12. J. S. Greene, "Neurasthenia: Its Causes and Its Home Treatment," *Boston Medical and Surgical Journal* 109 (1883): 76.

13. In many respects, Beard's class-conscious conception of neurasthenia resembled a disease described by George Cheyne in his 1733 treatise, *The English Malady*. As Roy Porter explains, "[N]ervous diseases were thus class-specific, affecting the cream, refined and delicate spirits, high flyers, those explained Cheyne, 'who have a great deal of sensibility, are quick thinkers, feel pleasure and pain the most readily, and are of the most lively imagination.'" Porter, *Mind Forg'd in Manacles,* 84.

14. Marrs, *Confessions,* 2.

15. McClain, "Psychology of Neurasthenia," 81–83.

16. Barbara Sicherman, *The Quest for Mental Health in America, 1880–1917* (New York: Arno Press, 1980), 175. Not all historians share this appraisal. Anson Rabinbach contends, "Clearly, fatigue was perceived as *both* a physical and a moral disorder—a sign of weakness and the absence of will." *The Human Motor: Energy, Fatigue, and the Origins of Modernity* (New York: Basic Books, 1990), 38–39. Rabinbach's use of the passive voice is problematic, however. Perceived by whom? As the above quotations make evident, many, in fact, regarded fatigue as a virtue of sorts—it implied that one was a hardworking "brain worker." See Haller, "Neurasthenia," 2489.

17. Beard, *Practical Treatise,* 81.

18. Paul Dubois, *The Psychic Treatment of Nervous Disorders,* trans. William Alanson White and Smith Ely Jelliffe (New York: Funk and Wagnalls, 1904), 18.

19. George Beard, *American Nervousness: Its Causes and Consequences, a Supplement to Nervous Exhaustion (Neurasthenia),* introd. Charles E. Rosenberg (New York: G. P. Putnam's Sons, 1881; New York: Arno Press, 1972), vi–vii.

20. Annie Payson Call, *Power Through Repose* (Boston: Roberts Brothers, 1891), 13.

21. George M. Beard, "Certain Symptoms of Nervous Exhaustion," *Virginia Medical Monthly* 5 (1878): 184.

22. Regarding the European context, Edward Shorter maintains, "The disease represented a way of bringing into the office of the nerve doctor rather than internists the lucrative clientele of middle-class businessmen." *From Paralysis,* 224.

23. Typically, the word *sex,* rather than the word *gender,* is used to denote

the "biological" rather than the "cultural" dimensions of various issues concerning the differences between males and females. Such a distinction, while certainly not arbitrary, nonetheless remains problematic. As Thomas Laqueur explains, "[On] the basis of historical evidence . . . almost everything one wants to *say* about sex—however sex is understood—already has in it a claim about gender." "So-called biological sex," Laqueur adds, "does not provide a solid foundation for the cultural category of gender, but constantly threats to subvert it." *Making Sex: Body and Gender from the Greeks to Freud* (Cambridge, Mass.: Harvard University Press, 1990), 11, 124.

24. For a discussion of the doctrine of separate spheres, see Rosalind Rosenberg, *Beyond Separate Spheres: The Intellectual Origins of Modern Feminism* (New Haven: Yale University Press, 1982).

25. Cowles, "The Mechanism of Insanity," 249.

26. H. C. Sharpe, "Neurasthenia and Its Treatment," *Journal of the American Medical Association* 32 (1899): 72. "To place a woman outside of a domestic setting, to train a woman to think and feel 'as a man,'" Carroll Smith-Rosenberg notes, "violated virtually every late-Victorian norm. It was literally to take her outside of conventional structures and social arrangements." "The New Women as Androgyne: Social Disorder and Gender Crisis, 1870–1936," in *Disorderly Conduct: Visions of Gender in Victorian America* (New York: Alfred A. Knopf, 1985), 252.

27. Lears, *No Place of Grace*, 51.

28. Beard, *American Nervousness*, 20.

29. J.S. Jewell, "Nervous Exhaustion, or Neurasthenia, in Its Bodily and Mental Relations," *Journal of Nervous and Mental Diseases* 6 (1879): 47.

30. Donald Meyer, *The Positive Thinkers: Religion as Pop Psychology from Mary Baker Eddy to Oral Roberts* (New York: Pantheon Books, 1965), 24.

31. Beard, *American Nervousness*, 10.

32. Beard, "Certain Symptoms," 182.

33. Thomas Stretch Dowse, *On Brain and Nerve Exhaustion (Neurasthenia) and on the Exhaustion of Influenza* (London: Bailliere, Tindall and Cox, 1892), 2.

34. John P. Savage, "Hints on Nervous Exhaustion (Neurasthenia)," *Cincinnati Lancet and Clinic* (1880): 153.

35. A.D. Rockwell, "Electricity in Neurasthenia and Other Functional Neuroses," *International Clinics* 2 (1891): 283.

36. C.P. Hughs, "Notes on Neurasthenia," *Alienist and Neurologist* 1 (1880): 439.

37. Louis Faugeres Bishop, "A Study of the Symptomatology of Neurasthenia in Women," *Medical News* 71 (1897): 71.

38. W.R. Gowers, *Diseases of the Nervous System* (Philadelphia: P. Blakiston, Son, 1889), 1341–1342. Emphasis in original.

39. Philip Coombs Knapp, "The Nature of Neurasthenia and Its Relation to Morbid Fears and Imperative Ideas," *Boston Medical and Surgical Journal* 135 (1896): 410.

40. Both Erwin Ackerknecht and Charles E. Rosenberg point out that the discovery of neurasthenia was partially attributable to interaction with a particular type of patient. Unlike asylum superintendents who saw predominantly in-

curable patients, Beard came across a number of men and women with whom he could work, and who appeared to benefit from medical intervention. See Ackerknecht, *A Short History of Psychiatry,* 2d ed. (New York: Hafner, 1968), 95, and Rosenberg, "George Beard," 98.

41. Henri Ellenberger attributes the first modern psychotherapeutic exploitation of the healer-patient rapport to Mesmer. "This term was used from the beginning by Mesmer and was handed down by generations of magnetizers and hypnotists to the beginning of the twentieth century while the concept was gradually being developed and perfected." Ellenberger, *Discovery of the Unconscious,* 152.

42. Russell C. Maulitz, " 'Physician versus Bacteriologist': The Ideology of Science in Clinical Medicine," in *The Therapeutic Revolution: Essays in the Social History of American Medicine,* ed. Charles E. Rosenberg and Morris J. Vogel (Philadelphia: University of Pennsylvania Press, 1970), 94–96.

43. John Harley Warner, *The Therapeutic Perspective: Medical Practice, Knowledge, and Identity in America, 1820–1885* (Cambridge, Mass.: Harvard University Press, 1986), 264; Maulitz makes the important point that " 'science,' in medicine, came to mean different things to different people." " 'Physician versus Bacteriologist,' " 104.

44. Martin S. Pernick, *A Calculus of Suffering: Pain, Professionalism, and Anesthesia in Nineteenth-Century America* (New York: Columbia University Press, 1985), 311 n.93; Warner, *The Therapeutic Perspective,* 247.

45. Pernick, *Calculus,* 143. Warner explains that "[the] movement in therapeutics from empiricism and specificity toward rationalism and universalism was accompanied by a growing belief that the quest for invariant therapeutic laws had again become a legitimate enterprise." Warner, *The Therapeutic Perspective,* 250.

46. See Gosling, *Before Freud.*

47. Warner, *The Therapeutic Perspective,* 250; Pernick, *Calculus,* 135–146.

48. Neurasthenic discourse is by no means the only example of this phenomena. An 1882 article, appearing in the *Boston Medical and Surgical Journal,* asserted that "[no] two patients have the same constitution or mental proclivities. No two instances of typhoid fever, or of any other disease, are precisely alike. The intelligent and efficient care of any case of illness demands a consideration of all the circumstances which are peculiar to itself and of the traits of the body and mind which are peculiar to the patient." "Routine Practice," *Boston Medical and Surgical Journal* 108 (1883): 42–43, quoted in Pernick, *Calculus,* 144.

49. T.W. Fisher, "Neurasthenia," *Boston Medical and Surgical Journal* 9 (1872): 72.

50. Howell T. Pershing, "The Treatment of Neurasthenia," *Colorado Medical Journal* 1 (1903–1904): 83.

51. Pritchard, "The American Disease," 19.

52. McClain, "Psychology of Neurasthenia," 81–83.

53. For an excellent and nuanced discussion of medical conservatives who championed the role accorded to the individual, see Pernick, *Calculus,* 135–141.

54. Warner, *The Therapeutic Perspective*, passim.

55. The significance that physicians attached to doctor-patient rapport was by no means confined to neurasthenia and other functional nervous diseases. It applied to various organic and structural diseases as well.

56. Pritchard, "The American Disease," 19–20.

57. John Punton, "Modern Aspects of Neurasthenia and Its Treatment," *Texas Journal of Medicine* 1 (1905–1906): 203.

58. William Harvey King, "Some Points in the Treatment of Neurasthenia," *Transactions of the American Homeopathic Association* (1901): 493. It is tempting to make more of King's phallic metaphor than he doubtless intended.

59. James Jackson Putnam, "Remarks on the Psychical Treatment of Neurasthenia," *Boston Medical and Surgical Journal* 132 (1895): 506.

60. Jeanne Cady Solis, "The Psychotherapeutics of Neurasthenia," *Physician and Surgeon* 27 (1905): 315.

61. William Broaddus Pritchard, "The American Disease: An Interpretation," *Canadian Journal of Medicine and Surgery* 18 (1905): 12.

62. Beard, *Practical Treatise*, 12.

63. Beard, *American Nervousness*, 276.

64. Cowles, "The Mechanism," 209.

65. Anna Hayward Johnson, "Neurasthenia," *Philadelphia Medical Times* (1881): 738.

66. Rabinbach, *The Human Motor*, 162.

67. The impact of alternative healing, and more particularly of the American mind cure movement, on the regular medical community is the subject of my next chapter. See Putnam, "Remarks," *Boston Medical and Surgical Journal* 132 (1895): 505.

68. Morton Prince, discussion following Putnam, "Remarks," 517.

69. Susan Leigh Star mistakenly attributes the wide array of somatic therapies designed to treat various nervous disorders to what she refers to as diagnostic uncertainty. "Clinicians responding to diagnostic uncertainty," she writes, "were forced to treat each patient with a wide variety of therapies. In the absence of simple testing procedures or pathognomonic signs, they had only the hope that by giving patients a number of different therapies one would succeed. Patients at Queen Square were massaged, electrified, and given steam baths and mud plaster, potassium bromide, 'metallotherapy' (an obscure treatment that involved placing metal disks over different parts of the body), and even leeches." Star, *Regions of the Mind: Brain Research and the Quest for Scientific Certainty* (Stanford: Stanford University Press, 1989), 76. What Star fails to appreciate is that for late-nineteenth-century physicians, even diagnostic certainty rarely inspired therapeutic certainty. It was rare indeed that the realm of diagnostics might affect the realm of treatment. In fact, the response to therapy was, and often still is, a key factor in diagnosis.

70. William F. Hutchinson, "Three Typical Cases of Neurasthenia," *Medical Record* 18 (1880): 399.

71. McClain, "The Psychology of Neurasthenia," 81–83.

72. A.D. Rockwell, "Neurasthenia and Its Relation to Other Disease," *Medical Record* 51 (1897): 307–310 (emphasis in original). For a contrary view,

see Ann Hayward Johnson, who contends, "The importance of making a correct differential diagnosis between functional and organic nervous disease cannot be overestimated. In general, prognosis and treatment are directly opposite." "Neurasthenia," 740.

73. Beard, "Neurasthenia, or Nervous Exhaustion," 217.

74. Rosenberg, "George Beard," 104.

75. Hale, *Freud and the Americans,* 67.

76. See Susan E. Cayleff, *Wash and Be Healed: The Water-Cure Movement and Women's Health* (Philadelphia: Temple University Press, 1987); for an excellent survey of the history of baleonology, see Roy Porter, ed., *The Medical History of Water and Spas* (London: Wellcome Institute for the History of Medicine, 1990). For a more detailed discussion of water cure in the United States, see Jane B. Donegan, *"Hydropathic Highway to Health": Women and Water-Cure in Antebellum America* (Westport, Conn.: Greenwood Press, 1986); and M. S. Legan "Hydropathy, or the Water-Cure," in *Pseudo-Science and Society in Nineteenth-Century America,* ed. A. Wroebel (Lexington: University Press of Kentucky, 1987), 74–99.

77. L. Reuben, "Imaginary Disease," *Water-Cure Journal* (1850): 120, quoted in Cayleff, *Wash and Be Healed,* 64–65. Emphasis in original.

78. Bernard Sachs, "Functional Nervous Troubles: Neurasthenia, Its Occurrence in Young and Old, Symptomatology, and Treatment," *International Clinics* 1 (1891): 241.

79. Harold N. Moyer, "The Treatment of Neurasthenia," *Journal of the American Medical Association* 37 (1901): 1568.

80. Solis, "Psychotherapeutics of Neurasthenia," 312–316.

81. G. Manley Ransom, "Neurasthenia—Its Cure by Thermal Therapy," *Medical Record* 47 (1895): 366.

82. Putnam, "Neurasthenia and Its Treatment," 21.

83. Daniel R. Brower, "The Treatment of Neurasthenia," *Journal of the American Medical Association* 36 (1901): 232–235.

84. Putnam, "Neurasthenia and Its Treatment," 21.

85. H.C. Patterson, "Practical Experience in the Treatment of Neurasthenia," *Medical Times* 29 (1901): 360.

86. Wharton Sinkler, "Use of Hydrotherapy in Neurasthenia and Other Nervous Affections," *Therapeutic Gazette* 25 (1901): 590.

87. Beard, "Certain Symptoms," 184.

88. Rockwell, "Neurasthenia and Its Relation to Other Disease," 306.

89. For an exception, see Morton Prince, "The Educational Treatment of Neurasthenia and Certain Hysterical States," *Boston Medical and Surgical Journal* 139 (1898): 333.

90. John D. Quackenbos, "Causes and Recent Treatment of Neurasthenia," *New Hampshire Medical Society* (1897–1898): 97.

91. C.F. Hodge, "A Microscopic Study of Changes Due to Functional Activity in Nerve Cells," reprinted from *Journal of Morphology* 7 (1892): 112–113.

92. Ibid., 158–159. Emphasis in original.

93. References to Hodge's work may be found in the following articles: H.C. Patterson, "Practical Experience in the Treatment of Neurasthenia," *Medical Times* 29 (1901): 360–362; Campbell Meyers, "Neurasthenia in Some

of Its Relations to Insanity," *Canadian Medical Journal* 16 (1904): 89–94; Solis, "The Psychotherapeutics of Neurasthenia," 312–316; and Punton, "Modern Aspects of Neurasthenia, 201–205.

94. Robert T. Edes, "The New England Invalid," *The Shattuck Lecture 1895* (Boston: David Clapp and Son, 1895), 32.

95. Quackenbos, "Causes and Recent Treatment," 97.

96. Moses Allen Starr, "The Toxic Origins of Neurasthenia and Melancholia," *Medical Record* 59 (1901): 721.

97. J.G. Biller, "Treatment of Neurasthenia," *Journal of the American Medical Association* 38 (1902): 4–6.

98. Archibald Church, "Treatment of Neurasthenia," *Chicago Medical Recorder* 20 (1901): 324.

99. George Beard, *Sexual Neurasthenia (Nervous Exhaustion): Its Hygiene, Causes, Symptoms and Treatment*, 5th ed. (New York: E.B. Treat, 1900), 271.

100. Ibid., 255–272.

101. Dowse, *On Brain and Nerve Exhaustion*, 61.

102. Margaret Rowbottom and Edward Susskind, *Electricity and Medicine: History of Their Interaction* (San Francisco: San Francisco Press, 1984); idem, "Psychiatric Treatment During the Nineteenth Century," *Bulletin of the History of Medicine* 22 (1948): 156–177; and Harry S. Holcombe, "Electrotherapy," *Journal of the History of Medicine and Allied Sciences* 22 (1967): 180–182.

103. Holcombe, "Electrotherapy," 180.

104. Rowbottom and Susskind, *Electricity*, 71–89.

105. Ibid., 113.

106. George M. Beard and A.D. Rockwell, *A Practical Treatise on the Medical and Surgical Uses of Electricity* (New York: William Wood, 1867).

107. Rowbottom and Susskind, *Electricity*, 113.

108. As early as 1846, John Galt referred to the clinical use of electricity. See John Galt, *The Treatment of Insanity* (New York, 1846), and S. Weir Mitchell, G.R. Morehouse, and W.E. Keen, *Gunshot Wounds and Other Injuries of Nerves* (Philadelphia, 1864).

109. Beard, "Neurasthenia or Nervous Exhaustion," 218.

110. Francis B. Bishop, "The Cause of Some Cases of Neurasthenia, and Their Treatment by Electricity," *Transactions of the American Electro-Therapeutic Association* (1901): 331.

111. Daniel R. Brower, "Cerebral Neurasthenia, or Failure of Brain Power, with Special Reference to Electrotherapeutics," *Transactions of the American Electro-Therapeutic Association* (1901): 337.

112. Rockwell, "Electricity in Neurasthenia," 282.

113. Margaret A. Cleaves, "Franklinization as a Therapeutic Measure in Neurasthenia," *Journal of the American Medical Association* 27 (1896): 1043.

114. W.F. Robinson, "The Electrical Treatment of Certain Phases of Neurasthenia," *Journal of Nervous and Mental Disease* 20 (1893): 34.

115. Robinson, "Electrical Treatment," 38.

116. Putnam, "Neurasthenia and Its Treatment," 22.

117. W.B. Miller, "Static Electrical Treatment of Neurasthenia," *Galliard's Southern Medicine* 83 (1905): 26.

118. Gerald N. Grob explains, "Medical intervention reflected shared faith

between patient and physician that assumed it would be effective. The alternative belief in therapeutic nihilism was never seriously entertained, partly because physicians rejected an approach that might impair their social legitimacy, and partly because these patients and families eagerly sought treatment." *Mental Illness and American Society,* 122.

119. Van Deusen, "Observation," 457.

120. For examples of medication recommended to treat neurasthenia, see Van Deusen, "Observation," 445–461; Beard, "Neurasthenia, or Nervous Exhaustion," 217–219; Beard, "Cases of Hysteria," 438–451; and Dana, "On the Pathology," 57–62.

121. Savage, "Hints on Nervous Exhaustion," 153–154.

122. J. P. C. Foster, "Suggestive and Hypnotic Treatment of Neurasthenia," *Yale Medical Journal* 8 (1901–1902): 14–22.

123. Greene, "Neurasthenia," 78.

124. Patterson, "Practical Experience," 361.

125. Harold N. Moyer, "The Treatment of Neurasthenia," *Journal of the American Medical Association* 37 (1901): 1657.

126. Beard, *American Nervousness,* 313.

127. See Beard, "Neurasthenia, or Nervous Exhaustion," 217–219; idem, *American Nervousness,* 253–277; William A. Hammond, *Cerebral Hyperaemia: The Result of Emotional Strain or Emotional Disturbance, the So-called Nervous Prostration of Neurasthenia* (Washington: G. P. Putnam's Sons, 1878); Savage, "Hints on Nervous Exhaustion," 153–154; Johnson, "Neurasthenia," 737–744; Greene, "Neurasthenia," 75–78; Cowles, "The Mechanism," 49–70; 209–252; Sachs, "Functional Nervous Troubles: Neurasthenia," 237–246; Putnam, "Neurasthenia and Its Treatment," 17–28; Quackenbos, "Causes and Recent Treatment," 92–103; Landon Carter Gray, "Neurasthenia: Its Symptoms and Treatment," *Medical News* 75 (1899): 788–791; Carlin Phillips, "The Etiology and Treatment of Neurasthenia: An Analysis of Three Hundred and Thirty-three Cases," *Medical Record* 55 (1899): 413–422; Frederick A. McGrew, "Neurasthenia and the Rest Cure," *Journal of the American Medical Association* 34 (1900): 1466–1468; Church, "Treatment of Neurasthenia," 320–325; King, "Some Points," 493–506; Patterson, "Practical Experience," 360–361; Moyer, "The Treatment of Neurasthenia, 1656–1658; Brower, "The Treatment of Neurasthenia," 232–235; Biller, "Treatment of Neurasthenia," 4–6; S. Weir Mitchell, "The Evolution of the Rest Treatment," *Journal of Nervous and Mental Disease* 31 (1904): 368–373; Pershing, "The Treatment of Neurasthenia," 82–87; and Solis, "The Psychotherapeutics of Neurasthenia," 312–316.

128. Mitchell, "Rest in Nervous Disease."

129. For biographical information on Mitchell, see Ernest Earnest, *S. Weir Mitchell, Novelist and Physician* (Philadelphia: University of Pennsylvania Press, 1950); D. M. Rein, *S. Weir Mitchell as a Psychiatric Novelist* (New York: International Universities Press, 1952).

130. Mitchell, "The Evolution of the Rest Treatment," 372.

131. Sicherman, "The Use of a Diagnosis," 40.

132. Mitchell, "Rest in Nervous Disease," 84.

133. Ibid., 85.

134. Ibid., 102.

135. Patterson, "Practical Experience," 360.

136. My use of feminine pronouns stems largely from the fact that most, though not certainly not all, rest cure patients were women.

137. Mitchell, *Fat and Blood,* 58.

138. Ibid., 59.

139. Mitchell, "Rest in Nervous Disease," 61.

140. Ibid., 95.

141. Ibid., 96.

142. Ibid.

143. Quackenbos, "Causes and Recent Treatment," 98.

144. Ann Douglas Wood may be correct when she asserts that "Mitchell's treatment depended in actuality not so much on the techniques of rest and overfeeding, as on the commanding personality and charismatic will of the physician." " 'The Fashionable Diseases.' " Little evidence exists, however, which can support the claim that Mitchell himself subscribed to such a belief. Although Mitchell readily conceded the role of the physician's personality in his "cure," he went to great lengths to emphasize the somatic aspects of his therapy. A similarly misplaced claim can be found in the writing of Kenneth Levin. "Without using the term 'unconscious,' " Levin proclaims, "Mitchell makes extensive use of the concept." True enough. But in making such a claim, Levin must rely on an anachronistic reading of Mitchell's writings that neglects to take seriously Mitchell's self-professed somaticism. Levin, "S. Weir Mitchell."

145. Smith-Rosenberg, "The Hysterical Woman," 195–216.

146. She continues: "Though much has been made recently of the painful procedure of cauterization for female complaints, it was actually a common therapy for venereal disease. Male genitals were cauterized by the same complacent physicians who cauterized their female patients." See Regina Morantz-Sanchez, "The Lady and Her Physicians," in *Clio's Consciousness Raised: New Perspectives on the History of Women,* ed. Mary S. Hartman and Lois Banner (New York: Octagon Books, 1976), 44.

147. Bromberg, *The Mind of Man,* 204.

148. Mitchell, "The Evolution of the Rest Treatment," 373.

149. Prince, "The Educational Treatment," 334.

150. McGrew, "Neurasthenia and the Rest Cure," 1466.

151. Church, "Treatment of Neurasthenia," 323.

152. Patterson, "Practical Experience," 362.

153. Arthur E. Mink, "Neurasthenia, with Special Reference to the Best Mode of Treatment," *Medical Bulletin* (Philadelphia) 20 (1898): 466.

154. Pritchard, "The American Disease," 22.

155. H.V. Halbert, "The Management of Neurasthenia," *Clinique* (Chicago) 24 (1903): 494–495.

156. Pritchard, "The American Disease," 22.

157. Herbert J. Hall, "The Systematic Use of Work as a Remedy in Neurasthenia and Allied Conditions," *Boston Medical and Surgical Journal* 152 (1905): 30.

158. King, "Some Points in the Treatment of Neurasthenia," 493.

159. Gray, "Neurasthenia: Its Symptoms and Treatment," 790.

160. For examples of works that make this mistake, see Kuttner, "Nerves"; Bunker, "From Beard to Freud"; Wiener, "G. M. Beard and Freud"; and Levin, "S. Weir Mitchell," 168–173.

Chapter 4

1. William James, *The Varieties of Religious Experience: A Study in Human Nature* (New York: Collier Books, 1961), 89.

2. John F. Teahan, "Warren Felt Evans and Mental Healing: Romantic Idealism and Practical Mysticism in Nineteenth-Century America," *Church History* 48 (1979): 74; Richard Weiss, *The American Myth of Success: From Horatio Alger to Norman Vincent Peale* (New York: Basic Books, 1969), 195–196.

3. This phrase, explains Stewart W. Holmes, "is preferable to that of 'scientific materialism' because a thorough understanding of modern science certainly does not necessarily make one mechanistically or grossly materialistic in his evaluation of the life process." "Phineus Parkhurst Quimby: Scientist of Transcendentalism," *New England Quarterly* 17 (1944): 356.

4. Martin S. Pernick, "Back from the Grave: Recurring Controversies over Defining and Diagnosing Death in History," in *Death: Beyond Whole-Brain Criteria*, ed. Richard M. Zaner (Dordrecht: Kluwer, 1988), 49.

5. James Turner, *Reckoning with the Beast: Animals, Pain, and Humanity in the Victorian Mind* (Baltimore: Johns Hopkins University Press, 1980), 83, 106.

6. James, *Varieties*, 90. Writing of the differences between Christian Science and New Thought, Richard M. Huber declares, "Though to an outsider Christian Science and New Thought seem practically indistinguishable, they differ sharply in two areas. Christian Science is closely organized and rigidly centralized with a unified doctrine and an absolute discipline over its practice. In matters of faith, the absolute idealism of Christian Science denies the existence of matter and the reality of suffering. The New Thought movement consists of independent sects loosely organized and is unified very casually in doctrine. Centering authority in no book or person, it permits the individual to roam freely in the world's literature and to develop his own beliefs. In matters of faith, the restrained idealism of New Thought does not deny the existence of sickness, sin, and poverty, but asserts that these evils can be overcome by right thinking." Huber, *The American Idea of Success* (New York: McGraw-Hill, 1971), 130.

7. In 1896 Horatio Dresser explained, "[The] mental healing world is split into two camps,—those who consistently carry out the law of love and those whose motive it is to support their leader at any cost. Concerted treatment to ruin the prospects and the business of those who fearlessly and charitably publish the truth about that leader is now a widely known and most deplorable fact. People hesitate to tell what they know lest they become the object of this underhand and most pernicious practice. They fear for themselves and their

friends. And thus aspersions are cast on the whole society of earnest truth-seekers whose sole object it is to win and promulgate impersonal truth." *The Life,* Kansas City, 22 January 1896.

8. Hale, *James Jackson Putnam,* 11. In his study of the origins of psychoanalysis in the United States, Hale adds that while "the mind cure cults [probably] forced New England physicians to develop psychotherapy, they discouraged physicians elsewhere. . . . As late as 1910 the New England interest in psychotherapy, especially of a religious nature, was regarded as a regional aberration." *Freud and the Americans,* 122. See also Weiss, *The American Myth of Success,* 197; Fuller, *Americans and the Unconscious,* 51.

9. Gardner Murphy and Robert O. Ballou, eds., *William James on Psychical Research* (New York: Viking Press, 1960), 10.

10. Richard Dewey, "Mental Therapeutics in Nervous and Mental Diseases," *American Journal of Insanity* 57 (1900–1901): 676.

11. Robert T. Edes, "Mind Cures from the Standpoint of the General Practitioner," *Boston Medical and Surgical Journal* 151 (18 August 1904): 173–179.

12. Edward W. Taylor, "The Attitude of the Medical Profession Toward the Therapeutic Movement," *Boston Medical and Surgical Journal* 157 (26 December 1907): 844.

13. Nancy B. Sherman, "Has Suggestion a Legitimate Place in Therapeutics?" *Transactions of the Fifty-second Session of the American Institute of Homeopathy* (1896): 651.

14. W.F. Hartford "Subjective Therapeutics," *Medical Record* 54 (1898): 158–159, quoted in John S. Haller, *American Medicine in Transition, 1840–1910* (Urbana: University of Illinois Press, 1981), 144–145.

15. Weiss, *The American Myth of Success,* 199; see Donald Meyer, "William James as the Authority," in *The Positive Thinkers: Religion as Pop Psychology from Mary Baker Eddy to Oral Roberts* (New York: Pantheon Books, 1965), 315–324.

16. Sydney E. Ahlstrom, "Harmonial Religion Since the Late Nineteenth Century," in *A Religious History of the American People* (Garden City: Image Books, 1975), 2:528; Ann Braude, *Radical Spirits: Spiritualism and Women's Rights in Nineteenth-Century America* (Boston: Beacon Press, 1989), 185.

17. See Haller, *American Medicine in Transition,* 100–149; Catherine L. Albanese, *Nature Religion in America: From the Algonkian Indians to the New Age* (Chicago: University of Chicago Press, 1990); idem, "Physic and Metaphysic in Nineteenth-Century America: Medical Sectarians and Religious History," *Church History* 55 (1986): 489–502; and James C. Whorton, *Crusaders for Fitness: The History of American Health Reformers* (Princeton: Princeton University Press, 1982).

18. Albanese, *Nature Religion,* 123

19. In addition to previously cited sources, see J. Stillson Judah, *The History and Philosophy of the Metaphysical Movement in America* (Philadelphia: Westminster Press, 1967); Ronald L. Numbers and Rennie B. Schoepflin, "Ministries of Healing: Mary Baker Eddy, Ellen G. White, and the Religion of Health," in *Women and Health in America,* ed. Judith Walzer Leavitt (Madison: University

of Wisconsin Press, 1984): 376–389; Rennie B. Schoepflin, "Christian Science Healing in America," in *Other Healers: Unorthodox Medicine in America,* ed. Norman Gevitz (Baltimore: Johns Hopkins University Press, 1988), 192–214; David Harrell, *All Things Are Possible: The Healing and Charismatic Movement in Modern America* (Bloomington: Indiana University Press, 1975); and R. Laurence Moore, *In Search of White Crows: Spiritualism, Parapsychology, and American Culture* (New York: Oxford University Press, 1977).

20. Meyer, *Positive Thinkers,* 312.

21. Gail Thain Parker, *Mind Cure in New England from the Civil War to World War One* (Hanover: University of New England Press, 1973), 32.

22. Horatio Dresser, "The Mental Cure in Its Relation to Modern Thought," *Arena* 16 (1896): 135.

23. For a fascinating and humorous tale of one man's quest for health, see William Taylor Marrs, *Confessions of a Neurasthenic* (Philadelphia: F.A. Davis, 1908).

24. While there is at present no biography of Phineus Parkhurst Quimby, there are a number of sources that discuss his life. He is listed in *Dictionary of American Biography* 15:304–305. The first historical treatment of Quimby occurred just two decades after his death when Julius A. Dresser published *The True History of Mental Science: The Facts Concerning the Discovery of Mental Healing* (Boston: Geo. H. Ellis, 1887). The following year, Quimby's son George published a brief biographical sketch that appeared in the *New England Magazine* 6 (1888): 267–276. A decade later, Annetta Gertrude Dresser published *The Philosophy of P. P. Quimby: With Selections from His Manuscripts and Sketch of His Life* (Boston: Geo. H. Ellis, 1895). Also see Georgine Milmine, *Mary Baker G. Eddy: The Story of Her Life and the History of Christian Science* (New York: Doubleday, Page, 1909); Horatio Dresser provides a biographical sketch in *The Quimby Manuscripts Showing the Discovery of Spiritual Healing and the Origins of Christian Science,* ed. Horatio W. Dresser (New York: Thomas Y. Crowell, 1921); Frank Podmore, *Mesmerism and Christian Science: A Short History of Mental Healing* (London: Methuen, 1909); Horatio Dresser, *A History of the New Thought Movement* (New York: Thomas Y. Crowell, 1919). For more recent sources, see Bromberg, *The Mind of Man,* 141–147; Holmes, "Phineus Parkhurst Quimby," 356–380; Charles Braden, *Spirits in Rebellion: The Rise and Development of New Thought* (Dallas: Southern Methodist University Press, 1963). Robert Peel has written extensively on Quimby in his biography of Mary Baker Eddy, *Mary Baker Eddy: The Years of Discovery* (New York: Holt, Rinehart and Winston, 1966), 151–192, 297–300. Also see Stephen Gottschalk, *The Emergence of Christian Science in American Religious Life* (Berkeley: University of California Press, 1973), 104–112; Robert C. Fuller, *Mesmerism and the American Cure of Souls* (Philadelphia: University of Pennsylvania Press, 1982); Errol Stafford Collie, *Quimby's Science of Happiness: A Non-Medical Scientific Explanation of the Cause and Cure of Disease* (Marina del Rey, Calif.: DeVorss, 1980). For Quimby's personal writings, see Earvin Seale, ed., *Phineus Parkhurst Quimby: The Complete Writings,* 3 vols. (Marina del Rey, Calif.: Devorss, 1988).

25. As quoted in Weiss, *The American Myth of Success,* 199–200.

26. Daniel Drake, a professor at the Louisville Medical Institute, was among the earliest American physicians to attribute mesmerism's power to suggestion. See Drake's *Analytical Report of a Series of Experiments in Mesmeric Somniquism* (1844).

27. For examples of "respectable" mesmeric literature, see "Wonderful Physical Manifestation," *Atlantic Monthly* (August 1868); Aaron S. Hayward, *Vital Magnetic Cure: An Exposition of Vital Magnetism, and Its Application to the Treatment of Mental and Physical Disease* (Boston: William White, 1871), and Frederick T. Parson, *Vital Magnetism: Its Power Over Disease—A Statement of the Facts Developed by Men Who Have Employed this Agenda Under Various Names as Animal Magnetism, Mesmerism, Hypnotism, Etc., from the Earliest Times Down to the Present* (New York: Adams, Victor, 1877).

28. Alan Gauld, *A History of Hypnotism* (Cambridge: Cambridge University Press, 1992), 193.

29. See Signe Toksvig, *Emanuel Swedenborg: Scientist and Mystic* (Freeport: Books for Library Press, 1948); Ralph Waldo Emerson, "Swedenborg: or, the Mystic," in *Representative Men* (Joseph Simon Publisher): 59–94.

30. Whitney Cross asserts that "mesmerism led to Swedenborgianism, and Swedenborgianism to Spiritualism, not because of the degree of intrinsic relationship between their propositions but because of the assumptions according to which their American adherents understood them." See Cross, *The Burned-over District: The Social and Intellectual History of Enthusiastic Religion in Western New York, 1800–1850* (New York: Octagon Books, 1981), 342.

31. John Humphrey Noyes, *History of American Socialism* (Philadelphia: J. B. Lippincott, 1870), 538–539; Robert C. Fuller, *Alternative Medicine and American Religious Life* (New York: Oxford University Press, 1989), 52.

32. Emerson, "Swedenborg," 59–94.

33. Fuller, *Unconscious*, 189. For biographical details of Grimes, see *Dictionary of American Biography* 4:630–631.

34. Fuller, *Unconscious*, 189.

35. Fuller, *Alternative*, 52; see George Bush, *Mesmer and Swedenborg; Or, The Relation of the Development of Mesmerism to the Doctrines and Disclosures of Swedenborg* (New York: John Allen, 1847). For details on Bush's life, see *Dictionary of American Biography* 2:347.

36. Bush, *Mesmer and Swedenborg*, v.

37. Ibid., 17.

38. See Janet Oppenheim, *The Other World and Beyond: Spiritualism and Psychical Research in England, 1850–1914* (Cambridge: Cambridge University Press, 1985).

39. Fuller, *Mesmerism*, 1982.

40. Dresser, *The Quimby Manuscripts Showing the Discovery of Spiritual Healing and the Origins of Christian Science*, 1921.

41. Quimby, *Phineus Parkhurst Quimby: The Complete Writings*, 319.

42. Ibid., 250.

43. Horatio Dresser provides a biographical sketch in *The Quimby Manuscripts*. For a more recent edition, see *Phineus Parkhurst Quimby: The Complete Writings*.

44. Dresser, *The Quimby Manuscripts*, 69, 263.

45. Ibid., 591.

46. Ibid., 194.

47. Ibid., 277.

48. Dresser, *The Philosophy of P. P. Quimby*, 23.

49. Ibid., 46.

50. Ibid., 96.

51. Quimby, *Phineus Parkhurst Quimby: The Complete Writings*, 288.

52. Julia Anderson Root, *Healing Power of Mind: A Treatise on Mind-Cure, with Original Views on the Subject and Complete Instructions for Practice and Self-Treatment*, 2d ed. (Peoria: H.S. Hill, 1886), 161.

53. Warren Felt Evans, *Divine Law of Cure* (Boston: H.H. Carter, 1884), 9.

54. Although there is no formal biography of Warren Felt Evans, the most detailed study of his life was prepared by William J. Leonard and presented in a prominent New Thought periodical. See William J. Leonard, "Warren Felt Evans, M.D.," *Practical Ideals* 10 (September–October 1905): 1–16; (November 1905): 1–23; (December 1905): 9–26; and (January 1906): 10–26. For a more recent discussion, see *Dictionary of American Biography* 3:213–214; and Teahan, "Warren Felt Evans and Mental Healing."

55. In 1862 Evans published his first book of significant length, *The Celestial Dawn*, in which he endeavored to promote Swedenborg's views without making any direct reference to the Swedish mystic. The book generated considerable dissatisfaction among his fellow ministers, and within months of its publication, Evans left the Methodist church and formally joined Swedenborg's New Church. See Leonard, "Warren Felt Evans" (September–October), 8–9.

56. Leonard, "Warren Felt Evans" (November), 14.

57. Warren Felt Evans, *The Mental Cure, Illustrating the Influence of the Mind on the Body, Both in Health and Disease, and the Psychological Method of Treatment*, 7th ed. (Boston: Colby and Rich, 1869). Over the course of the next decade and a half, Evans would write five additional books on the subject of mental healing: *Mental Medicine* (Boston, 1872), *Soul and Body* (Boston: Colby & Rich, 1876), *The Divine Law of Cure* (Boston: H.H. Carter, 1884), *The Primitive Mind Cure* (Boston. H.H. Carter, 1885), and *Esoteric Christianity, and Mental Therapeutics* (H.H. Carter & Karrick, 1886). The last work was a text that outlined the central principles of his system.

58. Evans, *Mental Cure*, 318.

59. Ibid., 38.

60. See Edwin Clarke and L.S. Jacyna, *Nineteenth-Century Origins of Neuroscientific Concepts* (Berkeley: University of California Press, 1987).

61. Evans, *Mental Cure*, 223.

62. Warren Felt Evans, "The Mental-Cure," *Mind Cure and Science of Life* 1 (1885): 141. Emphasis in original.

63. Evans, *Divine Law*, 203. Emphasis in original.

64. Ibid., 161. Emphasis in original.

65. Edna Heidbreder, *Seven Psychologies* (Englewood Cliffs, N.J.: Prentice Hall, 1933), 45.

66. Ibid., 44; Edwin G. Boring, *A History of Experimental Psychology*, 2d ed. (New York: Appleton-Century-Crofts, 1950), 181.

67. Boring, *A History,* 173, 185

68. Heidbreder, *Seven Psychologies,* 48. For a brief history of the law, see Robert Young, "Association of Ideas," in *Dictionary of the History of Ideas,* 1:111–118.

69. A notable exception, Evans acknowledged, could be found in the writing of James Mill. "I know of no writer on mental science who gives to it anything like the importance that belongs to it except Mr. James Mill." Indeed, Evans cited extensively from Mill's *Analysis of the Phenomena of the Human Mind* (1829). Evans, *Divine Law,* 287.

70. Evans, *Divine Law,* 293 (emphasis in original). For a splendid analysis of this issue in the British medical context, see Michael J. Clark, " 'Morbid Introspection,' Unsoundness of Mind and British Psychological Medicine, c. 1830–c. 1900," in *The Anatomy of Madness,* ed. W. F. Bynum, Roy Porter, and Michael Shepard (London: Routledge, 1988), 3:71–101.

71. Evans, *Mental Cure,* 252.

72. Evans, *Divine Law,* 205.

73. Evans, *Mental Cure,* 269.

74. Ibid., 277.

75. Ibid., 279.

76. Evans's understanding of the "law of sympathy" derived from his reading of Herman Boerhaave (1668–1738). "Boerhaave relates that the pupils of a squint-eyed schoolmaster near Leyden, after a while, exhibited the same obliquity of vision." *Mental Cure,* 276.

77. Ibid., 276.

78. Ibid., 277.

79. Ibid., 271–272.

80. The literature on Christian Science is vast. Much of it is polemical. A voluminous historiography exists concerning the life and work of Mary Baker Eddy alone. For contemporary commentary see James Monroe Buckley, *Faith-Healing, Christian Science and Kindred Phenomena* (New York: Century, 1887); Frederick W. Peabody, "A Complete Exposé of Eddyism or Christian Science and the Plain Truth in Plain Terms Regarding Mary Baker G. Eddy, Founder of Christian Science," an address delivered at Tremont Temple, Boston, on August 1, 1901; William A. Purrington, *Christian Science: An Exposition of Mrs. Eddy's Wonderful Discovery, Including Its Legal Aspects: A Plea for Children and Other Helpless Sick* (New York: E. B. Treat, 1900); Georgine Milmine, *Mary Baker G. Eddy: The Story of Her Life and the History of Christian Science* (New York: Doubleday, Page, 1909), which first appeared in serial form in *McClure's Magazine* (1907–1908); Mark Twain, *Christian Science* (New York: Harper and Brothers, 1907); Lyman P. Powell, *Christian Science: The Faith and Its Founder* (New York: G. P. Putnam's Sons, 1907); Frank Podmore, *Mesmerism,* chapter 16; James H. Snowden, *The Truth about Christian Science: The Founder and the Faith* (Philadelphia: Westminster Press, 1920). For more recent treatment, the best place to start is Bromberg, *Mind of Man,* 145–158, and Peel, *Mary Baker Eddy;* also see Marian King, *Mary Baker Eddy: Child of Promise* (Englewood Cliffs, N.J.: Prentice Hall, 1968). For balanced appraisals, see Gottschalk, *The Emergence;* Julius S. Silberger, Jr., *Mary Baker Eddy: An Interpretive Biography of the Founder of Christian Science* (Boston: Little, Brown,

1980); Schoepflin, "Christian Science Healing in America," 192–214; and Cassedy, *Medicine in America*, 100–101.

81. Schoepflin, "Christian Science Healing in America," 197–200.

82. Numbers and Schoepflin, "Ministries of Healing," 379.

83. Mary Baker Eddy was married several times and changed her name on numerous occasions. Her name at birth was Mary Morse Baker. In 1843 she married George Washington Glover and became Mary Baker Glover. Glover died within the decade, and in 1853 she married Dr. Daniel Patterson and became Mary Baker Patterson—this was her name when she visited Quimby in 1862. She later divorced Patterson and changed her name back to Mary Morse Glover. Finally, in 1877 she married Asa Gilbert Eddy and became and remained Mary Baker Eddy for the rest of her life. For purposes of narrative clarity, I have chosen to refer to her as Mary Baker Eddy except in those instances in which chronology compels me to do otherwise.

84. "Mary Baker Eddy," 3:9.

85. Ibid., 9.

86. Podmore, *Mesmerism*, 253.

87. Ibid., 268.

88. Mary Baker Eddy was certainly not unique in claiming that her theories of healing were entirely original. Earlier in the century, Sylvester Graham made no mention of his debt to Broussais. In his six major books on the subject of mental healing, Evans made only a single reference to Quimby. It appears in his second book, *Mental Medicine* (1872), 209. Ellen White, the prophetess of Seventh Day Adventism, likewise boasted that her views of health reform were divinely ordained. Numbers and Schoepflin, "Ministries of Healing," 376–389.

89. Mary Baker Glover Eddy, *Science and Health* (Boston: W.F. Brown, 1875), 72, 413.

90. My discussion focuses exclusively on the original 1875 edition.

91. "Mary Baker Eddy," 10.

92. Eddy, *Science and Health*, 334.

93. Ibid., 4.

94. Ibid., 330.

95. Ibid.

96. Ibid., 358.

97. Ibid., 334, 344, 361.

98. Ibid., 34.

99. Podmore, *Mesmerism*, 272.

100. In 1886, Mrs. Eddy's former student, Edward G. Arens, established "the University of the Science of the Spirit," which charged a tuition of only $100. The *Mind Cure Journal* reported, "We regret very much to see the spirit of mammon and avarice figure so prominent a part with *some* of the so-called Christian Scientists. Our objection is not general but limited to a very few. I know that $100 is a stiff sum to charge those who desire to learn this science, but when '$300' are charged it is the most shameful extortion." "Christian Science or Mammon," *The Mind Cure and Science of Life* 1 (1885): 109. Also see Buckley, *Faith-Healing*, 247.

101. Buckley, *Faith-Healing*, 242.

102. Schoepflin, "Christian Science," 197–200.

103. Numbers and Schoepflin, "Ministries of Healing," 381.

104. Rosenberg, *Beyond Separate Spheres.*

105. An article appearing in the *Boston Post* declared, "Mind Cure is called a Boston craze: no other city has developed the system to such an extent, and probably in no other place are there so many disciples of mental healing; a system claiming so many adherents, and recognized so largely by eminent men, deserves to be better understood than it is at present by the majority of people." Quoted in "A Fair Statement," *Mind Cure and Science of Life* 1 (1885): 79.

106. Gottschalk speculates that Julius Dresser's return to Boston was in large measure inspired by his having received news of Mrs. Eddy's success.

107. "A Fair Statement," 180.

108. Root, *Healing Power,* 165–169.

109. Swarts's journal chronicled the increasing national interest in mental healing. An editorial reported that "Mrs. Julia A. Root and others are sweeping the Pacific coast. Dr. Sawyer is holding guard over the Northwest with his Metaphysical Institute at Milwaukee, Wisconsin. Mrs. Mary H. Plunkett, and aids are flashing light at Detroit, Michigan, with the Mental Science College. "Mental-Cure Sanitarium," *Mind Cure and Science of Life* 2 (1886): 183.

110. The *Christian Science Journal* was narrower in its focus.

111. A. J. Swarts, "Defeat the Bill," *Mind Cure and Science of Life* 1 (28 January 1886): 114.

112. A. J. Swarts, "Metaphysics or Mind Cure," *Mind Cure and Science of Life* 1 (1885): 26.

113. Ibid., 27.

114. When it finally ceased publication in 1888, Katie Swarts recommended that subscribers switch to the *Christian Science Journal.*

115. *Journal of Christian Science* (February 1885), quoted in *Mind Cure and Science of Life Magazine* 1 (1885): 171.

116. For an excellent discussion of the issues confronting American Protestant ministers during the late nineteenth century, see Jon H. Roberts, *Darwinism and the Divine: Protestant Intellectuals and Organic Evolution, 1859–1900* (Madison: University of Wisconsin Press, 1988); also see Gottschalk, *The Emergence,* 188.

117. Buckley, *Faith-Healing.*

118. Ibid., 290.

119. Schoepflin, "Christian Science," 206; Ronald L. Numbers, "The Fall and Rise of American Medicine," in *The Professions in American History,* ed. and introd. Nathan O. Hatch (Notre Dame: University of Notre Dame Press, 1988), 64.

120. Purrington, *Christian Science,* 3.

121. Gottschalk correctly points out that prior to the mid-1890s non-Christian Science mental healers had yet to organize themselves as an effective opposition to Mrs. Eddy's church. The term New Thought does not appear until the mid-1890s.

122. Charles Brodie Patterson, *What Is New Thought? The Living Way* (New York: Thomas Y. Crowell, 1913), 14.

123. Braden, *Spirits*, 12-13.

124. W.J. Coleville, "The Ethics of Mental Healing," *Metaphysical Magazine* 1 (1895): 76.

125. Leander Edmund Whipple, *The Philosophy of Mental Healing* (New York: Metaphysical, 1893), 134.

126. Henry Wood, *The New Thought Simplified: How to Gain Harmony and Health* (Boston: Lee and Shepard, 1903), 150.

127. Henry Wood, *Ideal Suggestion Through Mental Photography: A Restorative System for Home and Private Use Preceded by a Study of the Laws of Mental Healing*, 10th ed. (Boston: Lea and Shepard Publishers, 1893), 21.

128. Henry Wood, *The New Old Healing* (Boston: Lothrop, Lea and Shepard, 1908), 234.

129. Joseph L. Hasbroucke, "Popular Fallacies Concerning Mind Cure," *Metaphysical Magazine* 1 (1895): 228.

130. Henry Wood, *The New Thought Simplified: How to Gain Harmony and Health* (Boston: Lea and Shepard, 1903), 159.

131. Ralph Waldo Trine, *In Tune with the Infinite or Fullness of Peace, Power, and Plenty* (New York: Thomas Y. Crowell, 1897), 51.

132. Wood, *The New Thought Simplified*, 93.

133. Josephine Curtis Woodbury, "Christian Science and Its Prophetess," *Arena* 21 (1899): 570.

134. Eddy, *Science and Health*, 342.

135. Joseph L. Hasbroucke, "Popular Fallacies Concerning Mind Cure," *Metaphysical Magazine* 1 (1895): 227.

136. Coleville, "The Ethics of Mental Healing," 81.

137. Hippolyte Bernheim, *Suggestive Therapeutics: A Treatise on the Nature and Uses of Hypnotism* (New York: G.P. Putnam's Sons, 1895).

138. W.J. Coleville, "The Educational Uses of Mental Suggestion," *Metaphysical Magazine* 1 (1895): 353-363; J. Elizabeth Hotchkiss, "The New Psychology," *Metaphysical Magazine* 1 (1895): 377-390; B.J. Fowler, "Hypnotism and Mental Suggestion," *Arena* 6 (1892): 208-218; Shelby Mamaugh, "The Philosophy of Psycho-Therapeutics," *Metaphysical Magazine* 3 (1896): 269-275.

139. W.H. Holcombe, "The Power of Thought," *Transactions of the Institute of Homeopathy* (1888): 603.

140. Patterson, *What Is New Thought?* 90.

141. Root, *Healing Power*, 9.

142. Wood, *Ideal Suggestion*, 79.

143. Ibid., 20.

144. "Thomas Jay Hudson," *Dictionary of American Biography* 9 : 341-342.

145. Thomas J. Hudson, *The Law of Psychic Phenomenon: A Working Hypothesis for the Systematic Study of Hypnotism, Spiritism, Mental Therapeutics, Etc.* 17th ed. (Chicago: A. C. McClurg, 1899), 150.

146. "Thomas J. Hudson," *Dictionary of American Biography*, 9 : 341-342.

147. Hudson, *Psychic Phenomenon*, 177.

148. Thomas J. Hudson, *The Law of Mental Medicine; and the Correlation of the Facts of Psychology and Histology in Their Relation to Mental Therapeutics* (London: G. P. Putnam's Sons, 1904), vii.

149. Ibid., 11, 14.

150. Shelby Mumaugh, "The Philosophy of Psycho-Therapeutics," *Metaphysical Magazine* 3 (1896): 271–272.

151. Ibid., 275.

152. Wood, *The New Old Healing*, 233.

153. Haller, *American Medicine*, 143.

154. Regular physicians had long challenged the claims of the Spiritualists. But prior to the 1870s, their efforts to discredit the movement typically consisted of isolated attempts to expose examples of fraud and deceit. This situation changed during the 1870s when neurologists began their own campaign to discredit the movement. Members of this novel medical specialty rejected Spiritualists' claims that the phenomena of somnambulism and trance were attributable to supernatural forces. George Beard regarded Spiritualism as one of history's greatest delusions. His views were echoed by several of his Anglo-American neurological colleagues. William Alexander Hammond linked the "disease" to the female reproductive system and sought to discredit the entire movement by arguing that Spiritualism was itself a form of mental illness In Great Britain, Henry Maudsley argued that belief in Spiritualism was the product of an inherited constitutional defect in the nerves and brain. See also George M. Beard, "The Psychology of Spiritualism," *North American Review* (July 1879): 75; William Alexander Hamilton, *The Physics and Physiology of Spiritualism* (New York: Appleton, 1871); and idem, *Spiritualism and Allied Causes of Nervous Derangement* (New York: G. P. Putnam's Sons, 1876). In addition, see Edward M. Brown "Neurology and Spiritualism in the 1870s," *Bulletin of the History of Medicine* 57 (1983): 563–577; S. E. D. Shortt, "Physicians and Psychics: The Anglo-American Medical Response to Spiritualism, 1870–1890," *Journal of the History of Medicine and Allied Sciences* 39 (1984): 339–355. For a comparative analysis of the situation in France, see Goldstein, *Console and Classify*, 257–263, 273.

155. Dresser, *History of New Thought*, 147.

156. T. L. Brown, "Metaphysical Healing versus Mental Science," *Transactions of the Institute of Homeopathy* (1886): 366–369.

157. Laura G. V. Mackie, "Psychotherapy, Its Use and Abuse," *Woman's Medical Journal* 19 (1909): 23.

158. Eliza Calvert Hall, "Mental Science and Homeopathy," *Metaphysical Magazine* 7 (1898): 350.

159. Eliza Calvert Hall, "The Evolution of Mental Science," *Metaphysical Magazine* 14 (1901): 174.

160. See William A. Purrington, *A Review of Recent Legal Decisions Affecting Physicians, Dentists, Druggists, and the Public Health together with a Brief for the Prosecution of Unlicensed Practitioners of Medicine, Dentistry, Pharmacy, with a Paper Upon Manslaughter, Christian Science and the Law and Other Matters* (New York: E. B. Treat, 1899); Samuel L. Baker, "Physician Licensure Laws in the United States, 1865–1915," *Journal of the History of Medicine and Allied Sciences* 39 (1984): 173.

161. For an analysis of the history of licensure laws, see Samuel L. Baker, "A Strange Case: The Physician Licensure Campaign in Massachusetts in 1880," *Journal of the History of Medicine and Allied Sciences* 40 (1984): 286–308;

Richard H. Shyrock, *Medical Licensing in America, 1650–1965* (Baltimore: Johns Hopkins University Press, 1967); Odin W. Anderson, *The Uneasy Equilibrium* (New Haven: Yale University Press, 1968); Rosemary Stevens, *American Medicine and Public Interest* (New Haven: Yale University Press, 1981); Numbers, "The Fall and Rise," 51–72; Burton J. Bledstein, *The Culture of Professionalism: The Middle Class and the Development of Higher Education in America* (New York: W. W. Norton, 1976), 97–99, 108–110; Samuel Haber, *The Quest for Authority and Honor in the American Professions, 1750–1900* (Chicago: University of Chicago Press, 1991), 329–331; and William G. Rothstein, *American Physicians in the Nineteenth Century: From Sects to Science* (Baltimore: Johns Hopkins University Press, 1972).

162. B. J. Fowler, "The Menace of Medical Monopoly," *Arena* 9 (1894): 400.

163. Henry Wood, "Medical Slavery," *Arena* 8 (1893): 681.

164. *Boston Evening Transcript*, 2 (March 1898), 7.

165. Ibid.

166. Ibid.

167. Ibid.

168. Ibid.

169. Ibid.

170. Murphy and Ballou, *William James on Psychical Research*, 10.

171. Letter from William James to James Jackson Putnam, 2 March 1898, cited in Hale, *James Jackson Putnam and Psychoanalysis*, 71.

172. Letter from William James to James Jackson Putnam, 4 March 1898, cited in Hale, *James Jackson Putnam and Psychoanalysis*, 73.

173. Letter from James Jackson Putnam to William James, 9 March 1898, cited in Hale, *James Jackson Putnam and Psychoanalysis*, 73–74.

174. Robert T. Edes, "The New England Invalid," *The Shattuck Lecture 1895* (Boston: David Clapp and Son, 1895), 48.

175. Robert T. Edes, "Points in the Diagnosis and Treatment of Some Common Neuroses," *Journal of the American Medical Association* 37 (1896): 1081.

176. Henry H. Goddard, "The Effects of Mind on Body as Evidenced by Faith Cures," *American Journal of Psychology* 10 (1899): 431–502.

177. Ibid., 491, 500.

178. Ibid., 499.

Chapter 5

1. See Roger Smith, *Inhibition: History and Meaning in the Sciences of the Mind and Brain* (Berkeley: University of California Press, 1992), 35; idem, "The Human Significance of Biology: Darwin, Carpenter, and the *versa causa*," in *Nature and the Victorian Imagination*, ed. U.C. Knoepflmacher and G.B. Tennyson (Berkeley: University of California Press, 1977), 219; and Clarke and Jacyna, *Nineteenth-Century Origins*, 128.

2. Speaking before the American Medico-Psychological Association in 1894, S. Weir Mitchell declared, "You were the first of the specialists and you have never come back into line. It is easy to see how this came about. You soon began to live apart, and you still do so. Your hospitals are not our hospitals; your ways are not our ways. You live out of the range of critical shot; you are not preceded and followed in your ward by clever rivals, or watched by able residents fresh with the learning of schools." Quoted in Gerald N. Grob, *The Mad Among Us: A History of the Care of America's Mentally Ill* (Cambridge, Mass.: Harvard University Press, 1994), 136.

3. Grob's discussion of psychoanalysis, a particular method of psychotherapy, can be applied to virtually all methods of psychotherapy. "For the bulk of institutionalized patients," Grob explains, "psychoanalytic therapy had little meaning. The number of mentally ill patients who were institutionalized would in any case have precluded its use within hospitals. Analysts, moreover, dealt mainly with what was known as the psychoneuroses; the hard-core psychoses remained largely outside psychoanalytic practice or theory." *Mental Illness and American Society*, 121, 179–200. See also Erwin Ackerknecht, *Short History of Psychiatry*, 82; and Françoise Castel, *The Psychiatric Society* (New York: Columbia University Press, 1982), 26.

4. The history of the reflex is long. The best places to start are Ruth Leys, *From Sympathy to Reflex: Marshall Hall and His Opponents* (New York: Garland, 1990); idem, "Background of the Reflex Controversy: William Alison and the Doctrine of Sympathy before Hall," *Studies in the History of Biology* 4 (1980): 1–66; see also Clarke and Jacyna, *Nineteenth-Century Origins*, 114–117, 124; and Shorter, *From Paralysis to Fatigue*, 40–68.

5. Quoted in Clarke and Jacyna, *Nineteenth-Century Origins*, 128. See also "Mid-Nineteenth-Century British Psycho-Physiology: A Neglected Chapter in the History of Psychology," in *The Problematic Science: Psychology in Nineteenth-Century Thought*, ed. William R. Woodward and Mitchell G. Ash (New York: Praeger, 1982), 124–125; Smith, *Inhibition*, 69.

6. L.S. Jacyna, "The Physiology of the Mind, the Unity of Nature, and the Moral Order in Victorian Thought," *British Journal of the History of Science* 14 (1981): 111.

7. William Carpenter, "On the Influence of Suggestion in Modifying and Directing Muscular Movement Independent of Volition," in *Nature and Man*, 170, quoted in Smith, "The Human Significance of Biology," 221.

8. Clarke and Jacyna, *Nineteenth-Century Origins*, 131, 147. Gregory Zilboorg notes, "It would be a mistake, of course, to consider this 'cerebromythological' trend nothing more than a rejection of psychology. It was a direct outgrowth of a narrowly conceived opposition to speculative psychology; it was a narrowly conceived attitude toward disease. But it was also a stimulus to further study of such organic diseases as general paralysis and to the deepening of the studies of various febrile exhaustive states, alcoholic mental disorders, and senile psychoses due to vascular changes in the brain." *History*, 442.

9. Cynthia Eagle Russett, *Sexual Science: The Victorian Construction of Womanhood* (Cambridge, Mass.: Harvard University Press, 1989), 109.

10. Quoted in Young, *Mind, Brain and Adaptation*, 208.

11. John P. Gray, "The Dependence of Insanity on Physical Disease," *Amer-*

ican Journal of Insanity 27 (1870–1871): 385–386. Although Gray represented the majority opinion of American psychiatrists, he was not without his critics. For an opposing view, see H. B. Wilbur, "Materialism In its Relations to the Causes, Conditions, and Treatment of Insanity," *Quarterly Journal of Psychological Medicine and Medical Jurisprudence* 6 (1872): 29–61. A reviewer contrasted the theories of Gray and Wilbur in the following manner: "The difference between Dr. Gray and Dr. Wilbur is this: The former . . . does not deny the agency of moral cause in producing insanity, but maintains that such causes first induce disease of the brain or of the system generally, and ultimately of the brain. . . . Dr. Wilbur maintains that moral causes induce a change in the immaterial entity mind, by which independently of any cerebral disease, its actions are disordered and insanity exists." T. H., "Is Insanity a Disease of the Mind, Or of the Body," *American Journal of Insanity* 29 (1872–1873): 884.

12. Clarke and Jacyna, *Nineteenth-Century Origins,* 213–214.

13. Its original German title was "Über die elektrische Erregbarkeit des Grosshirns," and it appeared in *Arch. f. Anat., Physiol. und wissenschaftl. Mediz.* (Leipzig) 37 (1970): 300–332. Much of my discussion follows from Young, *Mind, Brain and Adaptation,* 224–233.

14. Young, *Mind, Brain and Adaptation,* 229.

15. Quoted in Young, *Mind, Brain and Adaptation,* 232. Young notes that this particular sentence "raises the issue of the philosophic assumptions underlying Fritsch and Hitzig's experiments and their incompatibility with the assumptions of the associationist tradition to which Jackson and Ferrier belongs. Put simply, Fritsch and Hitzig were ontological dualists and believed in separate substances of mind and its mechanisms. The brain is the material substance of the immaterial soul, and the grey matter of the cortices constituted the 'first tools of the soul.' "

16. Ibid., 234.

17. Ibid., 134.

18. Kurt Danziger, "Mid-Nineteenth-Century British Psycho-Physiology: A Neglected Chapter in the History of Psychology." in *The Problematic Science: Psychology in Nineteenth-Century Thought,* ed. William R. Woodward and Michael G. Ash (New York: Praeger, 1982), 134. "In the mind of the medical man," explains Gregory Zilboorg, "mental disease became a purely physical disease long before he had the slightest conception of the anatomy of the brain or of the physiology of the glands of internal secretion. The scientific trends of all ages were brought to bear in order to justify the conviction rather than to explain the disease. This conviction has always been the most potent factor in the formation of purely somatological theories." *History,* 507.

19. John P. Gray, "Pathology of Insanity," *American Journal of Insanity* 31 (1874–1875): 13.

20. Shyrock, "Medical History of the American People," 21; Goldstein, *Console and Classify,* 332.

21. For an excellent discussion of the position held by nineteenth-century asylum superintendents, see Charles E. Rosenberg, *The Trial of Assassin Guiteau: Psychiatry and Law in the Gilded Age* (Chicago: University of Chicago Press, 1968).

22. King, *Transformations in American Medicine*, 174; Shyrock, "Medical History of the American People," 23.

23. Elaine Showalter, "Syphilis, Sexuality, and the Fiction of Fin de Siècle," in *Sex, Politics, and Science in the Nineteenth-Century Novel: Selected Papers from the English Institute, 1983–1984*, ed. Ruth Bernard Yeazell (Baltimore: Johns Hopkins University Press, 1986), 110.

24. Ibid. Showalter mistakenly fuses notions of organic models of mental illness with hereditary ones. While the two theories are not necessarily mutually exclusive, they are distinct. A germ that causes a disease is different from a gene that causes one. For clarification of this point, see Grob, "Rediscovering," 143.

25. Quetel, *History of Syphilis*, 161. Quetel's statement, while accurate, is exaggerated. The transformation of psychiatric medicine (i.e., of psychiatry and neurology) from its environmental to its organic orientation had begun long before Schaudinn's and Hoffmann's 1905 discovery of the *Treponema palladum*. Their discovery's significance to psychiatry was that it appeared to confirm a long-standing assumption regarding the somatic basis of certain states of insanity. See also Brandt, *No Magic Bullet*. The story of syphilis is obviously far more complex than I have presented. Because the disease owed itself to sexual activities and, often, sexual relations with prostitutes, morality frequently entered the discussion of the disease. Victims of syphilis were rarely accorded the same sympathy as, say, victims of cholera. See also Grob, *Mental Illness*, 112; Hideyo Noguchi and J.W. Moore, "Demonstration of *Treponema Palladum* In the Brain in Cases of General Paralysis" (1913), in *The Origins of Modern Psychiatry*, ed. C. Thompson (New York: John Wiley & Sons, 1987), 211–217.

26. For a concise biography of Daniel Hack Tuke, see Thompson, *Origins of Modern Psychiatry*, 53–58. According to the *Oxford English Dictionary*, Tuke is the first English-language speaker to employ the word *psychotherapeutics* (1872). Unlike later advocates of what came to be known as psychotherapy, Tuke did not conceive of psychotherapeutics as a method appropriate only for the treatment of mental disease. His aspirations were far more audacious. A proper understanding of the mind's impact on the body, he believed, would be useful in fighting not only functional but also organic disease. In this respect, his conception of psychotherapeutics bore a stark resemblance to the doctrines espoused by the leading exemplars of the American mind cure movement. For psychotherapy's etymology, see *Oxford English Dictionary*, 2d ed. (Oxford: Clarendon Press, 1989), 12:770–771.

27. Daniel Hack Tuke, *Of the Influences of the Mind Upon the Body in Health and Disease Designed to Elucidate the Actions of the Imagination* (London: J. & A. Churchill, 1872), vi.

28. Ibid., 381.

29. Oppenheim, *Shattered Nerves*. See also Clark, "The Rejection of Psychological Approaches," 281–282.

30. George Beard, "The Influence of the Mind in the Causation and Cure of Disease—The Potency of Definite Expectation," *Journal of Nervous and Mental Diseases* 1 (1876): 429–435.

31. Ibid., 429, 431.

32. Ibid., 432.

33. Hale recounts the hostile reception with which Beard's neurological colleagues greeted his 1876 paper on the subject of mental healing. See Hale, *Freud and the Americans,* 66; Andrew Scull, "Historical Sociology of Psychiatry," in *Social Order/Mental Disorder: Anglo-American Psychiatry in Historical Perspective* (Berkeley: University of California Press, 1989), 25.

34. Hale, *Freud and the Americans,* 66.

35. Beard, "The Influence of the Mind," 432.

36. Hale, *Freud and the Americans,* 67.

37. Ackerknecht, *Short History,* 82; see also Bockoven, *Moral Treatment in American Psychiatry,* 95.

38. Grob, *Mental Illness,* 111.

39. Ackerknecht, *Short History,* 82.

40. Sheldon Leavitt, *Psychotherapy in the Practice of Medicine and Surgery* (Chicago: Garner Press, 1903), 29.

41. Lewellys F. Barker, "Some Experiences with the Simpler Methods of Psychotherapy and Re-Education," *American Journal of the Medical Sciences* 132 (1906): 520.

42. Lewellys F. Barker, "Psychotherapy," *Journal of the American Medical Association* 51 (1 August 1908): 371.

43. Bernard Sachs, "Advances in Neurology and Their Relation to Psychiatry," *American Journal of Insanity* 54 (1898): 17.

44. Ibid., 18–19.

45. T.L. Brown, "Physical Causes of Nervous Diseases," *Transactions of the Institute of Homeopathy* (1884): 295.

46. For an excellent discussion of late-nineteenth- and early-twentieth-century medical optimism, see Haber, *Quest for Authority,* 326.

47. See Lewellys F. Barker, "On the Importance of Pathological and Bacteriological Laboratories in Connection with Hospitals for the Insane," *American Journal of Insanity* 57 (1900–1901): 515.

48. P.M. Wise, "Presidential Address," *American Journal of Insanity* 58 (1901–1902): 79 (italics added).

49. While discussions of heredity and its possible role in contributing to mental and nervous disorders were widespread, hereditary explanations had few, if any, therapeutic implications—at least for the growing number of anti-Lamarckians. For a fascinating study of the impact of hereditarian ideas, see Dowbiggin, *Inheriting Madness.*

50. Taylor, *William James on Exceptional Mental States,* 3.

51. Isador Coriat, "Some Personal Reminiscences of Psychoanalysis in Boston: An Autobiographical Note," *Psychoanalytic Review* 32 (January 1945): 2, 3.

52. George Gifford maintains, "At Harvard, psychologists William James and Hugo Münsterberg were part of the 'Boston Group' whose leader was J. J. Putnam and whose other members were: Josiah Royce, George A. Waterman, Boris Sidis, Morton Prince, and Edward Cowles. Later they were joined by Adolf Meyer. They met regularly to discuss patients and assess ideas stemming from the European literature, including those of Charcot, Janet, Bergson, and Freud." Gifford, *Psychoanalysis,* xix; Hoopes, *Consciousness in New England,* 237–243; see also Eugene Taylor, *William James on Consciousness beyond the Margin* (Princeton: Princeton University Press, 1996).

53. Kurt Danziger, "On the Threshold of the New Psychology: Situating Wundt and James," in *Wundt Studies: A Centennial Collection*, ed. Wolfgang G. Bringmann and Ryan O. Tweny (Toronto: C. J. Hogrefe, 1980): 365; quoted in Ruth Leys, "Adolf Meyer: A Biographical Note," in *Defining American Psychology: The Correspondence between Adolf Meyer and Edward Bradford Titchener*, ed. Ruth Leys and Rand B. Evans (Baltimore: Johns Hopkins University Press, 1990), 44.

54. Leys, "Adolf Meyer," 44.

55. Howard Feinstein suggests, "James was a mind that emphasized process and movement rather than inert categories, empirical evidence rather than process accepted canons, and the tensions, often actually painful for the young, between determinism (influence and historical possibilities) and the felt actuality of freedom of the will in the shaping of a life." *Becoming William James* (Ithaca: Cornell University Press, 1984), 15. Gerald Myers points out that, in James, one "finds . . . the struggle of the doctor, the psychologist, and the philosopher to solve that problem [i.e., the relationship between mind and body] in terms that satisfy all three; there is a tendency for the physiologist in James to solve it primarily through biology of the brain, for the psychologist in him to do it through sensations and experiences, and for the philosopher to resolve it through unusual concepts and arguments." See Gerald E. Myers, "Introduction: The Intellectual Context," in William James, *The Principles of Psychology* (Cambridge, Mass.: Harvard University Press, 1981), xii.

56. William James, *Talks to Teachers on Psychology and to Students on Some of Life's Ideals* (Cambridge, Mass.: Harvard University Press, 1983), 161.

57. See Kurt Danziger, "Mid-Nineteenth Century British Psycho-Physiology: A Neglected Chapter in the History of Psychology," in *The Problematic Science: Psychology in Nineteenth-Century Thought*, ed. William R. Woodward and Michael G. Ash (New York: Praeger, 1982), 130.

58. William James, "Habit," *Popular Science Monthly* 30 (1886–1887): 446.

59. William B. Carpenter, *Principles of Mental Physiology, with Their Application to the Training and Discipline of the Mind, and the Study of Its Morbid Condition* (New York: D. Aphelion, 1874); quoted in James, "Habit," 437.

60. James, *Talks to Teachers*, xi–xxvi.

61. For a brief introduction to James's *Talks to Teachers*, see the introduction prepared by Gerald E. Myers, xi–xxvi. See also "The Text of *Talks to Teachers on Psychology*," 234–287.

62. James, *Talks to Teachers*, 27, 48, 108.

63. James, "Habit," 447. Emphasis in original.

64. James, *Talks to Teachers*, 57.

65. Ibid., 57–58.

66. W. S. Taylor, *Morton Prince and Abnormal Psychology* (New York: D. Appleton, 1928). For biographical details on Prince's life, see Nathan G. Hale Jr., "Introductory Essay," in Morton Prince, *Psychopathology and Multiple Personality: Selected Essays* (Cambridge, Mass.: Harvard University Press, 1975) (hereafter cited as *P&MP*); and Otto Marx, "Morton Prince and Psychopathology," in George Gifford, *Psychoanalysis, Psychotherapy and the New England Medical Scene, 1894–1944* (New York: Science History Publications, 1978), 155–162.

67. Morton Prince, "Association Neuroses" (1891), in *P&MP*, 75.

68. Hale, "Introductory Essay," 2.

69. Morton Prince, *The Nature of the Mind and Human Automatism* (Philadelphia: J. B. Lippincott, 1885), 10.

70. Taylor, *Morton Prince*, 98.

71. Ibid., 97. For a brief discussion of the controversial history of hypnotism, see Ackerknecht, *Short History*, 83–91. For more extensive coverage, see Gauld, *History of Hypnotism*.

72. Morton Prince, "Hughlings Jackson on the Connection between the Mind and the Brain," in *Clinical and Experimental Studies in Personality* (Cambridge: Sci-Art Publishers, 1929), 515; quoted in Hale, "Introductory Essay," 5.

73. Prince, "Association Neuroses" (1891), in *P&MP*, 62–63. Association psychology has a long history dating back to John Locke and the late seventeenth century. For a brief background, see Robert Young, "Association of Ideas," in *Dictionary of the History of Ideas,* ed. Philip P. Wiener (New York: Charles Scribner's Sons, 1973), 1:111–118; Boring, *A History of Experimental Psychology;* Heidbreder, *Seven Psychologies;* L. S. Hearnshaw, *A Short History of British Psychology, 1840–1940* (Westport, Conn.: Greenwood Press, 1964).

74. Hale, "Introductory Essay," 5.

75. John Holland Mackenzie, "The Production of the So-Called 'Rose Cold' by Means of an Artificial Rose," *American Journal of the Medical Sciences* 91 (1886): 57; quoted in Hale, "Introductory Essay," 5.

76. Prince, "Association Neuroses" (1891), in *P&MP*, 65. Emphasis in original.

77. Ibid., 75.

78. Ibid., 63.

79. Hale, "Introductory Essay," 5.

80. Prince, "Association Neuroses" (1891), in *P&MP*, 82.

81. "Very largely due to Carpenter's advocacy," Hearnshaw explains, "the doctrine of unconscious cerebral functioning became generally accepted." Hearnshaw, *Short History of British Psychology,* 23.

82. Boring, *History,* 240.

83. Morton Prince, "The Educational Treatment of Neurasthenia and Certain Hysterical States," *Boston Medical and Surgical Journal* 139 (1898): 33.

84. Ibid., 335.

85. Ibid.

86. For a discussion of Putnam's views regarding neurasthenia, see chapter 2.

87. Hale, *James Jackson Putnam,* 11.

88. Ibid., 12.

89. Nathan G. Hale Jr., "James Jackson Putnam and Boston Neurology: 1877–1918," in *Psychoanalysis, Psychotherapy and the New England Medical Scene,* 149–154.

90. James Jackson Putnam, "Not the Disease Only, But Also the Man," *Boston Medical and Surgical Journal* (July 20, 1899): 53. Emphasis added.

91. Ibid., 54.

92. Boris Sidis, "The Nature and Principles of Psychology," *American Journal of Insanity* 56 (1899–1900): 41–52.

93. For biographical information on Sidis, see *Biographical Dictionary of American Psychology,* ed. Leonard Zusne (Westport, Conn.: Greenwood Press, 1984), 396.

94. Boris Sidis, *The Psychology of Suggestion: A Research into the Subconscious Nature of Man and Society* (New York: D. Appleton, 1898).

95. Boris Sidis and Simon P. Goodhart, *Multiple Personality: An Investigation into the Nature of Human Individuality* (New York: Greenwood Press, 1905).

96. H. Addington Bruce, *Scientific Mental Healing* (Boston: Little, Brown, 1911): 53.

97. For a succinct, intellectual biographical sketch of Meyer, see Ruth Leys, "Adolf Meyer," 39–57. See also Gerald N. Grob, "Adolf Meyer and American Psychiatry in 1895," *American Journal of Psychiatry* 119 (1963): 135–142; idem, *Mental Illness,* 112–118. See also Alfred Lief, ed., *The Commonsense Psychiatry of Dr. Adolf Meyer* (New York: McGraw-Hill, 1948); For Meyer's personal work, see *The Collected Papers of Adolf Meyer,* ed. Eunice E. Winters, 4 vols. (Baltimore: Johns Hopkins University Press, 1952) (hereafter cited as *CP*).

98. Ruth Leys, "Types of One: Adolf Meyer's Life Chart and the Representation of Individuality," *Representations* 34 (1991): 2.

99. Leys, "Adolf Meyer," 41. Meyer received his first appointment in the United States from Shobal Vail Clevenger, a leading proponent of a somatic interpretation of railway spine. See "Thirty-Five Years of Psychiatry" (1928–1929), *CP*, 2:2–3.

100. The word *pragmatism,* given its frequency of use, has not surprisingly taken on a multiplicity of meanings. Even those who pioneered the term did not always agree on its meaning. As James's biographer, Ralph Barton Perry, asserts, "Perhaps it would be correct, and just to all parties, to say that the modern movement known as pragmatism is largely the result of James's misunderstanding of Peirce." *The Thought and Character of William James* 2 (Boston: Little, Brown, 1935). Bruce Kuklick adds, "In time James diverged so radically from Peirce that the latter renounced the child that James had nurtured." *The Rise of American Philosophy: Cambridge, Massachusetts, 1860–1930* (New Haven: Yale University Press, 1977), 264. In a 1907 essay entitled, "What Pragmatism Means," James wrote,

Pragmatism is willing to take anything, to follow either logic or the senses and to count the humblest and most personal experience. She will count mystical experiences if they have practical consequences. She will take a God who lives in the very dirt of private fact—if that should seem a likely place to find him. Her only test of probable truth is what works best in the way of leading us, what fits every part of life best and combines with the collectivity of experience's demands, nothing being omitted. If theological ideas should do this, if the notion of God, in particular, should prove to do it, how could pragmatism possibly deny God's existence? She could see no meaning in treating as "not true" a notion that was pragmatically so successful. What other kind of truth could there be, for her, than all this agreement with concrete reality?

William James, "What Pragmatism Means" (1907), in *The American Intellectual Tradition: 1865 to the Present,* ed. David A. Hollinger and Charles Capper (New York: Oxford University Press, 1989), 2:110. See also Hollinger, "The Problem of Pragmatism in American History," in *In the American Province,*

23–43; S. P. Fullinwider, *Technicians of the Finite: The Rise and Decline of the Schizophrenic in American Thought, 1840–1960* (Westport, Conn.: Greenwood Press, 1982), 70.

101. Meyer, "The Problems of Mental Reaction Types, Mental Causes and Diseases" (1908), *CP*, 2:596. (italics added).

102. Ruth Leys explains that Meyer's conception of science was in part attributable to the "positivist or empiro-critical philosophy of the physicist Ernst Mach and the philosopher Richard Avenarius." Although he was exposed to Mach and Avenarius in the 1890s, Leys continues, "it was not until the early 1900s that Meyer came to appreciate fully the potential significance of those ideas for his own psychiatric work." "Correspondence Between Meyer and Titchener," 64–66. For a discussion of Mach's philosophy of science, see John T. Blackmore, *Ernst Mach: His Work, Life, and Influence* (Berkeley: University of California Press, 1972), 164–180. For a discussion of Avenarius's philosophy, see Wendall T. Bush, *Avenarius and the Standpoint of Pure Experience* (New York: Science Press, 1905), 34–59.

103. Meyer, "The Problems of Mental Reaction Types," 597.

104. Meyer's pragmatism was not without its limitations. As Ruth Leys explains:

Meyer's project was epistemologically incoherent on two closely related counts. First, as recent writers on the theory of interpretation have emphasized, the realm of facts cannot be imagined to precede the realm of interpretation in this way. A thoroughgoing pragmatism might rather have compelled Meyer to realize that the notion of an interpretatively neutral method was a chimera and that, inevitably, a particular interpretation inhered in the very procedures he advocated. . . . Second, conceding for a moment the possibility of such a method and hence the availability of a set of facts prior to the interpretation, Meyer's belief that the mere inspection of those facts would suffice to determine their correct interpretation was also problematic for either the facts in question were imagined as calling for one interpretation rather than another—in which case their neutrality became suspect—or they were genuinely neutral—in which case the choice of one interpretation over another could only be arbitrary.

See Leys, "The Correspondence between Adolf Meyer and E. B. Titchener," in *Defining American Psychology*, 88. In a later article, Leys says, "In spite of his professedly pragmatic orientation, Meyer's conception of science led him to conceive of the facts of a case as available *prior* to any particular interpretation—if only the investigator knew how to induce them and make them perspicuous." "Types of One," 6.

105. Meyer, "Problems of Mental Reaction Types," 597–598.

106. Ibid., 598.

107. Ibid., 599. Emphasis in original.

108. Leys, "Adolf Meyer," 45.

109. Ibid., 43. Meyer's early enthusiasm for hypnotism stemmed from his exposure to the theory and practice of Forel. "Thirty-Five Years of Psychiatry," 15; "The Scope of Psychopathology" (1916), *CP*, 2:618–623.

110. In the Index to the *Complete Papers,* there is not a single reference to either Christian Science or New Thought.

111. Leys, "Adolf Meyer," 43.

112. John Gach, "Culture and Complex: On the Early History of Psychoanalysis in America," in *Essays on the History of Psychiatry*, ed. Edwin R. Wallace IV and Lucius C. Pressley (Columbia: W.S. Hall Psychiatric Institute, 1980), 141.

113. Meyer, "The Dynamic Interpretation of Dementia Praecox" (1910), *CP*, 2:457.

114. James, *Varieties of Religious Experience*, 91.

115. Meyer, "A Few Trends in Modern Psychiatry," (1904), *CP*, 2: 386–404.

116. As Ruth Leys explains, "Meyer refined the method of history taking he had inherited from nineteenth-century hospital practice. First he formalized and standardized the method of examination so that it could be taught in a systematic fashion. He provided students with a basic outline to be followed, specifying the order of procedure, the essential psycho-biological data to be ascertained, the various tests to be used to determine the patient's mental and neurological states, and—most important—suggesting the actual questions to be asked the patient, something that had been lacking in previous handbooks of psychiatry. Leys, "Adolf Meyer," 71–72; "Types of One," 11–18.

117. See *Defining American Psychology*. See also Leys, "Type of One."

118. Adolf Meyer, "The Material of Human Nature and Conduct" (1935), *CP*, 3:49; quoted in Leys, "Adolf Meyer," 39. Meyer did not accept James's argument in *Variety of Religious Experiences* that while mind cure did not work for everyone, "[it] would surely be pedantic and over-scrupulous for those who *can* get their savage and primitive philosophy of mental healing verified in such experimental ways as this, to give us a work of command for more scientific therapies" (110). Indeed, Meyer wanted to do precisely this!

119. Meyer, "Misconceptions at the Bottom of Hopelessness of All Psychology," (1907), *CP*, 2:573–580.

120. Meyer, "Problems of Mental Reaction Types," 595.

121. Ibid., 596. Emphasis in original.

122. Ibid., 596–597.

123. Discussion following Ralph Layman Parson's paper on psychotherapy, *Transactions of the American Medico-Psychological Association* 10 (1903): 380.

124. Meyer, "Dynamic Interpretation," 443–458. Meyer's attitude on the inapplicability of the syphilis model was not typical. See Grob, *Mental Illness*, 347 n.5.

125. Meyer, "A Short Sketch of the Problems of Psychiatry," *CP*, 2: 273–282.

126. Ibid, 281.

127. For an example of Gray's somaticism, see John P. Gray, "Pathology of Insanity," *American Journal of Insanity* 31 (1874–1875): 13.

128. Meyer, "The Role of Mental Factors in Psychiatry" (1908), *CP*, 2: 581–590.

129. Ibid., 582. Emphasis in original.

130. Ibid., 582–583.

131. Ibid., 583.

132. Ibid., 583–584.

133. Ibid., 586.

134. Ibid.

135. Meyer, "A Few Trends," 386–404.

136. Beatrice M. Hinckle, M.D., "Psychotherapy, With Some of Its Results," *Journal of the American Medical Association* 50 (9 May 1908): 1496.

137. Both Hale and Burnham correctly note the impact of European neurology on American medicine. What neither author considers, however, is the relatively limited depth of its influence. While the "advanced guard" was doubtless aware of the latest neurological "breakthroughs" emanating from Paris, Berlin, Vienna, and other European capitals, the rank and file had little exposure to such ideas. Hale, *Freud in America;* John C. Burnham, *Psychoanalysis and American Medicine: 1894–1918* (New York: International Universities Press, 1967).

138. Edward Wylis Taylor, "The Attitude of the Medical Profession Toward the Psychotherapeutic Movement," *Boston Medical and Surgical Journal* 157 (26 December 1907): 843–850.

139. Ibid., 844.

140. Ibid., 847.

141. Ibid. Putnam had earlier asserted, "Through analytic case-histories, patiently recorded, it has been sought to picture the mental history of sufferers from such disorders as those enumerated, with the same sort of fidelity as is displayed in the descriptions of the anatomists." James Jackson Putnam, "A Consideration of Mental Therapeutics as Employed by Special Students of the Subject," *Boston Medical and Surgical Journal* 151 (1904): 179–183.

142. Discussion following E. W. Taylor, "The Attitude of the Medical Profession Toward the Psychotherapeutic Movement," *Journal of Nervous and Mental Diseases* (June 1908): 403. This article includes the discussion following the *Boston Medical and Surgical Journal* articles cited above.

143. Ibid., 403–404.

144. Ibid., 848, 850.

145. Ibid., 401.

146. Ibid., 403, 405, 406.

147. Ibid., 408, 410.

148. Ibid., 408, 413.

149. Ibid., 410.

Chapter 6

1. James Jackson Putnam Papers (hereafter referred to as JJPP), Countway Library, James Jackson Putnam to Richard C. Cabot, 5 November 1906.

2. "Emmanuel Movement Deplored by Eminent Physicians of Boston," *Boston Sunday Herald,* 27 December 1908.

3. Allen Bruce Fleming, "Psychology, Medicine, and Religion: A Form of Early Twentieth-Century American Psychotherapy (1905–09)" (Ph.D dissertation, Fuller Theological Seminary, School of Psychology, 1989), 29.

4. Several historians have written on the Emmanuel movement. Most focus primarily on the movement's religious and cultural impact. Described in a variety of fashions, this church-sponsored venture is rarely credited for its most enduring contribution. The Emmanuel movement was not merely "a variety of American religious experience," "a transition from the supernaturalism of the mind cure cults to scientific psychotherapy," "a defensive measure against the curists," or "a precursor to Freud." It was instead the primary agent responsible for the efflorescence of psychotherapy in the United States during the first decade of the twentieth century. See Raymond J. Cunningham, "Ministry of Healing: The Origins of the Psychosomatic Role of the American Churches" (Ph.D. dissertation, Johns Hopkins University, 1965); Fleming, *Psychology, Medicine, and Religion;* idem, "The Emmanuel Movement: A Variety of American Religious Experience," *American Quarterly* 14 (1964): 48–63; Brian Dean Smith, "The Moral Treatment of Psychological Disorder: A Historical and Conceptual Study of Selected Twentieth-Century Pastoral Psychologists" (Ph.D. dissertation, University of Washington, 1989); Robert Charles Powell, "Healing and Wholeness: Helen Flanders Dunbar (1902–59) and an Extra-Medical Origin of the American Psychosomatic Movement, 1906–36" (Ph.D. dissertation, Duke University, 1974); idem, "The 'Subliminal' versus the 'Subconscious' in the American Acceptance of Psychoanalysis, 1906–1910," *Journal of the History of the Behavioral Sciences* 15 (1979): 155–165; G. Allison Stokes, "The Rise of the Religion and Health Movement in American Protestantism, 1906–1945" (Ph.D. dissertation, Yale University, 1981); and Fuller, *Americans and the Unconscious,* 103. Notable exceptions to this line of analysis can be found in the work of John Gardner Greene and Katherine McCarthy. See Greene, "The Emmanuel Movement, 1906–1929," *New England Quarterly* 7 (1934): 532. More recently, McCarthy has suggested, "From today's perspective it appears that the medical profession won the territorial struggle essentially by co-opting the ideas that the Emmanuel clergy had demonstrated to have such popular appeal." "Psychotherapy and Religion: The Emmanuel Movement," *Journal of Religion and Health* 23 (1984): 102. See also Sanford Gifford, "Medical Psychotherapy and the Emmanuel Movement," in *Psychoanalysis, Psychotherapy and the New England Medical Scene, 1894–1944,* ed. George Gifford (New York: Science History Publications, 1978), 106–118; John C. Burnham, "Psychology and Counseling: Convergence into a Profession," in *The Professions in American History,* ed. and introd. Nathan O. Hatch (Notre Dame: University of Notre Dame Press, 1988), 181–198. For an example of a historian who appreciates the movement's impact on American medicine but lacks the requisite medical-historical background to frame his analysis effectively, see Stow Persons, *American Minds: A History of Ideas* (Huntington: Robert E. Krieger, 1958), 444–445. See also Hale, *Freud and the Americans,* 248; and Hoopes, *Consciousness in New England,* 261.

5. Fred Matthews, "The Americanization of Sigmund Freud: Adaptations of Psychoanalysis before 1917," *Journal of American Studies* 1 (1967): 45.

6. H. Addington Bruce, "Books and Men: Some Books on Mental Healing," *Forum* 43 (1910): 316–323.

7. Ray Stannard Baker, *New Ideas in Healing* (New York: Frederick A. Stokes, 1909), 51.

8. For some examples of medical opposition to the Emmanuel movement, see Clarence B. Farrar, "Psychotherapy and the Church," *Journal of Nervous and Mental Diseases* 36 (1909): 11–24; Allan McLane Hamilton, "The Religio-Medical Movements," *North American Review* 189 (February 1909): 223–232; W. Bunce, "The Emmanuel and Allied Movement," *Cleveland Medical Journal* 8 (1909): 254–263; Tom A. Williams, "Requisites for the Treatment of the Psycho-Neuroses: Psycho-Pathological Ignorance, and the Misuse of Psychotherapy by the Novice," *Old Dominion Journal of Medicine and Surgery* 8 (1909): 363–368; John J. Moren, "The Question of Therapeutics," *Louisville Monthly Journal of Medicine and Surgery* 16 (August 1909): 65–69; C. C. Beling, "Psychotherapy," *Journal of the Medical Society of New Jersey* 5 (May 1909): 617–619; and John K. Mitchell, "The Emmanuel Movement: Its Pretensions, Its Practice, Its Dangers," *American Journal of the Medical Sciences* (December 1909): 781–793. For examples of clerical opposition to the movement, see Harry Kimball, "A Little Excursion into Psychotherapy," *Congregationalist and Christian World* (January 30, 1909); George L. Parker, *The Other Side of Psychotherapy* (Boston: Salem D. Towne, 1908); James Monroe Buckley, "Dangers of the Emmanuel Movement: Reasons Why It Should Not Be Generally Adopted," *Century* 77 (February 1909): 631–635; Charles Reynolds Brown, *Faith and Health* (New York: Thomas Y. Crowell, 1910); and George A. Gordon, "The Practice of Medicine by the Unfit," *Congregationalist and Christian World* (February 13, 1909): 211–212.

9. See *Readers' Guide to Periodical Literature, 1905–1909,* 714. The next volume of the guide, which covers the years 1910–1914, lists only five articles under the heading Emmanuel Movement, four on Freud, and eleven on psychoanalysis. Volume 4, which covers the years from 1915 to 1918, lists eight articles on Freud and thirty-one on psychoanalysis. Volume 4 has no listing for the Emmanuel movement.

10. "Health and Happiness," *Good Housekeeping* 44 (1907): 405; quoted in Cunningham, *Ministry of Healing,* 147.

11. For an autobiographical sketch of Elwood Worcester, see *Life's Adventure: The Story of a Varied Career* (New York: Charles Scribner's Sons, 1932); see also Powell, *Healing and Wholeness,* and Cunningham, *Ministry of Healing,* 116–123.

12. My discussion of McComb derives from Cunningham, *Ministry of Healing,* 130; and William Macomber, *The History of the Emmanuel Movement from the Standpoint of a Patient* (Boston: Emmanuel Church, 1908).

13. Worcester, *Life's Adventure,* 162–166.

14. Powell, *Healing and Wholeness,* 167.

15. Worcester's claim regarding S. Weir Mitchell's influence served an important political function and thus helped to legitimate the movement in the eyes of many skeptical physicians. It is important to note, however, that Mitchell himself never came out in support of the movement. Indeed, by 1908 he had become an outspoken critic. See S. Weir Mitchell, "The Treatment by Rest, Seclusion, Etc., in Relation to Psychotherapy," *Journal of the American Medical Association* 50 (1908): 2033–2037.

16. As quoted in Greene, "The Emmanuel Movement, 1906–1929," 496.

·17. My discussion of Pratt follows largely from Powell, *Healing and Wholeness*, 171–173.

18. Powell, *Healing and Wholeness*, 172–173.

19. Powell, *Healing and Wholeness*, quoting Worcester, *Life's Adventure*, 1932A.

20. Worcester, *Life's Adventure*, 283.

21. Elwood Worcester, "The Emmanuel Movement," *Century* 78 (1909): 423.

22. Worcester, *Life's Adventure*, 278.

23. Ibid., 276.

24. Worcester "The Emmanuel Movement," 421–429.

25. Greene, "The Emmanuel Movement," 506.

26. Ibid.

27. Ibid., 507.

28. Worcester, *Life's Adventure*, 287. Emphasis added.

29. See Rollin Lynde Hart, " 'Christian Science' Without Mystery: Mental Healing on a Sound Basis as Practiced by the Emmanuel Episcopal Church, of Boston," *World's Work* 15 (December 1907): 9649.

30. Richard C. Cabot, "New Phases in the Relation of the Church to Health," *Outlook* (February 29, 1908): 504–508.

31. JJPP, James Jackson Putnam to Richard C. Cabot, 5 November 1906.

32. "Evening at the Emmanuel Church," *Good Housekeeping* 46 (February 1908): 200; Hart, " 'Christian Science' Without Mystery," 9649. Richard C. Cabot suggested the response of women was attributable to the fact that "most psychoneurotics are women . . . [and] [m]ost women care deeply for religion." Cabot, "The Literature of Psychotherapy," in *Psychotherapy: A Course Reading in Sound Psychology, Sound Medicine, and Sound Religion* 3, 24.

33. "Evening at the Emmanuel Church," 201.

34. Lyman P. Powell, "Psychotherapy at Northampton: An Account of Personal Experience," *Psychotherapy*, 66.

35. As quoted in Homer Gage, "The Emmanuel Movement from a Medical View Point," *Popular Science Monthly* 75 (October 1909): 363.

36. Elwood Worcester, Samuel McComb, and Isador H. Coriat, *Religion and Medicine: The Moral Control of Nervous Disorders* (New York: Moffat, Yard, 1908), 67.

37. "Emmanuel Clinics," *Good Housekeeping* 47 (October 1908): 361–363.

38. See Cunningham, *Ministry of Healing*.

39. Samuel Fallows and Helen M. Fallows, *Science of Health from the Viewpoint of the Newest Christian Thought* (Chicago: Our Daily Company, 1903); Cunningham, *Ministry of Healing*, 5.

40. Cunningham, *Ministry of Healing*, 151.

41. *The Emmanuel Movement: A Brief History of the New Cult, with Sermons from Prominent Ministers and Opinions of Laymen* (Brooklyn: Brooklyn Daily Eagle, 1908).

42. Samuel Fallows, *Health and Happiness; or Religious Therapeutics* (Chicago: A.C. McClurg, 1908).

43. Robert MacDonald, *Mind, Religion, and Health: With an Appreciation of the Emmanuel Movement* (New York and London: Funk & Wagnalls, 1908).

44. *The Emmanuel Movement: A Brief History,* 26.

45. In December 1906, a *Boston Journal* headline proclaimed, "At Auto-Suggestion Meeting Dr. Worcester Claims To Have Brought Dead Woman to Life Again." Reporting on the same alleged incident, the *Detroit News* declared, "That he himself had restored the dead to life—that he by prayer and faith had chased the grim destroyer from the bedside of a parishioner, some minutes after the soul had fled, was the statement by which Dr. Ellwood [*sic*] Worcester, whose auto-suggestion class at the fashionable Emanuel [*sic*] Church on Newbury Street is attracting much attention in society circles, electrified his hearers at the meeting last night. *Detroit Journal,* 16 December 1906, quoted in Greene, "The Emmanuel Movement." Worcester responded to these charges almost immediately. The respectable *Boston Transcript* reported that the woman had not died; she had merely lost consciousness, which she regained on hearing the rector's voice. "Dr. Worcester states emphatically that he did not ascribe her change to the power of prayer at all." *Boston Transcript,* 13 December 1906, quoted in Greene, "The Emmanuel Movement."

46. Worcester, *Life's Adventure,* 287.

47. Powell, *Healing and Wholeness,* 183.

48. Samuel McComb, "The Moral Treatment of Nervous Diseases," *Good Housekeeping* 44 (March 1907): 269 (italics added).

49. Ibid., 269–271.

50. "This Department and the Emmanuel Church Movement," *Good Housekeeping* 44 (April 1907): 405.

51. "Results at Emmanuel," *Good Housekeeping* 45 (November 1907): 504, 507, 508.

52. The *Readers' Guide to Periodical Literature, 1905–1909,* lists only two articles on the movement for the year 1907.

53. Hart, "'Christian Science' Without Mystery," 9648, 9652.

54. Cabot, "New Phases," 504–508.

55. Ibid., 506.

56. Samuel McComb, "Christianity and Health: An Experiment in Practical Religion," *Century* 75 (March 1908): 795.

57. Cunningham, *Ministry of Healing,* 154.

58. For an excellent summary of the traveling experiences of Worcester and McComb, see Cunningham, "A Parish Church Only in Name," chapter 5 in *Ministry of Healing,* 150–189.

59. Worcester, *Life's Adventure,* 293.

60. Cunningham, *Ministry of Healing,* 154.

61. "Report of the Committee Appointed to Consider and Report on the Subject of Ministries of Healing: (a) The Unction of the Sick; (b) Faith Healing and 'Christian Science,'" in *Six Lam Beth Conferences,* edited by Davidson, 390–393.

62. *New York Times,* 22 November 1908.

63. Cunningham, *Ministry of Healing,* 162.

64. Samuel McComb, *The Healing Ministry of the Church* (Boston: Emmanuel Church, 1908); Macomber, *History of the Emmanuel Movement;* William James, "Energies of Man" (from *American Magazine* October 1907) (New York: Moffat, Yard, 1908); J. Warren Achorn, *Some Physical Disorders Having Mental Origin* (Boston: Emmanuel Church, 1908); Isador H. Coriat, *Some Familiar Forms of Nervousness* (New York: Moffat, Yard, 1908); James G. Mumford, *Some End-Results of Surgery* (New York: Moffat, Yard, 1908); and Cabot, *Psychotherapy in Its Relation to Religion*.

65. *Index Catalogue of the Library of the Surgeon-General's Office*, 2d ser., 14 (1909): 42.

66. "The Greatest Modern Discovery," *Current Literature* 45 (September 1908): 304–307.

67. *New York Times*, 18 July 1908.

68. H. Addington Bruce, "Review of *Religion and Medicine*," *Outlook* (November 1908): 72.

69. Greene, "The Emmanuel Movement," 518.

70. Worcester, McComb, and Coriat, *Religion and Medicine*, 13.

71. Ibid., 52.

72. Ibid., 7.

73. Charles L. Dana, "Psychotherapy," *Journal of Nervous and Mental Diseases* 35 (1908): 389.

74. Ibid., 389.

75. Farrar, "Psychotherapy and the Church," 11–24.

76. Ibid., 11.

77. Ibid., 13.

78. Ibid., 14.

79. Ibid., 18.

80. Charles K. Mills, M.D., "Psychotherapy: Its Scope and Limitations," *Monthly Cyclopedia and Medical Bulletin* 1 (1908): 329.

81. Ibid., 340 (italics added).

82. Mitchell, "The Treatment by Rest, Seclusion, Etc.," 2033–2037.

83. Ibid., 2035.

84. Discussion following S. Weir Mitchell's paper, "Rest Treatment in Relation to Psychotherapy," *Transactions of the American Neurological Association* 37 (1909): 215–218.

85. Ibid., 218, 219.

86. Ibid., 217.

87. JJPP, James Jackson Putnam to Elwood Worcester, 12 September 1908.

88. Ibid. (italics added).

89. Worcester, *Life's Adventure*, 295.

90. Cunningham, *Ministry of Healing*, 163; see Elwood Worcester, "The Results of the Emmanuel Movement," *Ladies Home Journal* 25 (November 1908): 7–8; 26 (December 1908): 9–10; (January 1909): 17–18; (February 1909): 15–16; idem, "The Emmanuel Church Tuberculosis Class," (March 1909): 17–18. Despite the editors' claim that Worcester would not respond to any mail, Worcester received close to five thousand letters, most of which he

answered. "These articles, more than anything else," Worcester recounted, "brought our work before the whole country." *Life's Adventure*, 296.

91. *Psychotherapy: A Course Reading in Sound Psychology, Sound Medicine, and Sound Religion* 1 (New York: Centre, 1908).

92. In a letter to Putnam dated 19 August 1908, William James spoke highly of the venture: "Your program for Parker takes my breath away. It is truly grand to see you in extreme old age renewing your mighty youth and planning yourself for flights to which those of the newest airships are as sparrows fluttering in the gutter! Go in, dear Jim! It is magnificent. It won't be easy work, but it has got to be done by someone. The program you sketch is, I think, the form which the more spiritualistic philosophy of the future is bound more and more to assume, thou I fancy it will always be dogged more or less by a more materialistic or mechanistic-deterministic enemy." William James to James Jackson Putnam, 19 August 1908 in *James Jackson Putnam and Psychoanalysis: Letters between Putnam and Sigmund Freud, Ernest Jones, William James, Sandor Ferenczi, and Morton Prince, 1877–1917*, ed. Nathan G. Hale, Jr. (Cambridge, Mass.: Harvard University Press, 1971), 74.

93. From "Announcement of the Course," *Psychotherapy—A Course of Readings in Sound Psychology, Sound Medicine, and Sound Religion*, ed. William B. Parker (New York: Centre, 1908) appearing in *Outlook*.

94. Over twenty men and women published articles in *Psychotherapy*. James Jackson Putnam, Richard C. Cabot, and John Warren Achorn all contributed to the general section. The physiological section contained articles by Frederick Peterson, E.E. Southard, Beatrice Hinckle, Frederick T. Simpson, John E. Donley, M.A. Bliss, Frank K. Hallock, and Isador Coriat. The psychological section included pieces by Josiah Royce, R.S. Woodworth, James R. Angell, Joseph Jastrow, J.M. Bramwell, Charles Lloyd Tuckey, and Paul Dubois. Parker had also intended to include an article by Sigmund Freud in this section but was forced instead to rely on one furnished by Ernest Jones. The historical section was composed of Reverend Loring W. Batten, Reverend Joseph Cullen Ayer, Reverend Curtis Manning Geer, Max Eastman, and I.W. Bevan, the associate editor of the *Churchman*. Finally, the Religious section contained articles by Samuel Fallows, Lyman Powell, Albert Shields, and Dickinson S. Miller. For an excellent analysis of *Psychotherapy*, see Fleming, *Psychology, Medicine, and Religion*.

95. JJPP, W.B. Parker to James Jackson Putnam, 15 August 1908.

96. Ibid.

97. Ibid.

98. Ibid.

99. Loring W. Batten, *The Relief of Pain by Mental Suggestion: A Study of the Moral and Religious Forces of Healing* (New York: Moffat, Yard, 1917), preface.

100. "Emmanuel Clinics," *Good Housekeeping* 47 (October 1908): 361.

101. Ibid.

102. Joseph Collins, "Some Fundamental Principles in the Treatment of Functional Nervous Disease, with Especial Reference to Psychotherapy," *American Journal of Medical Science* 135 (February 1908): 169.

103. Ibid., 170.

104. *New York Times*, 10 November 1908.

105. *New York Times*, 8 November 1908.

106. Ibid.

107. Ibid., 13 November 1908.

108. Ibid., 24 November 1908.

109. Ibid., 26 November 1908.

110. "Clerical Healing," *Medical Record* 74 (1908): 840.

111. Ibid.

112. "Medical Practice and Medical Record," *New York Medical Journal* 84 (November 14, 1908). As quoted in Cunningham, *Ministry of Healing*.

113. *Boston Herald*, 21 November 1908.

114. Ibid.

115. *Boston Herald*, 22 November 1908.

116. Ibid.

117. "The Emmanuel Movement of Mental Healing," *Boston Medical and Surgical Journal* 159 (26 November 1908): 730–732.

118. Ibid., 731.

119. *New Jersey Herald*, 30 November 1908.

120. "The Emmanuel Movement: A Rejoinder," *Boston Medical and Surgical Journal* 159 (December 31, 1908): 9.

121. Ibid., 10.

122. Robert T. Edes, "The Present Relations of Psychotherapy," *Journal of the American Medical Association* 52 (9 January 1909): 96.

123. See "An Advisory Board for the Emmanuel Movement," *Boston Medical and Surgical Journal* 160 (January 21, 1909): 90–91; "The Emmanuel Movement: An Explanation," *Boston Medical and Surgical Journal* 160 (28 January 1909): 123.

124. Hamilton, "The Religio-Medical Movements," 225.

125. "Religion and Medicine: The Emmanuel Movement," *Old Dominion Journal of Medicine and Surgery* 8 (February 1909): 122, 123.

126. *Psychotherapeutics: A Symposium* (Boston: R. G. Badger, 1910).

127. For a brief discussion of the New Haven conference, see Hale, *Freud and the Americans*.

128. *Psychotherapeutics: A Symposium*, 9.

129. Ibid., 118.

130. *Boston Transcript*, 11 September 1909.

131. Mitchell, "The Emmanuel Movement," 781.

132. "Dangers of the New Therapeutic Movement," *Current Literature* 44 (April 1908): 634–635.

133. Chauncey Hawkins, "Psychotherapy and the Church: Some Guiding Principles," *Congregationalist and Christian World* (October 10, 1908).

134. Parker, *The Other Side of Psychotherapy*, 23, 24.

135. Buckley, "Dangers of the Emmanuel Movement," 635.

136. Gordon, "The Practice of Medicine by the Unfit," 211–212.

137. "The Practice of Psychotherapy: Some Counter Considerations," *Congregationalist and Christian World* (6 March 1909): 308.

138. Ibid., 308.

139. Brown, *Faith and Health*, 167.

140. Lightner Witmer, "Review and Criticism: Mental Healing and the Emmanuel Movement," *Psychological Clinic* 2 (15 December 1908, 15 January 1909, 15 February 1909): 212–224, 239–250, 282–300.

141. Ibid., 249–250.

142. Henry Rutgers Marshall, "Psychotherapy and Religion," *Hibbert Journal* 7 (January 1909): 300. For a reply to Marshall's critique, see Samuel McComb, "The Christian Religion as a Healing Power," *Hibbert Journal* 7 (October 1909): 10–27.

143. Hugo Münsterberg, *Psychotherapy* (New York: Moffat, Yard, 1909), 346. For an excellent biography of Münsterberg, see Matthew Hale, *Human Science and Social Order: Hugo Münsterberg and the Origins of Applied Psychology* (Philadelphia: Temple University Press, 1980).

144. Münsterberg, *Psychotherapy*, 10.

145. James Jackson Putnam, "The Service to Nervous Invalids of the Physician and of the Minister," *Harvard Theological Review* 2 (April 1909): 239.

146. Elwood Worcester and Samuel McComb, *Christian Religion as a Healing Power: A Defense and Exposition of the Emmanuel Movement* (New York: Moffat, Yard, 1909). An abridged version of this work appeared in *Century* magazine. See Worcester, "The Emmanuel Movement," 421–429.

147. Worcester, "The Emmanuel Movement," 421.

148. McComb and Worcester, *Christian Religion as a Healing Power*, 96–97.

149. Worcester, "The Emmanuel Movement," 422.

150. McComb and Worcester, *Christian Religion as a Healing Power*, 54–56.

151. Brown, *Faith and Health*, 157–158.

152. Worcester, *Life's Adventure*, 289.

153. Greene, "The Emmanuel Movement," 525.

154. See *Readers' Guide to Periodical Literature*, 1910–1914. The article of note is by Ralph Wallace Reed, M.D. (visiting neurologist to the Bethesda Hospital and the Ohio Hospital for Women and Children), Cincinnati, Ohio, in a letter to *Everybody's* 22 (May 1910): 713–714.

155. Greene, "The Emmanuel Movement," 525. Although they ceased to publicize their work, Worcester and McComb did not abandon their venture altogether. No longer in the public spotlight, the program assumed a far more modest scope. Worcester and McComb continued to write on topics germane to psychotherapy, but they ceased to present their views in the popular press. In 1917, McComb published *The New Life: The Secret of Happiness and Power* (New York: Harper and Brothers, 1917). Three years later, Worcester published *The Subconscious Mind: Its Nature and Value for the Cure of Nervous Disorders by Means of Suggestion and Auto-Suggestion* (London: K.P. Trench, Trubner, 1920). In 1931, Worcester and McComb coauthored *Body, Mind and Spirit* (Boston: Marshall Jones, 1931).

156. John C. Fisher, "The Emmanuel Work from the Physician's Viewpoint," *Review of Reviews* 39 (May 1909): 586.

157. Homer Gage, "The Emmanuel Movement from a Medical View-Point," *Popular Science Monthly* 75 (October 1909): 369.

158. H. Addington Bruce, review of *The Christian Religion as a Healing Power*.

Conclusion

1. For a brilliant discussion of professional boundaries, see Andrew Delano Abbott, *The System of Professions: An Essay on the Division of Expert Labor* (Chicago: University of Chicago Press, 1988).

2. See the discussion in chapter 4 concerning the response to George Beard's "The Influence of the Mind in the Causation and Cure of Disease—The Potency of Definite Expectation" *Journal of Nervous and Mental Diseases* 1 (1876): 429–435.

3. For phrenology, see Roger Cooter, *The Cultural Meaning of Popular Science: Phrenology and the Organization of Consent in Nineteenth-Century Britain* (Cambridge: Cambridge University Press, 1985); idem, "Phrenology: The Provocation of Progress," *History of Science* 14 (1976): 211–234. For a discussion of the American scene, see John D. Davies, *Phrenology Fad and Science: A 19th-Century American Crusade* (New Haven: Yale University Press, 1955); and Eric T. Carlson, "The Influence of Phrenology on Early American Psychiatric Thought," *American Journal of Psychiatry* 115 (1958): 535–538. For a discussion of mesmerism, see Gauld, *A History of Hypnotism*. For a discussion of spiritualism, see Edward M. Brown, "Neurology and Spiritualism in the 1870s," *Bulletin of the History of Medicine* 57 (1983): 563–577; Shortt, "Physicians and Psychics."

4. See Burnham, *Psychoanalysis and American Medicine; Freud and the Americans;* and F. H. Matthews, "The Americanization of Sigmund Freud: Adaptations of Psychoanalysis before 1917," *Journal of American Studies* 1 (1967): 39–62.

5. Prior to 1910 the *Readers' Guide to Periodical Literature* does not list a single article on either Freud or psychoanalysis. The third volume, which covers the years 1910–1914, lists 4 articles on Freud and 11 on psychoanalysis. Volume 4, 1915–1918, lists 8 articles on Freud and 31 on psychoanalysis. Some of the more prominent articles are Charles F. Ousler, "Behind the Madman's Dreams," *Technical World* 21 (April 1914): 205–207; James Jackson Putnam, "The Psycho-Analytic Movement," *Scientific American Supplement* 78 (19 December 1914): 391; Max Eastman, "Exploring the Soul and Healing the Body," *Everybody's* 32 (1915): 741–750; idem, "Mr.-er-er- Oh! What's His Name? Ever Say That?" *Everybody's* 33 (1915): 95–103; Peter Clark Macfarlane, "Diagnosis by Dreams," *Good Housekeeping* 60 (1915): 125–133, 278–286; Lucian Cary, "Escaping Your Past," *Technical World* 23 (August 1915): 730–735; Walter Lippmann, "Freud and the Layman," *New Republic* 2 (April 17, 1915): 9–10; Floyd Dell, "Speaking of Psycho-Analysis: The New Boon for Dinner

Table Conversationalists," *Vanity Fair* 5 (December 1915): 53; John. B. Watson, "The Psychology of Wish Fulfillment," *Scientific American* 3 (November 1916): 479–487; Joseph Jastrow, "The Psycho-Analyzed Self," *Dial* 62 (3 May 1917): 395–398; and John P. Toohey, "How We All Reveal Our Soul Secrets," *Ladies' Home Journal* 34 (November 1917): 97; William H.W. Chase, "Freud's Theories of the Unconscious," *Popular Science Monthly* 78 (1 April 1911): 355–363; Edward M. Weyer, "The New Art of Interpreting Dreams," *Forum* 15 (May 1911): 589–600; "Freud's Discovery of the Lowest Chamber of the Soul," *Current Literature* 50 (May 1911): 512–514; H. Addington Bruce, "The Nature of Dreams," *Outlook* (August 1911): 875–881; idem, "Dreams and the Supernatural," *Outlook* (December 1911): 862–871; idem, "The Marvels of Dream Analysis," *McClure's* 40 (November 1912): 113–119; Stephen S. Colvin, "Real Mind Reading," *Independent* 71 (7 December 1911): 1258–1261; Samuel McComb, "The New Interpretation of Dreams," *Century* 34 (September 1912): 663–669; Edwin Tenney Brewster, "Dreams and Forgetting: New Discoveries in Dream Psychology," *McClure's* 39 (October 1912): 714–719.

6. For a discussion of the popular press's role in early-twentieth-century American medicine, see James H. Cassedy, "Muckraking and Medicine: Samuel Hopkins Adams," *American Quarterly* 16 (1964): 85–99.

7. See Catherine Lucille Covert, "Freud on the Front Page: Transmission of Freudian Ideas in the American Newspaper of the 1920s" (Ph.D. dissertation, Syracuse University, 1975).

8. The contribution of the refugee psychoanalysts who fled Europe in the 1930s played an important role in transforming both the style and the practice of psychoanalysis in the United States. I would argue, however, that as with the first wave of psychoanalysis, the second was susceptible to the overarching inflence of American culture.

9. Nathan G. Hale, Jr., *The Rise and Crisis of Psychoanalysis in the United States: Freud and the Americans, 1917–1985* (New York: Oxford University Press, 1995), 355.

10. For a fascinating discussion of these and other somatic therapies, see Andrew Scull, "Psychiatrists and Historical 'Facts' Part One: The Historiography of Somatic Treatments," *History of Psychiatry* 6 (1995): 225–241. For lobotomy, see Eliot S. Valenstein, *Great and Desperate Cures: The Rise and Decline of Psychosurgery and Other Radical Treatments for Mental Illness* (New York: Basic Books, 1986); Jack Pressman, *Last Resort: Psychosurgery and the Limits of Medicine* (Cambridge: Cambridge University Press, 1998). For a broad overview of somatic therapies, see Edward Shorter, *A History of Psychiatry: From the Era of the Asylum to the Age of Prozac* (New York: John Wiley and Sons, 1997), 190–238.

Selected Bibliography

Unpublished Sources

Abbott, Andrew Delano. "The Emergence of American Psychiatry, 1880–1930." Ph.D. dissertation, University of Chicago, 1982.

Cunningham, Raymond J. "Ministry of Healing: The Origins of the Psychosomatic Role of the American Churches." Ph.D. dissertation, Johns Hopkins University, 1965.

Fleming, Allen Bruce. "Psychology, Medicine, and Religion: A Form of Early Twentieth-Century American Psychotherapy (1905–1909)." Ph.D. dissertation, Fuller Theological Seminary, School of Psychology, 1989.

Micale, Mark S. "Diagnostic Discrimination: Jean-Martin Charcot and the Nineteenth-Century Idea of Masculine Hysterical Neurosis." Ph.D. dissertation, Yale University, 1987.

Pitts, John Albert. "The Association of Medical Superintendents of American Institutions for the Insane, 1844–1892: A Case Study of Specialism in American Medicine." Ph.D. dissertation, University of Pennsylvania, 1981.

Powell, Robert Charles. "Healing and Wholeness: Helen Flanders Dunbar (1902–59) and an Extra-Medical Origin of the American Psychosomatic Movement, 1906–36." Ph.D. dissertation, Duke University, 1974.

Smith, Brian Dean. "The Moral Treatment of Psychological Disorders: A Historical and Conceptual Study of Selected Twentieth-Century Pastoral Psychologists." Ph.D. dissertation, University of Washington, 1989.

Stokes, G. Allison. "The Rise of the Religion and Health Movement in American Protestantism, 1906–1945." Ph.D. dissertation, Yale University, 1981.

Wilkerson, Stephen Young. "James Jackson Putnam and the Impact of Neurology on Psychotherapy in Late Nineteenth-Century America." Ph.D. dissertation, Duke University, 1978.

Primary Periodicals

Albany Annals of Medicine
Alienist and Neurologist
American Journal of Insanity
American Journal of Medical Sciences
American Journal of Neurology and Psychiatry
American Journal of Psychology
American Journal of Psychiatry
American Law Review
American Journal of Neurology and Psychiatry
Arena
Boston Medical and Surgical Journal
British Medical Journal
Canadian Journal of Medicine and Surgery
Century
Chicago Journal of Nervous and Mental Diseases
Chicago Medical Recorder
Christian Science Journal
Cincinnati Lancet and Clinic
Cleveland Medical Journal
Clinique
Colorado Medical Journal
Colorado Medicine
Congregationalist and Christian World
Current Literature
Detroit Medical Journal
Fort Wayne Journal of the Medical Sciences
Galliard's Southern Medicine
Good Housekeeping
Harvard Theological Review
Hibbert Journal
Illinois Medical Journal
Independent
International Clinics
International Journal of Railway Surgery
International Journal of Surgery
Journal of Abnormal Psychology
Journal of Christian Science
Journal of Morphology
Journal of Nervous and Mental Diseases
Journal of the American Medical Association
Journal of the Medical Society of New Jersey
Lancet

Louisville Monthly Journal of Medicine and Surgery
Medical Bulletin (Philadelphia)
Medical News
Medical Record
Medical Times and Gazette
Medical-Legal Journal
Metaphysical Magazine
Mind Cure and Science of Life
Mind Cure Journal
Monthly Cyclopedia and Medical Bulletin
National Association of Railway Surgeons Journal
New Hampshire Medical Society
New York Medical Journal
North American Review
Old Dominion Journal of Medicine and Surgery
Outlook
Philadelphia Medical Times
Physician and Surgeon
Popular Science Monthly
Practical Ideals
Proceedings of the Society for Psychical Research
Psychological Clinic
Psychotherapy: A Course Reading in Sound Psychology, Sound Medicine and Sound Religion
Quarterly Journal of Psychological Medicine and Medical Jurisprudence
Railway Age
Railway Surgeon: Official Journal of the National Association of Railway Surgeons
Railway Surgery
Texas Journal of Medicine
Texas Sanitarian
Transactions and Studies of the College of Physicians of Philadelphia
Transactions of the American Homeopathic Association
Transactions of the American Medico-Psychological Association
Transactions of the American Neurological Association
Transactions of the Electro-Therapeutics Association
Transactions of the Institute of Homeopathy
Transactions of the Iowa State Medical Society
Virginia Medical Monthly
Water-Cure Journal
Water-Cure World
Women's Medical Journal
World's Word
Yale Medical Journal

Primary Books

Baker, Ray Stannard. *New Ideas in Healing*. New York: Frederick A. Stokes, 1909.

Batten, Loring W. *The Relief of Pain by Mental Suggestion: A Study of the Moral and Religious Forces of Healing*. New York: Moffat, Yard, 1917.

Beard, George. *American Nervousness: Its Causes and Consequences, a Supplement to Nervous Exhaustion (Neurasthenia)*. Introduction by Charles E. Rosenberg. New York: G. P. Putnam's Sons, 1881.

———. *Practical Treatise on Nervous Exhaustion (Neurasthenia): Its Symptoms, Nature, Sequences, and Treatment*. New York: William Wood, 1880.

———. *Sexual Neurasthenia (Nervous Exhaustion): Its Hygiene, Causes, Symptoms and Treatment*, 5th ed. New York: E. B. Treat, 1900.

Beard, George Miller, and A. D. Rockwell. *A Practical Treatise on the Medical and Surgical Uses of Electricity*. New York: William Wood, 1867.

Bernheim, Hippolyte. *Hypnosis and Suggestion in Psychotherapy: A Treatise on the Nature and Use of Hypnotism*. Translated by Christian A. Herter. New York: Jason Aronson, 1973.

———. *New Studies in Hypnotism*. Translated by Richard S. Sandor. New York: International Universities Press, 1980.

———. *Suggestive Therapeutics: A Treatise on the Nature and Uses of Hypnotism*. New York: G. P. Putnam's Sons, 1895.

Brown, Charles Reynolds. *Faith and Health*. New York: Thomas Y. Crowell, 1910.

Bruce, H. Addington. *Scientific Mental Healing*. Boston: Little, Brown, 1911.

Buckley, James Monroe. *Faith-Healing, Christian Science and Kindred Phenomena*. New York: Century, 1887.

Bush, George. *Mesmer and Swedenborg; Or, The Relation of the Development of Mesmerism to the Doctrines and Disclosures of Swedenborg*. New York: John Allen, 1847.

Camps, William. *Railway Accidents or Collisions: Their Effects upon the Nervous System*. London: H. K. Lewis, 1866.

Carpenter, William B. *Principles of Mental Physiology, with Their Application to the Training and Discipline of the Mind, and the Study of Its Morbid Conditions*. New York: D. Appleton, 1894.

Charcot, J. M. *Clinical Lectures on Certain Diseases of the Nervous System*. Translated by E. P. Hurt. Detroit: George S. Davis, 1888.

Clarke, Edward H. *Sex in Education, or a Fair Chance for the Girls*. Boston: Robert Brothers, 1873.

Clevenger, Shobal Vail. *Spinal Concussion: Surgically Considered as a Cause of Spinal Injury, and Neurologically Restricted to a Certain Symptom Group, for which Is Suggested the Designation Erichsen's Disease, as One Form of the Traumatic Neuroses*. Philadelphia: F. A. Davis, 1889.

Dercum, Francis X. *Hysteria and Accident Compensation: Nature of Hysteria and the Lesson of Post-Litigation Results*. Philadelphia: Geo. T. Bisel, 1916.

————, ed. *Text Book on Nervous Disease by American Authors,* New York: Lea Brothers, 1895.

Dods, John Bovee. *The Philosophy of Electrical Psychology: In a Course of Twelve Lectures.* New York: Fowler and Wells, 1854.

————. *Six Lectures on Electrical Psychology.* New York: Fowler and Wells, 1854.

Dowse, Thomas Stretch. *On Brain and Nerve Exhaustion (Neurasthenia) and on the Exhaustion of Influenza.* London: Bailliere, Tindall and Cox, 1892.

Dresser, Annetta Gertrude. *The Philosophy of P. P. Quimby: With Selections from His Manuscripts and Sketch of His Life.* Boston: Geo. H. Ellis, 1895.

Dresser, Horatio. *A History of the New Thought Movement.* New York: Thomas Y. Crowell, 1919.

————, ed. *The Quimby Manuscripts Showing the Discovery of Spiritual Healing and the Origins of Christian Science.* New York: Thomas Y. Crowell, 1921.

Dubois, Paul. *The Psychic Treatment of Nervous Disorders.* Translated by William Alanson White and Smith Ely Jelliffe. New York: Funk and Wagnalls, 1904.

Eddy, Mary Baker Glover. *Science and Health.* Boston: W. F. Brown, 1875.

Edes, Robert T. *The New England Invalid.* Boston: David Clapp & Son, 1895.

Erichsen, John Eric. *On Concussion of the Spine, Nervous Shock, and Other Obscure Injuries to the Nervous System in Their Clinical and Medico-Legal Aspects.* New York: William Wood, 1883.

————. *On Railway and Other Injuries of the Nervous System.* London: Walton and Maberly, 1866.

Evans, Warren Felt. *Divine Law of Cure.* Boston: H. H. Carter, 1884.

————. *Esoteric Christianity, and Mental Therapeutics.* Boston: H. H. Carter and Karrick, 1886.

————. *The Mental Cure, Illustrating the Influence of the Mind on the Body, Both in Health and Disease, and the Psychological Method of Treatment.* 7th. ed. Boston: Colby and Rich, 1869.

————. *Mental Medicine.* Boston: Colby and Rich, 1872.

————. *Soul and Body.* Boston: Colby and Rich, 1876.

Fallows, Samuel. *Health and Happiness: or Religious Therapeutics.* Chicago: A. C. McClurg, 1908.

Fallows, Samuel, and Helen Fallows. *Science of Health from the Viewpoint of the Newest Christian Thought.* Chicago: Our Daily Company, 1903.

Freud, Sigmund, and Joseph Breuer. *Studies on Hysteria.* New York: Basic Books, 1957.

Galt, John. *The Treatment of Insanity.* New York, 1846.

Gerrish, Frederick H., ed. *Psychotherapeutics: A Symposium.* Boston: R. G. Badger, 1910.

Gowers, W. R. *Diseases of the Nervous System.* Philadelphia: P. Blakiston, Son, 1889.

Hamilton, Allan McClane. *A Manual of Medical Jurisprudence with Special Reference to Diseases and Injuries of the Nervous System.* New York: Bermingham, 1883.

————. *Railway and Other Accidents with Relation to Injury and Disease of the Nervous System: A Book for Court Use.* New York: William Wood, 1904.

Hamilton, Allan McClane, and Lawrence Godkin, eds. *A System of Legal Medicine*. 2d ed. New York: E.B. Treat, 1894.

Hamilton, William Alexander. *The Physics and Physiology of Spiritualism*. New York: Appleton, 1871.

———. *Spiritualism and Allied Causes of Nervous Derangement*. New York: G. P. Putnam's Sons, 1876.

Hammond, William A. *Cerebral Hyperaemia: The Result of Emotional Strain or Emotional Disturbance, the So-called Nervous Prostration of Neurasthenia*. Washington: G.P. Putnam's Sons, 1878.

Hayward, Aaron S. *Vital Magnetic Cure: An Exposition of Vital Magnetism, and Its Application to the Treatment of Mental and Physical Disease*. Boston: William White, 1871.

Holmes, Oliver Wendell. *Medical Essays, 1842–1882*. Boston: Houghton Mifflin, 1891.

Hudson, Thomas J. *The Law of Mental Medicine; and the Correlation of the Facts of Psychology and Histology in Their Relation to Mental Therapeutics*. London: G.P. Putnam's Sons, 1904.

———. *The Law of Psychic Phenomenon: A Working Hypothesis for the Systematic Study of Hypnotism, Spiritism, Mental Therapeutics, Etc*. 17th ed. Chicago: A.C. McClurg, 1899.

Jackson, John Hughlings. *Selected Writings of John Hughlings Jackson*. Edited by J. Taylor, G. Holmes and F.M.R. Walsh J. Taylor. London: Hodder and Stoughton, 1932.

James, William. *Principles of Psychology*. Cambridge, Mass.: Harvard University Press, 1982.

———. *Talks to Teachers on Psychology and to Students on Some of Life's Ideals*. Cambridge, Mass.: Harvard University Press, 1983.

———. *The Varieties of Religious Experience: A Study in Human Nature*. New York: Collier Books, 1961.

Jastrow, Joseph. *The Subconscious*. Boston: Houghton Mifflin, 1906.

Leavitt, Sheldon. *Psychotherapy in the Practice of Medicine and Surgery*. Chicago: Garner Press, 1903.

McComb, Samuel. *The New Life: The Secret of Happiness and Power*. New York: Harper and Brothers, 1917.

MacDonald, Robert. *Mind, Religion and Health: With an Appreciation of the Emmanuel Movement*. New York: Funk and Wagnalls, 1908.

Marrs, William Taylor. *Confessions of a Neurasthenic*. Philadelphia: F.A. Davis, 1908.

Meyer, Adolf. *The Collected Papers of Adolf Meyer*. 4 vols. Edited by Eunice Winters. Baltimore: Johns Hopkins University Press, 1952.

———. *The Commonsense Psychiatry of Dr. Adolf Meyer*. Edited by Alfred Lief. New York: McGraw-Hill, 1948.

Mitchell, S. Weir. *Fat and Blood: An Essay on the Treatment of Certain Forms of Neurasthenia and Hysteria*. 4th ed. Philadelphia: J.B. Lippincott, 1888.

———. *Wear and Tear or Hints for the Overworked*. Philadelphia: J.B. Lippincott, 1872.

Mitchell, S. Weir, G.R. Morehouse, and W.E. Keen. *Gunshot Wounds and Other Injuries of Nerves*. Philadelphia, 1864.

Münsterberg, Hugo. *Psychotherapy.* New York: Moffat, Yard, 1909.

Page, Herbert. *Injuries of the Spine and Spinal Cord Without Apparent Mechanical Lesion and Nervous Shock in Their Surgical and Medico-Legal Aspect.* London: J. & A. Churchill, 1883.

Paget, James. "Nervous Mimicry." In *Clinical Lectures and Essays.* London: Longmans, Green, 1875.

Parker, George L. *The Other Side of Psychotherapy.* Boston: Salem D. Towne, 1908.

Parson, Frederick T. *Vital Magnetism: Its Power Over Disease—A Statement of the Facts Developed by Men Who Have Employed this Agenda Under Various Names as Animal Magnetism, Mesmerism, Hypnotism, Etc., from the Earliest Times Down to the Present.* New York: Adams, Victor, 1877.

Patterson, Christopher Stuart. *Railway Accident Law, the Liability of Railways for Injuries to the Person.* Philadelphia: T. & W. Johnson, 1886.

Powell, Lyman P. *Christian Science: The Faith and Its Founder.* New York: G.P. Putnam's Sons, 1907.

———. *The Emmanuel Movement in a Small New England Town.* New York: G.P. Putnam's Sons, 1909.

Prince, Morton. *The Nature of the Mind and Human Automatism.* Philadelphia: J.B. Lippincott, 1885.

———. *Psychopathology and Multiple Personality: Selected Essays.* Edited by Nathan G. Hale, Jr. Cambridge, Mass.: Harvard University Press, 1975.

Purrington, William A. *Christian Science: An Exposition of Mrs. Eddy's Wonderful Discovery, Including Its Legal Aspects: A Pleas for Children and Other Helpless Sick.* New York: E.B. Treat, 1900.

———. *A Review of Recent Legal Decisions Affecting Physicians, Dentists, Druggists, and the Public Health Together with a Brief for the Prosecution of Unlicensed Practitioners of Medicine, Dentistry, Pharmacy with a Paper Upon Manslaughter, Christian Science and the Law and other Matters.* New York: E.B. Treat, 1899.

Root, Julia Anderson. *Healing Power of Mind: A Treatise on Mind-Cure, with Original Views on the Subject and Complete Instruction for the Practice and Self Treatment.* 2d ed. Peoria: H.S. Hill, 1886.

Rush, Benjamin. *Benjamin Rush's Lectures on the Mind.* Edited by Jeffrey L. Wollock, Patricia S. Noel, and Eric T. Carlson. Philadelphia: American Philosophical Society, 1981.

Seguin, E.C. *Opera Minora.* New York: G.P. Putnam's Sons, 1884.

Sidis, Boris. *The Psychology of Suggestion: A Research into the Subconscious Nature of Man and Society.* New York: D. Appleton, 1898.

Sidis, Boris, and Simon P. Goodhart. *Multiple Personality: An Investigation into the Nature of Human Individuality.* New York: Greenwood Press, 1905.

Trine, Ralph Waldo. *In Tune with the Infinite or Fullness of Peace, Power, and Plenty.* New York: Thomas Y. Crowell, 1897.

Tuke, Daniel Hack. *Dictionary of Psychological Medicine.* Philadelphia: Blakiston, Son, 1892.

———. *Of the Influences of the Mind Upon the Body in Health and Disease Designed to Elucidate the Actions of the Imagination.* London: J. &. A. Churchill, 1872.

Twain, Mark. *Christian Science.* New York: Harper and Brothers, 1907.

Wells, David W. *Psychology Applied to Medicine*. Philadelphia: F.A. Davis, 1907.

Whipple, Leander Edmund. *The Philosophy of Mental Healing*. New York: Metaphysical, 1893.

Witthaus, R.A., and Tracy C. Becker, eds. *Medical Jurisprudence: Forensic Medicine and Toxicology*. 2d ed. New York: William Wood, 1894.

Wood, Henry. *Ideal Suggestion Through Mental Photography: A Restorative System for Home and Private Use Preceded by a Study of the Laws of Mental Healing*. 10th ed. Boston: Lea and Shepard, 1893.

————. *The New Old Healing*. Boston: Lothrop, Lea and Shepard, 1908.

————. *The New Thought Simplified: How to Gain Harmony and Health*. Boston: Lea and Shepard, 1903.

Worcester, Elwood, and Samuel McComb. *Body, Mind, and Spirit*. Boston: Marshall Jones, 1931.

————. *The Christian Religion as a Healing Power: A Defense of the Emmanuel Movement*. New York: Moffat, Yard, 1909.

Worcester, Elwood. *Life's Adventure: The Story of a Varied Career*. New York: Charles Scribner's Sons, 1932.

————. *The Subconscious Mind: Its Nature and Value for the Cure of Nervous Disorders by Means of Suggestion and Auto-Suggestion*. London: K.P. Trench, Truber, 1920.

Worcester, Elwood, Samuel McComb, and Isador Coriat. *Religion and Medicine: The Moral Control of Nervous Disorders*. New York: Moffat, Yard, 1908.

Secondary Books

Abbott, Andrew Delano. *The System of Professions: An Essay on the Division of Expert Labor*. Chicago: University of Chicago Press, 1988.

Abse, Wilfred, George Kriegman, and Robert Gardner, eds. *American Psychiatry: Past, Present and Future*. Charlottesville: University of Virginia Press, 1975.

Ackerknecht, Erwin. *A Short History of Psychiatry*. 2d ed. New York: Hafner, 1968.

Ahlstrom, Sydney E. *A Religious History of the American People*. 2 vols. Garden City: Image Books, 1975.

Albanese, Catherine L. *Nature Religion in America: From the Algonkian Indians to the New Age*. Chicago: University of Chicago Press, 1990.

Alexander, Franz, and Sheldon T. Selesnick. *The History of Psychiatry: An Evaluation of Psychiatric Thought and Practice from Prehistoric Times to the Present*. New York: Harper and Row, 1966.

Anderson, Odin W. *The Uneasy Equilibrium*. New Haven: Yale University Press, 1968.

Anderson, Ola. *Studies in the Prehistory of Psychoanalysis: The Etiology of Psychoneuroses and Some Related Themes in Sigmund Freud's Scientific Writings and Letters, 1866–1896*. n.p.: Scandinavian University Books, 1962.

Avrich, Paul. *The Haymarket Tragedy*. Princeton: Princeton University Press, 1984.

Berman, Jeffrey. *Narcissism and the Novel*. New York: New York University Press, 1990.

————. *The Talking Cure: Literary Representations of Psychoanalysis*. New York: New York University Press, 1985.

Blackmore, John T. *Ernst Mach: His Work, Life, and Influence*. Berkeley: University of California Press, 1972.

Bledstein, Burton. *The Culture of Professionalism and the Development of Higher Education in America*. New York: W.W. Norton, 1976.

Blustein, Bonnie Ellen. *Preserve Your Love for Science: Life of William Alexander Hammond, American Neurologist*. Cambridge: Cambridge University Press, 1991.

Bockoven, J. Sanbourne. *Moral Treatment in American Psychiatry*. New York: Springer, 1963.

Boring, Edwin. *A History of Experimental Psychology*. 2d ed. New York: Appleton-Century-Crofts, 1950.

Braden, Charles. *Spirits in Rebellion: The Rise and Development of New Thought*. Dallas: Southern Methodist University Press, 1963.

Brandt, Allan M. *No Magic Bullet: A Social History of Venereal Disease in the United States since 1880*. New York: Oxford University Press, 1985.

Braude, Ann. *Radical Spirits: Spiritualism and Women's Rights in Nineteenth-Century America*. Boston: Beacon Press, 1989.

Brend, William A. *Traumatic Mental Disorder in Courts of Law with a General Survey of Medical Evidence and Procedure in Civil Action*. London: William Heinemann (Medical Books), 1938.

Bromberg, Walter. *From Shaman to Psychotherapist: A History of the Treatment of Mental Illness*. Chicago: Henry Regnery, 1975.

————. *The Mind of Man: The Story of Man's Conquest of Mental Illness*. New York: Harper & Brothers, 1937.

Brumberg, Joan Jacobs. *Fasting Girls: The History of Anorexia Nervosa*. New York: Plume Books, 1988.

Buckley, Kerry W. *Mechanical Man: John Broadus Watson and the Beginnings of Behaviorism*. New York: Guilford Press, 1989.

Burnham, John C. *Paths into American Culture: Psychology, Medicine, and Morals*. Philadelphia: Temple University Press, 1988.

————. *Psychoanalysis and American Medicine, 1894–1918*. New York: International Universities Press, 1967.

Bush, Wendall T. *Avenarius and the Standpoint of Pure Experience*. New York: Science Press, 1905.

Bynum, W.F., Roy Porter, and Michael Shepard, eds. *The Anatomy of Madness: Essays in the History of Psychiatry*. 3 vols. Cambridge: Cambridge University Press, 1988.

Cassedy, James H. *American Medicine and Statistical Thinking, 1800–1860*. Cambridge, Mass.: Harvard University Press, 1984.

————. *Medicine and American Growth, 1800–1860*. Madison: University of Wisconsin Press, 1986.

————. *Medicine in America: A Short History.* Baltimore: Johns Hopkins University Press, 1991.

Cayleff, Susan E. *Wash and Be Healed: The Water-Cure Movement and Women's Health.* Philadelphia: Temple University Press, 1987.

Chesler, Phyllis. *Women and Madness.* London: Allen Lane, 1974.

Clarke, Edwin, and L. S. Jacyna. *Nineteenth-Century Origins of Neuroscientific Concepts.* Berkeley: University of California Press, 1987.

Cohen, R. Robert. *Traumatic Neuroses and Personal Injury Cases.* Washington: Trial Lawyers Service Co., 1970.

Collie, Errol Stafford. *Quimby's Science of Happiness: A Non-Medical Scientific Explanation of the Cause and Cure of Disease.* Marina del Rey, Calif.: DeVorss, 1980.

Cooper, David Graham. *Psychiatry and Anti-Psychiatry.* London: Tavistock, 1967.

Cooter, Roger. *The Cultural Meaning of Popular Science: Phrenology and the Organization of Consent in Nineteenth-Century Britain.* Cambridge: Cambridge University Press, 1985.

Crabtree, Adam. *From Mesmer to Freud: Magnetic Sleep and the Roots of Psychological Healing.* New Haven: Yale University Press, 1993.

Cross, Whitney. *The Burned-over District: The Social and Intellectual History of Enthusiastic Religion in Western New York, 1800–1850.* New York: Octagon Books, 1981.

Cushman, Philip. *Constructing the Self, Constructing America: A Cultural History of Psychotherapy.* Reading, Mass.: Addison-Wesley, 1995.

Dain, Norman. *Clifford W. Beers, Advocate for the Insane.* Pittsburgh: University of Pittsburgh Press, 1980.

————. *Concepts of Insanity in the United States, 1789–1865.* New Brunswick: Rutgers University Press, 1964.

Darnton, Robert. *Mesmerism and the End of the Enlightenment in France.* Cambridge, Mass.: Harvard University Press, 1968.

Davies, John D. *Phrenology Fad and Science: A 19th-Century American Crusade.* New Haven: Yale University Press, 1955.

de Kruif, Paul. *The Microbe Hunters.* New York: Harcourt Brace Jovanovich, 1964.

Degler, Carl N. *In Search of Human Nature: The Decline and Revival of Darwinism in American Social Thought.* New York: Oxford University Press, 1991.

Dembe, Allard. *Occupation and Disease: How Social Factors Affect the Conception of Work-related Disorders.* New Haven: Yale University Press, 1996.

Deutsch, Albert. *The Mentally Ill in America: A History of Their Care and Treatment from Colonial Times.* Garden City: Doubleday, Doran, 1937.

Dictionary of American Biography. New York: Charles Scribner's Sons, 1964.

Dictionary of American Medical Biography: Lives of Eminent Physicians of the United States and Canada, from the Earliest Times. Edited by Howard A. Kelly and Walter L. Burrage. Boston: Milford House, 1971.

Digby, Ann. *Madness, Morality, and Medicine: A Study of the York Retreat, 1796–1914.* Cambridge: Cambridge University Press, 1985.

Donegan, Jane B. *"Hydropathic Highway to Health": Women and Water-Cure in Antebellum America*. Westport, Conn.: Greenwood Press, 1986.

Donnelly, Michael. *Managing the Mind: A Study of Medical Psychology in Early Nineteenth-Century Britain*. London: Tavistock, 1983.

Dowbiggin, Ian. *Inheriting Madness: Professionalization and Psychiatric Knowledge in Nineteenth-Century France*. Berkeley: University of California Press, 1991.

Drinka, George Frederick. *The Birth of Neurosis*. New York: Simon and Schuster, 1984.

Dubos, Rene. *The White Plague: Tuberculosis, Man, and Society*. New Brunswick: Rutgers University Press, 1987.

Duffy, John. *The Healers: A History of American Medicine*. New York: McGraw-Hill, 1976.

———. *The Sanitarians: A History of American Public Health*. Urbana: University of Illinois Press, 1990.

Earnest, Ernest. *S. Weir Mitchell, Novelist and Physician*. Philadelphia: University of Pennsylvania Press, 1950.

Ehrenreich, Barbara, and Deidre English. *For Her Own Good: 150 Years of the Experts' Advice to Women*. New York: Anchor Books, 1978.

Ellenberger, Henri F. *The Discovery of the Unconscious: The History and Evolution of Dynamic Psychiatry*. New York: Basic Books, 1970.

English, Peter. *Shock, Physiological Surgery, and George Washington Crile: Medical Innovation in the Progressive Era*. Westport, Conn.: Greenwood, 1980.

Etheridge, Elizabeth W. *The Butterfly Caste: A Social History of Pellagra in the South*. Westport, Conn.: Greenwood, 1972.

Feinstein, Howard. *Becoming William James*. Ithaca: Cornell University Press, 1984.

Foucault, Michel. *Discipline and Punish: The Birth of the Prison*. New York: Vintage Books, 1977.

———. *Madness and Civilization: A History of Insanity in the Age of Reason*. Translated by Richard Howard. New York: Vintage Books, 1973.

Fox, Daniel, and Christopher Lawrence. *Photographing Medicine: Images and Power in Britain and America Since 1840*. New York: Greenwood Press, 1988.

Fox, Richard Wightman. *So Far Disordered in Mind: Insanity in California, 1870–1930*. Berkeley: University of California Press, 1978.

Frederickson, George. *The Inner Civil War: Northern Intellectuals and the Crisis of the Union*. New York: Harper and Row, 1965.

Freedheim, Donald K., ed. *History of Psychotherapy: A Century of Change*. Washington, D.C.: American Psychological Association, 1992.

Friedman, Lawrence J. *Menninger: The Family and the Clinic*. New York: Alfred A. Knopf, 1990.

Friedman, Lawrence M. *A History of American Law*. 2d ed. New York: Touchstone Books, 1985.

Friedson, Eliot. *Professional Dominance: The Social Structure of Medical Care*. New York: Atherton Press, 1970.

Frohock, Fred M. *Healing Powers: Alternative Medicine, Spiritual Communities, and the State*. Chicago: University of Chicago Press, 1992.

Fuller, Robert C. *Alternative Medicine and American Religious Life*. New York: Oxford University Press, 1989.

———. *Americans and the Unconscious*. New York: Oxford University Press, 1986.

———. *Mesmerism and the American Cure of Souls*. Philadelphia: University of Pennsylvania Press, 1982.

Fullinwider, S. P. *Technicians of the Finite: The Rise and Decline of the Schizophrenic in American Thought*. Westport, Conn.: Greenwood Press, 1982.

Galdston, Iago, ed. *Historic Derivations of Modern Psychiatry*. New York: McGraw-Hill, 1969.

Gauld, Alan. *The Founders of Psychical Research*. London: Routledge & Kegan Paul, 1968.

———. *A History of Hypnotism*. Cambridge: Cambridge University Press, 1992.

Gay, Peter. *Freud: A Life for Our Time*. New York: W. W. Norton, 1988.

Gevitz, Norman. *The D.O.'s: Osteopathic Medicine in America*. Baltimore: Johns Hopkins University Press, 1982.

———, ed. *Other Healers: Unorthodox Medicine in America*. Baltimore: Johns Hopkins University Press, 1988.

Gifford, George, ed. *Psychoanalysis, Psychotherapy and the New England Medical Scene, 1894–1944*. New York: Science History, 1978.

Gilman, Sander L. *The Case of Sigmund Freud: Medicine and Identity at the Fin de Siècle*. Baltimore: Johns Hopkins University Press, 1993.

———. *Difference and Pathology: Stereotypes of Sexuality, Race, and Madness*. Ithaca: Cornell University Press, 1985.

———. *Disease and Its Representations: Images of Illness from Madness to AIDS*. Ithaca: Cornell University Press, 1988.

———. *Freud, Race, and Gender*. Princeton: Princeton University Press, 1993.

———. *Seeing the Insane*. New York: John Wiley, 1982.

Goldstein, Jan Ellen. *Console and Classify: The French Psychiatric Profession in the Nineteenth Century*. New York: Cambridge University Press, 1987.

Goshen, Charles E. *Documentary History of Psychiatry: A Source Book on Historical Principles*. New York: Philosophical Library, 1967.

Gosling, Francis G. *Before Freud: Neurasthenia and the American Medical Community, 1870–1910*. Urbana: University of Illinois Press, 1987.

Gottschalk, Stephen. *The Emergence of Christian Science in American Religious Life*. Berkeley: University of California Press, 1973.

Grob, Gerald N. *From Asylum to Community: Mental Health Policy in Modern America*. Princeton: Princeton University Press, 1992.

———. *The Mad Among Us: A History of the Care of America's Mentally Ill*. Cambridge, Mass.: Harvard University Press, 1994.

———. *Mental Illness and American Society, 1875–1940*. Princeton: Princeton University Press, 1983.

Grosskurth, Phyllis. *Havelock Ellis: A Biography*. New York: New York University Press, 1985.

———. *Melanie Klein: Her Word and Her Work*. New York: Alfred A. Knopf, 1986.

Haber, Samuel. *The Quest for Authority and Honor in the American Professions, 1750–1900*. Chicago: University of Chicago Press, 1991.

Hacking, Ian. *Rewriting the Soul: Multiple Personality and the Sciences of Memory.* Princeton: Princeton University Press, 1995.

Hale, Nathan G., Jr. *Freud and the Americans: The Beginnings of Psychoanalysis in the United States, 1876–1917.* New York: Oxford University Press, 1971.

———. *James Jackson Putnam and Psychoanalysis.* Cambridge, Mass.: Harvard University Press, 1971.

———. *The Rise and Crisis of Psychoanalysis in the United States: Freud and the Americans, 1917–1985.* New York: Oxford University Press, 1995.

Hall, David D. *Worlds of Wonder, Days of Judgment: Popular Religious Belief in Early New England.* Cambridge, Mass.: Harvard University Press, 1990.

Hall, Kermit L., ed. *Tort Law in American History.* New York: Garland, 1987.

Haller, John S. *American Medicine in Transition, 1840–1910.* Urbana: University of Illinois Press, 1981.

Haller, John S., Jr., and Robin M. Haller. *The Physicians and Sexuality in Victorian America.* Urbana: University of Illinois Press, 1974.

Harrell, David. *All Things Are Possible: The Healing and Charismatic Movement in Modern America.* Bloomington: Indiana University Press, 1975.

Harrington, Anne. *Medicine, Mind, and the Double Brain: A Study in Nineteenth-Century Thought.* Princeton: Princeton University Press, 1989.

Hartman, Mary S., and Lois Banner, eds. *Clio's Consciousness Raised: New Perspectives in the History of Women.* New York: Octagon Books, 1976.

Haskall, Thomas. *The Emergence of Professional Social Science.* Urbana: University of Illinois Press, 1977.

Hatch, Nathan O., ed. *The Professions in American History.* Notre Dame: University of Notre Dame Press, 1988.

Hearnshaw, L.S. *A Short History of British Psychology, 1840–1940.* Westport, Conn.: Greenwood Press, 1964.

Heidbreder, Edna. *Seven Psychologies.* Englewood Cliffs, N.J.: Prentice Hall, 1933.

Herman, Judith Lewis. *Trauma and Recovery: The Aftermath of Violence—From Domestic Abuse to Political Terror.* New York: Basic Books, 1992.

Herrmann, Frederick M. *Dorothea Dix and the Politics of Institutional Reform.* Trenton: New Jersey Historical Commission, 1981.

Hollinger, David A. *In the American Province: Studies in the History and Historiography of Ideas.* Bloomington: Indiana University Press, 1985.

Hoopes, James. *Consciousness in New England: From Puritanism and Ideas to Psychoanalysis and Semiotics.* Baltimore: Johns Hopkins University Press, 1989.

Horwitz, Morton J. *The Transformation of American Law, 1780–1860.* Cambridge, Mass.: Harvard University Press, 1977.

———. *The Transformation of American Law, 1870–1960: The Crisis of Legal Orthodoxy.* New York: Oxford University Press, 1992.

Howe, Daniel Walker. *The Political Culture of American Whigs.* Chicago: University of Chicago Press, 1979.

Huber, Richard M. *The American Idea of Success.* New York: McGraw-Hill, 1971.

Issac, Rael Jean, and Virginia C. Armat. *Madness in the Streets: How Psychiatry and the Law Abandoned the Mentally Ill.* New York: Free Press, 1990.

Jimenez, Mary Ann. *Changing Face of Madness: Early American Attitudes and Treatment of the Insane*. Hanover: University of New England Press, 1987.

Jones, Anne Hudson, ed. *Images of Healers*. Albany: State University of New York Press, 1983.

———. *Images of Nurses: Perspectives from History, Art, and Literature*. Philadelphia: University of Pennsylvania Press, 1988.

Jones, Ernest. *The Life and Work of Sigmund Freud*. 3 vols. New York: Basic Books, 1953.

Judah, J. Stillson. *The History and Philosophy of the Metaphysical Movement in America*. Philadelphia: Westminster Press, 1967.

Kaminer, Wendy. *I'm Dysfunctional, You're Dysfunctional: The Recovery Movement and Other Self-Help Fashions*. New York: Vintage Books, 1993.

Kaufmann, Martin F. *Homeopathy in America: The Rise and Fall of a Medical Heresy*. Baltimore: Johns Hopkins University Press, 1971.

Keiser, Lester. *The Traumatic Neurosis*. Philadelphia: J.B. Lippincott, 1968.

Kett, Joseph K. *The Formation of the American Medical Profession: The Role of Institutions, 1780–1860*. New Haven: Yale University Press, 1968.

King, Lester S. *Transformations in American Medicine: From Benjamin Rush to William Osler*. Baltimore: Johns Hopkins University Press, 1991.

King, Marian. *Mary Baker Eddy: Child of Promise*. Englewood Cliffs, N.J.: Prentice Hall, 1968.

Kuhn, Thomas S. *The Structure of Scientific Revolutions*. 2d ed. Chicago: University of Chicago Press, 1970.

Kuklick, Bruce. *The Rise of American Philosophy: Cambridge, Massachusetts, 1860–1930*. New Haven: Yale University Press, 1977.

Laqueur, Thomas. *Making Sex: Body and Gender from the Greeks to Freud*. Cambridge, Mass.: Harvard University Press, 1990.

Larson, Magali Sarfatti. *The Rise of Professionalism: A Sociological Analysis*. Berkeley: University of California Press, 1977.

Lasch, Christopher. *The World of Nations: Reflections on American History, Politics, and Culture*. New York: Alfred A. Knopf, 1973.

Lears, T. Jackson. *No Place of Grace: Anti-Modernism and the Transformation of American Culture, 1880–1920*. New York: Pantheon Books, 1981.

Leavitt, Judith Walzer. *Brought to Bed: Childbearing in America, 1750–1950*. New York: Oxford University Press, 1986.

Levin, Kenneth. *Freud's Early Psychology of the Neuroses: A Historical Perspective*. Pittsburgh: University of Pittsburgh Press, 1978.

Leys, Ruth. *From Sympathy to Reflex: Marshall Hall and His Opponents*. New York: Garland, 1990.

Leys, Ruth, and Rand B. Evans, eds. *Defining American Psychiatry: The Correspondence between Adolf Meyer and Edward Bradford Titchener*. Baltimore: Johns Hopkins University Press, 1990.

Licht, Walter. *Working for the Railroad: The Organization of Work in the Nineteenth Century*. Princeton: Princeton University Press, 1983.

Lubove, Roy. *The Professional Altruist: The Emergence of Social Work as a Career, 1880–1930*. Cambridge, Mass.: Harvard University Press, 1965.

Lunbeck, Elizabeth. *The Psychiatric Persuasion: Knowledge, Gender, and Power in Modern America*. Princeton: Princeton University Press, 1994.

Lutz, Tom. *American Nervousness, 1903: An Anecdotal History*. Ithaca: Cornell University Press, 1991.

MacAlpine, Ida, and Richard Hunter. *George III and the Mad-Business*. London: Allen Lane, 1969.

MacDonald, Michael. *Mystical Bedlam: Madness, Anxiety and Healing in Seventeenth-Century England*. Cambridge: Cambridge University Press, 1981.

McGovern, Constance M. *Masters of Madness: Social Origins of the American Psychiatric Profession*. Hanover: University of New England Press, 1985.

McGrath, William J. *Freud's Discovery of Psychoanalysis*. Ithaca: Cornell University Press, 1986.

Malmsheimer, Richard. *Doctors Only: The Evolving Image of the American Physician*. New York: Greenwood Press, 1988.

Marshall, Helen E. *Dorothea Dix: Forgotten Samaritan*. Chapel Hill: University of North Carolina Press, 1937.

Martin, Albro. *Railroads Triumphant: The Growth, Rejection, and Rebirth of a Vital American Force*. New York: Oxford University Press, 1992.

May, Henry. *The Enlightenment in America*. New York: Oxford University Press, 1976.

Meyer, Donald. *The Positive Thinkers: Religion as Pop Psychology from Mary Baker Eddy to Oral Roberts*. New York: Pantheon Books, 1965.

Milmine, Georgine. *Mary Baker G. Eddy: The Story of Her Life and the History of Christian Science*. New York: Doubleday, Page, 1909.

Mohr, James. *Doctors and the Law: Medical Jurisprudence in Nineteenth-Century America*. New York: Oxford University Press, 1993.

Moore, R. Laurence. *In Search of White Crows: Spiritualism, Parapsychology, and American Culture*. New York: Oxford University Press, 1977.

Murphy, Gardner, and Robert O. Ballou, eds. *William James on Psychical Research*. New York: Viking Press, 1960.

Napoli, Donald. *Architects of Adjustment: The History of the Psychological Profession in the United States*. Port Washington: International University Publications, 1981.

Nissenbaum, Stephen. *Sex, Diet, and Debility in Jacksonian America: Sylvester Graham and Health Reform*. Westport, Conn.: Greenwood Press, 1980.

Noyes, John Humphrey. *History of American Socialism*. Philadelphia: J.B. Lippincott, 1870.

Numbers, Ronald L. *Prophetess of Health: A Study of Ellen G. White*. New York: Harper and Row.

O'Donnell, John. *The Origins of Behaviorism: American Psychology, 1870–1920*. New York: New York University Press, 1985.

Oppenheim, Janet. *The Other World and Beyond: Spiritualism and Psychical Research in England, 1850–1914*. New York: Cambridge University Press, 1985.

———. *Shattered Nerves: Doctors, Patients and Depression in Victorian England*. New York: Oxford University Press, 1991.

Parker, Gail Thain. *Mind Cure in New England from the Civil War to World War One*. Hanover: University of New England Press, 1973.

Parry-Jones, William L. *The Trade in Lunacy*. London: Routledge & Kegan Paul, 1972.

Peel, Robert. *Mary Baker Eddy: The Years of Discovery*. New York: Holt, Rinehart and Winston, 1966.

Pernick, Martin S. *A Calculus of Suffering: Pain, Professionalism, and Anesthesia in Nineteenth-Century America*. New York: Columbia University Press, 1985.

Perry, Ralph Barton. *The Thought and Character of William James*. Boston: Little, Brown, 1935.

Persons, Stow. *American Minds: A History of Ideas*. Huntington, N.Y.: Robert E. Krieger, 1958.

———. *Free Religion, an American Faith*. New Haven: Yale University Press, 1947.

Peterson, Kirtland C. *Post-Traumatic Stress Disorder: A Clinician's Guide*. New York: Plenum Press, 1991.

Plarr's Lives of the Fellows of the Royal College of Surgeons of England. 2 vols. Bristol: John Wright & Sons, 1930.

Podmore, Frank. *Mesmerism and Christian Science: A Short History of Mental Healing*. London: Methuen, 1909.

Porter, Roy, ed. *The Medical History of Water and Spas*. London: Wellcome Institute for the History of Medicine, 1990.

———. *Mind Forg'd in Manacles: A History of Madness in England from the Restoration to the Regency*. Cambridge, Mass.: Harvard University Press, 1987.

Quen, Jacques M., ed. *Split Minds/Split Brains: Historical and Current Perspectives*. New York: New York University Press, 1986.

Quen, Jacques M., and Eric T. Carlson, eds. *American Psychoanalysis: Origins and Development*. New York: Brunner Mazel, 1978.

Quetel, Claude. *History of Syphilis*. Translated by Judith Braddock and Brian Pike. Baltimore: Johns Hopkins University Press, 1990.

Rabinbach, Anson. *The Human Motor: Energy, Fatigue, and the Origins of Modernity*. New York: Basic Books, 1990.

Rance, Nicholas. *Wilkie Collins and Other Sensation Novelists*. Rutherford: Farleigh Dickinson University Press, 1991.

Rein, David M. *S. Weir Mitchell as a Psychiatric Novelist*. New York: International Universities Press, 1952.

Reverby, Susan, and David Rosner, eds. *Health Care in America: Essays in Social History*. Philadelphia: Temple University Press, 1979.

Richards, Robert John. *Darwin and the Emergence of Evolutionary Theories of Mind and Behavior*. Chicago: University of Chicago Press, 1987.

Roazen, Paul. *Freud and His Followers*. New York: New York University Press, 1984.

Roberts, Jon H. *Darwinism and the Divine: Protestant Intellectuals and Organic Evolution, 1859–1900*. Madison: University of Wisconsin Press, 1988.

Roberts, Shirley. *Sir James Paget: The Rise of Clinical Surgery*. London: Royal Society of Medicine, 1989.

Roe, Daphne A. *A Plague of Corn: The Social History of Pellagra*. Ithaca: Cornell University Press, 1973.

Rosenberg, Charles E. *The Care of Strangers: The Rise of America's Hospital System*. New York: Basic Books, 1987.

——. *The Cholera Years*. Chicago: University of Chicago Press, 1987.

——. *The Trial of Assassin Guiteau: Psychiatry and Law in the Gilded Age*. Chicago: University of Chicago Press, 1968.

Rosenberg, Charles E., and Janet Golden, eds. *Framing Disease: Studies in Cultural History*. New Brunswick: Rutgers University Press, 1992.

Rosenberg, Charles E., and Morris J. Vogel, eds. *The Therapeutic Revolution: Essays in the Social History of American Medicine*. Philadelphia: University of Pennsylvania Press, 1979.

Rosenberg, Rosalind. *Beyond Separate Spheres: The Intellectual Origins of Modern Feminism*. New Haven: Yale University Press, 1982.

Rosner, David, and Gerald Markowitz, eds. *Dying for Work: Workers' Safety and Health in Twentieth-Century America*, Bloomington: Indiana University Press, 1987.

Rothman, David. *Conscience and Convenience: The Asylum and Its Alternatives in Progressive America*. Boston: Little, Brown, 1980.

——. *The Discovery of the Asylum: Social Order and Disorder in the New Republic*. Boston: Little, Brown, 1971.

Rothstein, William G. *American Physicians in the Nineteenth Century: From Sects to Science*. Baltimore: Johns Hopkins University Press, 1972.

Rowbottom, Margaret, and Edward Susskind. *Electricity and Medicine: History of Their Interaction*. San Francisco: San Francisco Press, 1984.

Russett, Cynthia Eagle. *Sexual Science: The Victorian Construction of Womanhood*. Cambridge, Mass.: Harvard University Press, 1989.

Sass, Louis A. *Madness and Medicine: Insanity in the Light of Modern Art, Literature, and Thought*. New York: Basic Books, 1992.

Scarborough, Elizabeth, and Laurel Furumoto. *Untold Lives: The First Generation of American Women Psychologists*. New York: Columbia University Press, 1987.

Schiebinger, Londa. *The Mind Has No Sex? Women in the Origins of Modern Science*. Cambridge, Mass.: Harvard University Press, 1989.

Schivelbusch, Wolfgang. *Railway Journey: The Industrialization of Time and Space in the 19th Century*. Berkeley: University of California Press, 1989.

Scull, Andrew. *Museums of Madness: The Social Organization of Insanity in Nineteenth-Century England*. London: Allen Lane, 1979.

——. *Social Order/Mental Disorder: Anglo-American Psychiatry in Historical Perspective*. Berkeley: University of California Press, 1989.

——, eds. *Madhouses, Mad-Doctors, and Madmen: The Social History of Psychiatry in the Victorian Era*. Philadelphia: University of Pennsylvania Press, 1981.

Searle, Jonathan R. *The Rediscovery of the Mind*. Cambridge: MIT Press, 1992.

Shaw, Robert B. *A History of Railroad Accidents, Safety Precautions and Operating Practices*. n.p.: Vail-Ballou Press, 1978.

Shorter, Edward. *From Paralysis to Fatigue: A History of Psychosomatic Illness in the Modern Era*. New York: Free Press, 1992.

————. *From the Mind into the Body: The Cultural Origins of Psychosomatic Symptoms*. New York: Free Press, 1994.

————. *A History of Psychiatry: From the Era of the Asylum to the Age of Prozac*. New York: John Wiley and Sons, 1997.

Shortt, S.E.D. *Victorian Lunacy: Richard M. Burke and the Practice of Late Nineteenth-Century Psychiatry*. London: Cambridge University Press, 1986.

Showalter, Elaine. *The Female Malady: Women, Madness, and English Culture, 1830–1980*. New York: Penguin Books, 1985.

————. *Sexual Anarchy: Gender and Culture at the Fin de Siècle*. New York: Viking Press, 1990.

Shyrock, Richard Harrison. *The Development of Modern Medicine*. New York: Alfred A. Knopf, 1947.

————. *Medical Licensing in America, 1650–1965*. Baltimore: Johns Hopkins University Press, 1967.

Sicherman, Barbara. *The Quest for Mental Health in America, 1870–1917*. New York: Arno Press, 1980.

Silberger, Julius S., Jr. *Mary Baker Eddy: An Interpretive Biography of the Founder of Christian Science*. Boston: Little, Brown, 1980.

Smith, Laurence D. *Behaviorism and Logical Positivism: A Reassessment of the Alliance*. Stanford: Stanford University Press, 1986.

Smith, Roger. *Inhibition: History and Meaning in the Sciences of the Mind and Brain*. Berkeley: University of California Press, 1992.

Smith-Rosenberg, Carroll. *Disorderly Conduct: Visions of Gender in Victorian America*. New York: Alfred A. Knopf, 1985.

Snowden, James H. *The Truth about Christian Science: The Founder and the Faith*. Philadelphia: Westminster Press, 1920.

Stage, Sarah. *Female Complaints: Lydia Pinkham and the Business of Women's Medicine*. New York: W. W. Norton, 1979.

Star, Susan Leigh. *Regions of the Mind: Brain Research and the Quest for Scientific Certainty*. Stanford: Stanford University Press, 1989.

Starr, Paul. *The Transformation of American Medicine: The Rise of a Sovereign Profession and the Making of a Vast Industry*. New York: Basic Books, 1982.

Stevens, Rosemary. *American Medicine and Public Interest*. New Haven: Yale University Press, 1981.

Still, Andrew, and Irving Velody, eds. *Rewriting the History of Madness: Studies in Foucault's Histoire de Folie*. London: Routledge, 1992.

Strouse, Jean. *Alice James: A Biography*. Boston: Houghton Mifflin, 1980.

Sulloway, Frank J. *Freud, Biologist of the Mind: Beyond the Psychoanalytic Legend*. New York: Basic Books, 1979.

Sutton, S.B. *Crossroads in Psychiatry: A History of the McLean Hospital*. Washington, D.C.: American Psychiatric Press, 1986.

Taylor, Eugene. *William James on Consciousness beyond the Margin*. Princeton: Princeton University Press, 1996.

————. *William James on Exceptional Mental States: The 1898 Lowell Lectures*. New York: Charles Scribner's Sons, 1984.

Taylor, Jenny Bourne. *In the Secret Theatre of Home: Wilkie Collins, Sensation Narrative, and Nineteenth-Century Psychology*. London: Routledge, 1988.

Taylor, W. S. *Morton Prince and Abnormal Psychology*. New York: D. Appleton, 1928.

Timms, Edward, and Naomi Segal, eds. *Freud in Exile: Psychoanalysis and Its Vicissitudes*. New Haven: Yale University Press, 1988.

Toksvig, Signe. *Emmanual Swedenborg: Scientist and Mystic*. Freeport: Books for Library Press, 1948.

Tomes, Nancy. *A Generous Confidence: Thomas Kirkbride and the Art of Asylum-keeping, 1840–1883*. Cambridge: Cambridge University Press, 1984.

Trimble, Michael R. *Post-Traumatic Neurosis: From Railway Spine to Whiplash*. New York: John Wiley and Sons, 1981.

Turner, James. *Reckoning with the Beast: Animals, Pain, and Humanity in the Victorian Mind*. Baltimore: Johns Hopkins University Press, 1980.

———. *Without God, Without Creed*. Baltimore: Johns Hopkins University Press, 1983.

Valenstein, Elliot S. *Great and Desperate Cures: The Rise and Decline of Psychosurgery and Other Radical Treatments for Mental Illness*. New York: Basic Books, 1986.

Veith, Ilza. *Hysteria: The History of a Disease*. Chicago: University of Chicago Press, 1965.

Wallace, Edward R., and Lucius Pressley, eds. *Essays on the History of Psychiatry*. Columbia: Wm. S. Hall Psychiatric Institute, 1980.

Walters, Ronald G. *American Reformers, 1815–1865*. New York: Hill and Wang, 1978.

Warner, John Harley. *The Therapeutic Perspective: Medical Practice, Knowledge, and Identity in America, 1820–1885*. Cambridge, Mass.: Harvard University Press, 1986.

Weiss, Richard. *The American Myth of Success: From Horatio Alger to Norman Vincent Peale*. New York: Basic Books, 1969.

Whorton, James C. *Crusaders for Fitness: The History of American Health Reformers*. Princeton: Princeton University Press, 1982.

Wilson, Dorothy Clark. *Stranger and Traveler: The Story of Dorothea Dix, American Reformer*. Boston: Little, Brown, 1975.

Woodward, William R., and Mitchell G. Ash, eds. *The Problematic Science: Psychiatry in Nineteenth-Century Thought*. New York: Praeger, 1982.

Wroebel, A., ed. *Pseudo-Science in Nineteenth-Century America*. Lexington: University Press of Kentucky, 1987.

Young, Allan. *The Harmony of Illusions: Inventing Post-Traumatic Stress Disorder*. Princeton: Princeton University Press, 1995.

Young, Robert. *Mind, Brain and Adaptation in the Nineteenth Century: Cerebral Localization and Its Biological Context from Gall to Ferrier*. Oxford: Oxford University Press, 1970.

Young-Bruehl, Elizabeth. *Anna Freud: A Biography*. New York: Summit Books, 1988.

Zilboorg, Gregory, in collaboration with George W. Henry. *A History of Medical Psychology*. New York: W. W. Norton, 1941.

Secondary Articles

Abby, Susan E., and Paul Garfinkle. "Neurasthenia and Chronic Fatigue Syndrome: The Role of Culture in the Making of a Diagnosis." *American Journal of Psychiatry* 148 (1991): 1638–1646.

Albanese, Catherine L. "Physic and Metaphysic in Nineteenth-Century America: Medical Sectarians and Religious History." *Church History* 55 (1986): 489–502.

Baker, Samuel L. "Physician Licensure Laws in the United States." *Journal of the History of Medicine and Allied Sciences* 39 (1984): 173–197.

———. "A Strange Case: The Physician Licensure Campaign in Massachusetts in 1880." *Journal of the History of Medicine and Allied Sciences* 40 (1984): 286–308.

Blustein, Bonnie Ellen. "'A Hollow Square of Psychology Science': American Neurologists and Psychiatrists in Conflict." In *Madhouses, Mad-Doctors, and Madmen,* edited by Andrew Scull, 241–270. Philadelphia: University of Pennsylvania Press, 1981.

———. "The Brief Career of 'Cerebral Hyperaemia': William A. Hammond and His Insomnia Patients, 1854–1890." *Journal of the History of Medicine and Allied Sciences* 41 (1986): 24–51.

———. "New York Neurologists and the Specialization of American Medicine." *Bulletin of the History of Medicine* 53 (1979): 170–183.

Brown, Edward M. "Neurology and Spiritualism in the 1870s." *Bulletin of the History of Medicine* 57 (1983): 563–577.

———. "Regulating Damage Claims for Emotional Injuries before the First World War." *Behavioral Sciences and the Law* 8 (1990): 421–434.

Bunker, Henry Alden, Jr. "From Beard to Freud: A Brief History of the Concept of Neurasthenia." *Medical Review of Reviews* 36 (1930): 108–114.

Burnham, John C. "Psychology and Counseling: Convergence into a Profession." In *The Professions in American History,* edited and with an introduction by Nathan O. Hatch, 181–198. Notre Dame: University of Notre Dame Press, 1988.

Bynum, William F., Jr. "Rationales for Therapy in British Psychiatry, 1780–1835." In *Madhouses, Mad-Doctors, and Madmen: The Social History of Psychiatry in the Victorian Era,* edited by Andrew Scull, 35–57. Philadelphia: University of Pennsylvania Press, 1981.

Carlson, Eric T. "George Beard and Neurasthenia." In *Essays on the History of Psychiatry,* edited by Edwin R. Wallace IV and Lucius C. Pressley, 50–57. Columbia: W.S. Hall Psychiatric Institute, 1980.

———. "The Influence of Phrenology in Early American Psychiatric Thought." *American Journal of Psychiatry* 115 (1958): 535–538.

Cayleff, Susan E. "'Prisoners of Their Own Feebleness': Women, Nerves, and Western Medicine—A Historical Overview." *Social Science and Medicine* 26 (1988): 1199–1208.

Chertok, Leon. "Hysteria, Hypnosis, Psychopathology." *Journal of Nervous and Mental Diseases* 161 (1975): 367–378.

———. "On Objectivity in the History of Psychotherapy." *Journal of Nervous and Mental Diseases* 153 (1971): 73–78.

Clark, Michael J. "The Rejection of Psychological Approaches to Mental Disorders in Late Nineteenth-Century British Psychiatry." In *Madhouses, Mad-Doctors, and Madmen: The Social History of Psychiatry in the Victorian Era,* edited by Andrew Scull, 271–312. Philadelphia: University of Pennsylvania Press, 1981.

Cooter, Roger. "Phrenology: The Provocation of Progress." *History of Science* 14 (1976): 211–234.

———. "Phrenology and the British Alienists, ca. 1825–1845." In *Madhouses, Mad-Doctors, and Madmen: The Social History of Psychiatry in the Victorian Era,* edited by Andrew Scull, 58–104. Philadelphia: University of Pennsylvania Press, 1981.

Cunningham, Raymond J. "The Emmanuel Movement: A Variety of Religious Experience." *American Quarterly* 14 (1964): 46–83.

Dain, Norman. "American Psychiatry in the Eighteenth Century." In *American Psychiatry: Past Present and Future,* edited by Robert Gardener, Wilfred Abse, and George Kriegman, 15–27. Charlottesville: University of Virginia Press, 1975.

Dain, Norman, and Eric T. Carlson. "Milieu Therapy in the Nineteenth Century: Patient Care at the Friend's Asylum, Frankford, Pennsylvania, 1817–1861." *Journal of Nervous and Mental Disease* 131 (October 1960): 277–290.

———. "Social Class and Psychological Medicine in the United States, 1789–1824." *Bulletin of the History of Medicine* 33 (1959): 454–465.

Dana, Charles. "Dr. George M. Beard: A Sketch of His Life and Character, with Some Personal Reminiscences." *Archives of Neurology and Psychiatry* 10 (1923): 427–435.

Danziger, Kurt. "Mid-Nineteenth Century British Psycho-Physiology: A Neglected Chapter in the History of Psychology." In *The Problematic Science: Psychology in Nineteenth-Century Thought,* edited by William R. Woodward and Michael G. Ash. New York: Praeger, 1982.

———. "On the Threshold of the New Psychology: Situating Wundt and James." In *Wundt Studies: A Centennial Collection,* edited by Wolfgang G. Bringman and Ryan O. Tweny. Toronto: C. J. Hogrefe, 1980.

Daston, Lorraine J. "British Responses to Psycho-Physiology, 1860–1900." *Isis* 69 (1978): 192–208.

———. "The Theory of Will versus the Science of Mind." In *The Problematic Science: Psychology in Nineteenth-Century Thought,* edited by William R. Woodward and Mitchell G. Ash, 88–115. New York: Praeger, 1982.

Diethelm, Oskar. "An Historical View of Somatic Treatment in Psychiatry." *American Journal of Psychiatry* 95 (1939): 1165–1179.

Dowbiggin, Ian. "French Psychiatry, Hereditarianism, and Professional Legitimacy, 1840–1900." *Research in Law, Deviancy, and Social Control* 7 (1985): 135–165.

Englehardt, H. Tristram, Jr. "John Hughlings Jackson and the Mind-Body Relation." *Bulletin of the History of Medicine* 49 (1975): 131–151.

Fox, Claire Gilbride. "The Madness of Mankind." In *Essays on the History of Psychology,* edited by Edwin R. Wallace and Lucius C. Pressley, 30–49. Columbia: W.S. Hall Psychiatric Institute, 1980.

Fox, Richard Wightman. "Beyond 'Social Control': Institutions and Disorder in Bourgeois Society." *History of Education Quarterly* 16 (1976): 203–204.

Gach, John. "Culture and Complex: On the Early History of Psychoanalysis in the United States." In *Essays on the History of Psychiatry,* edited by Edwin R. Wallace IV and Lucius C. Pressley. Columbia: W.S. Hall Psychiatric Institute, 1980.

Gifford, Sanford. "Medical Psychotherapy and the Emmanuel Movement." In *Psychoanalysis, Psychotherapy and the New England Medical Scene, 1894–1944,* edited by George Gifford, 106–118. New York: Science History Publications, 1978.

Gilman, Sander L. "The Image of the Hysteric." In *Hysteria Beyond Freud,* edited by Sander L. Gilman, 345–453. Berkeley: University of California Press, 1993.

Goldstein, Jan Ellen. " 'The Lively Sensibility of the Frenchmen': Some Reflections on the Place of France in Foucault's *Histoire de la Folie.*" In *Rewriting the History of Madness: Studies in Foucault's* Histoire de la Folie, edited by Andrew Still and Irving Velody, 69–77. London: Routledge, 1992.

Gosling, Francis, and J.M. Ray. "The Right to be Sick: American Physicians and Nervous Patients." *Journal of Social History* 20 (1986): 286–301.

Greene, John Gardner. "The Emmanuel Movement, 1906–1929." *New England Quarterly* 7 (1934): 506–532.

Grob, Gerald N. "Adolf Meyer and American Psychiatry in 1895." *American Journal of Psychiatry* 119 (1963): 135–142.

———. "Rediscovering Asylums: The Unhistorical History of the Asylum." In *The Therapeutic Revolution: Essays in the Social History of American Medicine,* edited by Morris J. Vogel and Charles E. Rosenberg, 135–157. Philadelphia: University of Pennsylvania Press, 1979.

Haller, John S., Jr. "Neurasthenia: Medical Profession and Urban 'Blahs.'" *New York State Journal of Medicine* 473 (1970): 2489–2496.

———. "Neurasthenia: The Medical Profession and the 'New Woman' of the Late Nineteenth Century." *New York State Journal of Medicine* 474 (1971): 473–482.

Harrington, Anne. "Hysteria, Hypnotism, and the Lure of the Invisible: The Rise of Neo-Mesmerism in Fin-de-Siècle French Psychiatry." In *The Anatomy of Madness: Essays on the History of Psychiatry,* edited by Roy Porter, Michael Shepard, and Walter F. Bynum, 226–246. London: Cambridge University Press, 1988.

Hillman, Robert G. "A Scientific Study of Mystery: The Role of the Medical and Popular Press in the Nancy-Salpêtrière Controversy on Hypnotism." *Bulletin of the History of Medicine* 39 (1965): 163–182.

Holcombe, Harry S. "Electrotherapy." *Journal of the History of Medicine and Allied Sciences* 22 (1967): 180–182.

Hollinger, David A. "The Problem of Pragmatism in American History." In *In the American Province: Studies in the History and Historiography of Ideas*, 23–43. Bloomington: Indiana University Press, 1985.

———. "T. S. Kuhn's Theory of Science and Its Implications for History." In *In the American Province: Studies in the History and Historiography of Ideas*, 105–129. Bloomington: Indiana University Press, 1985.

Holmes, Stewart W. "Phineus Parkhurst Quimby: Scientist of Transcendentalism." *New England Quarterly* 17 (1944): 356–380.

Jacyna, L.S. "The Physiology of the Mind, the Unity of Nature, and the Moral Order in Victorian Thought." *British Journal of the History of Science* 14 (1981): 109–132.

Kaufmann, Martin F. "The American Anti-Vaccinationists and Their Arguments." *Bulletin of the History of Medicine* 41 (1967): 463–478.

———. "Homeopathy in America: The Rise and Fall and Persistence of a Medical Heresy." In *Other Healers: Unorthodox Medicine in America*, edited by Norman Gevitz, 99–123. Baltimore: Johns Hopkins University Press, 1988.

King, Helen. "Once Upon a Text: Hysteria from Hippocrates." In *Hysteria Beyond Freud*, edited by Sander L. Gilman, 3–91. Berkeley: University of California Press, 1993.

Kuttner, Alfred Booth. "Nerves." In *Civilization in the United States*, edited by Harold Stearns, 427–442. New York: Harcourt, Brace, 1922.

Legan, M.S. "Hydropathy, or the Water Cure." In *Pseudo-Science and Society in Nineteenth-Century America*, edited by A. Wroebel, 74–99. Lexington: University Press of Kentucky, 1987.

Levin, Kenneth. "Freud's Paper 'On Male Hysteria' and the Conflict Between Anatomical and Physiological Models." *Bulletin of the History of Medicine* 48 (1974): 377–397.

———. "S. Weir Mitchell: Investigation and Insights in Neurasthenia and Hysteria." *Transactions and Studies of the College of Physicians of Philadelphia* 38 (1970): 168–173.

Leys, Ruth. "Background of the Reflex Controversy: William Alison and the Doctrine of Sympathy before Hall." *Studies in the History of Biology* 4 (1980): 1–66.

Malone, Web. "The Formative Era of Contributory Negligence." In *Tort Law in American History*, edited and with an introduction by Kermit L. Hall. New York: Garland, 1987.

Marx, Otto. "Morton Prince and Psychopathology." In *Psychoanalysis, Psychotherapy, and the New England Medical Scene, 1894–1944*, edited by George Gifford, 163–180. New York: Science History Publications, 1978.

———. "What Is the History of Psychiatry?" *American Journal of Orthopsychiatry* 40 (1970): 593–605.

Matthews, Fred. "The Americanization of Sigmund Freud: Adaptations of Psychoanalysis before 1917." *Journal of American Studies* 1 (1967): 45–79.

McCandless, Peter. "Liberty and Lunacy: The Victorians and Wrongful Confinement." In *Madhouses, Mad-Doctors, and Madmen: The Social History of Psychiatry in the Victorian Era*, edited by Andrew Scull, 280–299. Philadelphia: University of Pennsylvania Press, 1981.

McCarthy, Katherine. "Psychotherapy and Religion: The Emmanuel Movement." *Journal of Religion and Health* 23 (1984): 100–114.

Micale, Mark S. "Hysteria and Its Historiography: A Review of Past and Present Writings (I and II)." *History of Science* 27 (1989): 223–261, 319–351.

———. "Hysteria Male/Hysteria Female: Reflection on Comparative Gender Construction in Nineteenth-Century France and Britain." In *Science and Sensibility: Gender and Scientific Inquiry, 1780–1945,* edited by Marina Benjamin, 363–411. Oxford: Basil Blackwood, 1990.

Morantz-Sanchez, Regina. "The Lady and Her Physicians." In *Clio's Consciousness Raised: New Perspectives on the History of Women,* edited by Mary S. Hartman and Lois Banner, 38–53. New York: Octagon Books, 1976.

Noel, P. S., and Eric T. Carlson. "Origins of the Word, 'Phrenology.'" *American Journal of Psychiatry* 127 (1970): 694–697.

Numbers, Ronald L. "The Fall and Rise of American Medicine." In *The Professions in American History,* edited and with an introduction by Nathan O. Hatch, 51–72. Notre Dame: University of Notre Dame Press, 1988.

Numbers, Ronald L., and Rennie B. Schoepflin. "Ministries of Healing: Mary Baker Eddy, Ellen G. White, and the Religion of Health." In *Women and Health in America,* edited by Judith Walzer Leavitt, 376–389. Madison: University of Wisconsin Press, 1984.

Numbers, Ronald L., and John H. Warner. "The Maturation of American Medical Science." In *Sickness and Health in America: Readings in the History of Medicine and Public Health,* 2d ed., edited by Judith Walzer Leavitt and Ronald L. Numbers, 113–129. Madison: University of Wisconsin Press, 1985.

Pernick, Martin S. "Back from the Grave: Recurring Controversies over Defining and Diagnosing Death in History." In *Death: Beyond Whole-Brain Criteria,* edited by Richard M. Zaner, 17–74. Dordrecht: Kluwer, 1988.

———. "The Calculus of Suffering in 19th-Century Surgery." In *Sickness and Health in America: Readings in the History of Medicine and Public Health,* 2d ed., edited by Judith Walzer Leavitt and Ronald L. Numbers. Madison: University of Wisconsin Press, 1985.

Poirier, Suzanne. "The Weir Mitchell Rest Cure: Doctors and Patients." *Women's Studies* 10 (1983): 15–40.

Porter, Roy. "The Body and the Mind, the Doctor and the Patient: Negotiating Hysteria." In *Hysteria Beyond Freud,* edited by Sander L. Gilman, 225–285. Berkeley: University of California Press,

———. "Foucault's Great Confinement." In *Rewriting the History of Madness: Studies in Foucault's* Histoire de la Folie, edited by Andrew Still and Irving Velody, 119–125. London: Routledge, 1992.

———. "Shutting People Up." *Social Studies of Science* 12 (1982): 467–476.

Posner, Richard. "A Theory of Negligence." *Journal of Legal Studies* 1 (January 1972): 29–96.

Powell, Robert Charles. "The 'Subliminal' versus the 'Subconscious' in the American Acceptance of Psychoanalysis." *Journal of the History of the Behavioral Sciences* 15 (1979): 155–165.

Quen, Jacques M. "Asylum Psychiatry, Neurology, Social Work, and Mental Hygiene: An Exploratory Interprofessional History." *Journal of the History of the Behavioral Sciences* 13 (1977): 3–11.

Riese, Walter. "The Neuropsychologic Phase in the History of Psychiatric Thought." In *Historic Derivations of Modern Psychiatry*, edited by Iago Galdston, 104–112. New York: McGraw-Hill, 1969.

Rosenberg, Charles E. "The Bitter Fruit: Heredity, Disease, and Social Thought." In *No Other Gods: On Science and Social Thought*, 25–53. Baltimore: Johns Hopkins University Press, 1976.

———. "Body and Mind in Nineteenth-Century Medicine: Some Clinical Origins of the Neurosis Construct." *Bulletin of the History of Medicine* 63 (1989): 185–197.

———. "George M. Beard and American Nervousness." In *No Other Gods: On Science and American Social Thought*, 98–109. Baltimore: Johns Hopkins University Press, 1976.

———. "The Therapeutic Revolution: Medicine, Meaning, and Social Change in Nineteenth-Century America." In *The Therapeutic Revolution: Essays in the Social History of American Medicine*, edited by Charles E. Rosenberg and Morris J. Vogel. Philadelphia: University of Pennsylvania Press, 1979.

Rosenberg, Charles E., and Carroll Smith-Rosenberg. "The Female Animal: Medical and Biological Reviews of Woman and Her Role in Nineteenth-Century America." *Journal of American History* 60 (1973): 332–356.

Ross, Barbara. "William James: A Prime Mover of the Psychoanalytic Movement in America." In *Psychoanalysis, Psychotherapy, and the New England Medical Scene, 1894–1944*, edited by George Gifford, 10–23. New York: Science History Publications, 1978.

Rousseau, G. S. "'A Strange Pathology': Hysteria in the Early Modern World, 1500–1800." In *Hysteria Beyond Freud*, edited by Sander L. Gilman, 91–221. Berkeley: University of California Press, 1993.

Rothman, David. "Social Control: The Uses and Abuses of the Concept in the History of Incarceration." In *Social Control and the State*, edited by Stanley Cohen and Andrew Scull, 106–117. New York: St. Martin's Press, 1981.

Schneck, Jerome M. "Jean-Martin Charcot and the History of Experimental Hypnosis." *Journal of the History of Medicine and Allied Sciences* 16 (1961): 297–300.

Schoepflin, Rennie B. "Christian Science Healing in America." In *Other Healers: Unorthodox Medicine in America*, edited by Norman Gevitz, 192–214. Baltimore: Johns Hopkins University Press, 1988.

Schwartz, Gary Y. "Tort Law and the Economy in Nineteenth-Century America: A Reinterpretation." *Yale Law Journal* 90 (July 1981): 1717–1775.

Scott, Joan W. "Gender: A Useful Category of Historical Analysis." *American Historical Review* 91 (1986): 1053–1076.

Scull, Andrew. "The Discovery of the Asylum Revisited." In *Madhouses, Mad-Doctors, and Madmen: The Social History of Psychiatry in the Victorian Era*, edited by Andrew Scull, 144–165. Philadelphia: University of Pennsylvania Press, 1981.

————. "Madness and Segregative Control: The Rise of the Insane Asylum." *Social Problems* 24 (1977): 338–351.

————. "Psychiatry and Its Historians." *History of Psychiatry* 2 (1991): 229–250.

Shortt, S.E.D. "Physicians and Psychics: The Anglo-American Medical Response to Spiritualism, 1870–1890." *Journal of the History of Medicine and Allied Sciences* 39 (1984): 339–355.

Showalter, Elaine. "Hysteria, Feminism, and Gender." In *Hysteria Beyond Freud*, edited by Sander L. Gilman, 286–344. Berkeley: University of California Press, 1993.

————. *Hystories: Hysterical Epidemics and Modern Media*. New York: Columbia University Press, 1997.

————. "Syphilis, Sexuality, and the Fiction of Fin de Siècle." In *Sex, Politics, and Science in the Nineteenth-Century Novel: Selected Papers from the English Institute, 1983–1984*, edited by Ruth B. Yeazell. Baltimore: Johns Hopkins University Press, 1986.

Shyrock, Richard Harrison. "The Advent of Modern Medicine in Philadelphia, 1800–1850." In *Medicine in America: Historical Essays*, 203–232. Baltimore: Johns Hopkins University Press, 1966.

————. "Benjamin Rush from the Perspective of the Twentieth Century." In *Medicine in America: Historical Essays*, 233–251. Baltimore: Johns Hopkins University Press, 1966.

————. "The Medical History of the American People." In *Medicine in America: Historical Essays*. Baltimore: Johns Hopkins University Press, 1966.

Sicherman, Barbara. "The New Psychiatry: Medical and Behavioral Science, 1895–1921." In *American Psychoanalysis: Origins and Development*, edited by Jacques M. Quen and Eric T. Carlson. New York: Brunner Mazel, 1978.

————. "The Paradox of Prudence: Mental Health in the Gilded Age." In *Madhouses, Mad-Doctors and Madmen: The Social History of Psychiatry in the Victorian Era*, edited by Andrew Scull, 201–217. Philadelphia: University of Pennsylvania Press, 1981.

————. "The Use of Diagnosis: Doctors, Patients, and Neurasthenia." *Journal of the History of Medicine and Allied Sciences* 32 (1977): 33–54.

Smith, Roger. "The Human Significance of Biology: Darwin, Carpenter and the *versa causa*." In *Nature and the Victorian Imagination*, edited by U.C. Knoepflmacher and G.B. Tennyson. Berkeley: University of California Press, 1977.

Smith-Rosenberg, Carroll. "The Hysterical Woman: Sex Roles and Role Conflict in Nineteenth-Century America," in *Disorderly Conduct: Visions of Gender in Victorian America*, 195–216. New York: Alfred A. Knopf, 1985.

Teahan, John F. "Warren Felt Evans and Mental Healing: Romantic Idealism and Practical Mysticism in Nineteenth-Century America." *Church History* 48 (1979): 63–80.

Thielman, Samuel B. "Madness and Medicine: Trends in American Medical Therapeutics for Insanity, 1820–1860." *Bulletin of the History of Medicine* 61 (1987): 25–46.

Wiener, Philip. "G.M. Beard and Freud on 'American Nervousness.'" *Journal of the History of Ideas* 17 (1956): 269–274.

Wood, Ann Douglas. "'The Fashionable Diseases': Women's Complaints and Their Treatment in Nineteenth-Century America." In *Clio's Consciousness Raised: New Perspectives in the History of Women,* edited by Mary S. Hartman and Lois Banner, 1–22. New York: Octagon Books, 1976.

Young, Robert. "Association of Ideas." In *Dictionary of the History of Ideas,* edited by Philip P. Wiener, 111–118. New York: Charles Scribner's Sons, 1968.

Index